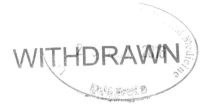
Food and health in Europe:
a new basis for action

WHO Library Cataloguing in Publication Data

Food and health in Europe : a new basis for action

    (WHO regional publications. European series ; No. 96)

    1.Nutrition 2.Food supply 3.Food contamination - prevention and control
    4.Nutritional requirements 5.Nutrition policy 6.Intersectoral cooperation
    7.Sustainability 8.Europe
    I.Series

    ISBN 92 890 1363 X   (NLM Classification: WA 695)
    ISSN 0378-2255

Text editing: Mary Stewart Burgher

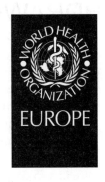

Food and health in Europe:
a new basis for action

Edited by:
Aileen Robertson, Cristina Tirado,
Tim Lobstein, Marco Jermini,
Cecile Knai, Jørgen H. Jensen,
Anna Ferro-Luzzi and W.P.T. James

WHO Regional Publications, European Series, No. 96

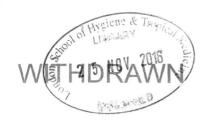

ISBN 92 890 1363 X
ISSN 0378-2255

Address requests for copies of publications of the WHO Regional Office to publicationrequests@euro.who.int; for permission to reproduce them to permissions@euro.who.int; and for permission to translate them to pubrights@euro.who.int; or contact Publications, WHO Regional Office for Europe, Scherfigsvej 8, DK-2100 Copenhagen Ø, Denmark, (tel.: +45 3917 1717; fax: +45 3917 1818; web site: http://www.euro.who.int).

Contents

	Page
Contents	v
Acknowledgements	vii
Editors	xii
Abbreviations	xiii
Foreword	xv
Introduction: the need for action on food and nutrition in Europe	1
Overview of the book	2
WHO activities	6
1. Diet and disease	7
Diet-related diseases: the principal health burden in Europe	7
Variations in CVD: the fundamental role of diet	23
Diet's role in limiting the development of cancer	32
Epidemic of overweight and obesity	35
Type 2 diabetes and excessive weight gain	38
Impact of physical inactivity on health	38
Impaired infant and child development from micronutrient deficiency	40
Pregnancy and fetal development	45
Feeding of infants and young children	50
Dental health	55
The health of the ageing population of Europe	57
Nutritional health of vulnerable groups	64
Social inequalities and poverty	66
References	73
2. Food safety	91
Food safety and food control	91
Causes of foodborne disease	92
Effects of foodborne disease	93
Extent of foodborne disease	94

Trends in foodborne disease   98
The burden of foodborne disease   101
Microbial hazards in food.   104
Chemical hazards in the food chain   112
Risk assessment   115
Food safety, diet and nutrition   116
Inequality in food safety.   119
Case studies   121
Emerging food control issues   140
WHO and food safety   142
References   144

3. Food security and sustainable development   155
Food security   155
Food production and health policies.   156
Food and nutrition insecurity.   158
Current trends in food supply   168
Agricultural policies and diet   182
Policies for food and nutrition security.   196
References   210

4. Policies and strategies   221
WHO Action Plan on Food and Nutrition Policy   221
Need for integrated and comprehensive food and nutrition policies   222
Food and nutrition policies in the European Region.   230
Nutrition policy.   231
Food control policy   255
Food security and sustainable development policy   270
Mechanisms to help health ministries set priorities for future action   277
References   297

5. Conclusion.   309
References   310

Annex 1. The First Action Plan for Food and Nutrition Policy,
WHO European Region, 2000–2005   313

Annex 2. International and selected national recommendations
on nutrient intake values   341

Acknowledgements

This publication was prepared by the nutrition and food security and the food safety programmes of the WHO Regional Office for Europe. We, the editors, gratefully acknowledge the financial support provided by the Government of the Netherlands. We are particularly grateful to the following people for helping us with the conceptual framework: Dr Eric Brunner (University College London, United Kingdom), Dr Raymond Ellard (Food Safety Authority of Ireland, Dublin, Ireland), Professor Tim Lang (Thames Valley University, London, United Kingdom), Professor Martin McKee (London School of Hygiene and Tropical Medicine, United Kingdom), Dr Mike Rayner (British Heart Foundation Health Promotion Research Group, Oxford, United Kingdom) and Dr Alan Lopez (Evidence and Information for Policy, WHO headquarters).

It is impossible to give individual credit for all the ideas and inspiration included in this book. We give references for the evidence we present, but the thinking and the arguments that allow us to interpret the evidence have come from many sources. We acknowledge the help we have received from a wide array of experts who contributed to individual sections or reviewed the draft text. These generous people have provided information and given their comments and support without any question of charge or any attempt to exchange favours. For this, we and WHO are immensely grateful.

For personal contributions and additional research, we are indebted to (in alphabetical order): Dr Martin Adams (University of Surrey, Guildford, United Kingdom), Dr Brian Ardy (South Bank University, London, United Kingdom), Dr Paolo Aureli (Istituto Superiore di Sanità, Rome, Italy), Dr Bruno de Benoist (Department of Nutrition for Health and Development, WHO headquarters), Dr Elisabeth Dowler (University of Warwick, United Kingdom), Dr Margaret Douglas (Common Services Agency for the National Health Service (NHS) Scotland, Edinburgh, United Kingdom), Dr Robert Goodland (World Bank, Washington, DC, United States of America), Dr Jens Gundgaard (University of Southern Denmark, Odense, Denmark), Dr Corinna Hawkes (Sustain: the alliance for better food and farming, London, United Kingdom), Dr Annemein Haveman-Nies (National Institute of Public Health and the Environment (RIVM), Bilthoven, Netherlands), Dr Anne Käsbohrer (Bundesinstituts für gesundheitlichen Verbraucherschutz und

Veterinärmedizin (BgVV), Berlin, Germany), Dr Alan Kerbey (International Obesity TaskForce, London, United Kingdom), Dr Marion Koopmans (Research Laboratory for Infectious Diseases, Bilthoven, Netherlands), Dr Karen Lock (London School of Hygiene and Tropical Medicine), Professor Jim Mann (University of Otago, Dunedin, New Zealand), Dr Eric Millstone (University of Sussex, Brighton, United Kingdom), Dr Gerald Moy (Department of Food Safety, WHO headquarters), Dr Joceline Pomerleau (London School of Hygiene and Tropical Medicine, United Kingdom), Dr Elio Riboli (International Agency for Research on Cancer, Lyon, France), Dr Maura Ricketts (Communicable Disease Surveillance and Response, WHO headquarters), Dr Jocelyn Rocourt (Department of Food Safety, WHO headquarters), Dr Katrin Schmidt (Bundesinstituts für gesundheitlichen Verbraucherschutz und Veterinärmedizin (BgVV), Berlin, Germany), Professor Aubrey Sheiham (University College London, United Kingdom) and Professor Leigh Sparks (University of Stirling, United Kingdom).

For assistance with reading and commenting on drafts of the text, we express our appreciation and gratitude to (in alphabetical order): Dr Martin Adams (University of Surrey, Guildford, United Kingdom), Dr Carlos Alvarez-Dardet (University of Alicante, San Vicente del Raspeig, Spain), Dr Dieter Arnold (Bundesinstituts für gesundheitlichen Verbraucherschutz und Veterinärmedizin (BgVV), Berlin, Germany), Dr Paolo Aureli (Istituto Superiore di Sanità, Rome, Italy), Dr Sue Barlow (Institute for Environment and Health, University of Leicester, United Kingdom), Dr Wolfgang Barth (Centre for Epidemiology and Health Research, Zepernick, Germany), Dr Bruno de Benoist (Department of Nutrition for Health and Development, WHO headquarters), Dr Carsten Bindslev-Jensen (Allergy Centre, Odense University Hospital, Denmark), Dr Gunn-Elin Bjørneboe (National Nutrition Council, Oslo, Norway), Dr Zsuzsanna Brazdova (Masaryk University, Brno, Czech Republic), Dr Eric Brunner (University College London, United Kingdom), Dr Caroline Codrington (University of Crete, Heraklion, Greece), Professor Finn Diderichsen (Karolinska Institute, Stockholm, Sweden), Dr Carlos Dora (European Centre for the Environment and Health, Rome, WHO Regional Office for Europe), Dr Elisabeth Dowler (University of Warwick, United Kingdom), Dr Guy van den Eede (European Commission Joint Research Centre, Institute for Health and Consumer Protection, Ispra, Italy), Dr Raymond Ellard (Food Safety Authority of Ireland, Dublin, Ireland), Dr Maria Ellul (Health Promotion Department, Floriana, Malta), Dr Gino Farchi (Istituto Superiore di Sanità, Rome, Italy), Dr Peter Fürst (Chemical and Veterinary Control Laboratory, Münster, Germany), Professor Igor Glasunov (State Research Centre for Preventive Medicine, Moscow, Russian

Federation), Dr Robert Goodland (World Bank, Washington, DC, United States of America), Professor Vilius Grabauskas (Kaunas University of Medicine, Lithuania), Dr Donato Greco (Istituto Superiore di Sanità, Rome, Italy), Dr Jens Gundgaard (University of Southern Denmark, Odense, Denmark), Dr Elizabeth Guttenstein (WWF European Policy Office, Brussels, Belgium), Dr Ranate Hans (Bundesinstituts für gesundheitlichen Verbraucherschutz und Veterinärmedizin (BgVV), Berlin, Germany), Dr Annemein Haveman-Nies (National Institute of Public Health and the Environment (RIVM), Bilthoven, Netherlands), Dr Serge Hercberg (Institut nationale de la santé et de la recherche médicale (INSERM), Paris, France), Dr Vicki Hird (Sustain: the alliance for better food and farming, London, United Kingdom), Professor Alan Jackson (University of Southampton, United Kingdom), Dr Anthony Kafatos (University of Crete, Heraklion, Greece), Dr Dorit Nitzan Kaluski (Ministry of Health, Jerusalem, Israel), Dr Ilona Koupilova (London School of Hygiene and Tropical Medicine, United Kingdom), Dr Alan Kerbey (International Obesity TaskForce, London, United Kingdom), Dr Marion Koopmans (Research Laboratory for Infectious Diseases, Bilthoven, Netherlands), Professor Daan Kromhout (National Institute of Public Health and the Environment (RIVM), Bilthoven, Netherlands), Dr Anne Käsbohrer (Bundesinstituts für gesundheitlichen Verbraucherschutz und Veterinärmedizin (BgVV), Berlin, Germany), Dr Denis Lairon (Institut nationale de la santé et de la recherché médicale (INSERM), Paris, France), Ms Hanne Larsen (Veterinary and Food Administration, Ministry of Food, Agriculture and Fisheries, Copenhagen, Denmark), Ms Lisa Lefferts (Comsumers Union, Washington, DC, United States of America), Dr Karen Lock (London School of Hygiene and Tropical Medicine, United Kingdom), Dr Susanne Logstrup (European Heart Network, Brussels, Belgium), Jeannette Longfield (Sustain: the alliance for better food and farming, London, United Kingdom), Dr Fabio Luelmo (tuberculosis consultant, WHO headquarters), Dr Ian MacArthur (Chartered Institute of Environmental Health, London, United Kingdom), Professor Lea Maes (University of Ghent, Belgium), Dr Rainer Malisch (State Institute for Chemical and Veterinary Analysis of Food, Freiburg, Germany)Professor Jim Mann (University of Otago, Dunedin, New Zealand), Professor Barrie Margetts (University of Southampton, United Kingdom), Ms Karen McColl (International Obesity TaskForce, London, United Kingdom), Professor Martin McKee (London School of Hygiene and Tropical Medicine, United Kingdom), Professor Anthony McMicheal (London School of Hygiene and Tropical Medicine, United Kingdom), Dr Bettina Menne (Technical Officer, Global Change and Health, WHO Regional Office for Europe), Dr Eric Millstone (University of Sussex, Brighton, United

Kingdom), Dr Gerald Moy (Department of Food Safety, WHO headquarters), Dr Paula Moynihan (University of Newcastle upon Tyne, United Kingdom), Professor Aulikki Nissinen (National Public Health Institute, Helsinki, Finland), Professor Andreu Palou (University of the Balearic Islands, Palma de Mallorca, Spain), Dr Carmen Perez-Rodrigo (Department of Public Health, Bilbao, Spain), Ms Annette Perge (Veterinary and Food Administration, Ministry of Food, Agriculture and Fisheries, Copenhagen, Denmark), Professor Janina Petkeviciene (Kaunas Medical University, Lithuania), Dr Stefka Petrova (National Centre of Hygiene, Medical Ecology and Nutrition, Sofia, Bulgaria), Dr Pirjo Pietenen (National Public Health Institute, Helsinki, Finland), Professor David Pimentel (Cornell University, Ithaca, New York, United States of America), Dr Joceline Pomerleau (London School of Hygiene and Tropical Medicine, United Kingdom), Professor Ritva Prättälä (National Public Health Institute, Helsinki, Finland), Professor Jules Pretty (University of Essex, Colchester, United Kingdom), Dr Iveta Pudule (Health Promotion Centre, Riga, Latvia), Professor Pekka Puska (Noncommunicable Diseases and Mental Health, WHO headquarters), Dr Mike Rayner (British Heart Foundation Health Promotion Research Group, Oxford, United Kingdom), Dr Allan Reilly (Food Safety Authority of Ireland, Dublin, Ireland), Dr Anton Reinl (Rechts und Steuerpolitik Präsidentenkonferenz der landwirtschaftskammern österreichs, Vienna, Austria), Professor Andrew Renwick (University of Southampton, United Kingdom), Dr Elio Riboli (International Agency for Research on Cancer, Lyon, France), Dr Maura Ricketts (Communicable Disease Surveillance and Response, WHO headquarters), Dr Anna Ritsatakis (former Head, WHO European Centre for Health Policy, WHO Regional Office for Europe), Dr Jocelyn Rocourt (Department of Food Safety, WHO headquarters), Professor A.J. Rugg-Gunn (WHO Collaborating Centre for Nutrition and Oral Health, University of Newcastle upon Tyne, United Kingdom), Professor Hugh Sampson (Jaffe Food Allergy Institute, Mount Sinai School of Medicine, New York, New York, United States of America), Dr Jørgen Schlundt (Department of Food Safety, WHO headquarters), Professor Liselotte Schäfer Elinder (National Institute of Public Health, Stockholm, Sweden), Professor Lluis Serra-Majem (University of Las Palmas de Gran Canaria, Spain), Professor Aubrey Sheiham (University College London, United Kingdom), Dr Prakash Shetty (Food and Agriculture Organization of the United Nations, Rome, Italy), Professor Leigh Sparks (University of Stirling, United Kingdom), Dr Sylvie Stachenko (former Head, Non-Communicable Diseases and Mental Health, WHO Regional Office for Europe), Professor Elizaveta Stikova (Republic Institute for Health Protection, Skopje, The former Yugoslav Republic of Macedonia), Dr Boyd Swinburn (Deakin University, Melbourne, Australia), Professor Andrew Tompkins (Institute of Child Health, London, United Kingdom), Professor Antonia Trichopoulou (WHO Collaborating Centre for Nutrition, University of Athens, Greece), Dr Sirje Vaask (Ministry of Social Affairs, Tallinn, Estonia), Professor Paolo Vineis (University of Turin, Italy), Dr Mathilde de Wit (Protection of the Human Environment/Food Safety, WHO headquarters), Professor Alicja Wolk (Karolinska Institute, Stockholm, Sweden) and Dr Gabor Zajkas (National Institute of Food Hygiene and Nutrition, Budapest, Hungary).

For their assistance in the production of this book, we are also very much in debt to staff of the WHO Regional Office for Europe (Ms Sally Charnley, Ms Elena Critselis, Ms Madeleine Nell Freeman, Ms Gillian Holm, Ms Carina Madsen and Ms Nina Roth) and the International Obesity TaskForce (Ms Rachel Jackson Leach, Dr Neville Rigby and Dr Maryam Shayeghi), who have helped in the production of this book.

Aileen Robertson, Cristina Tirado,
Tim Lobstein, Marco Jermini, Cecile Knai, Jørgen H. Jensen,
Anna Ferro-Luzzi and W.P.T. James

Editors

Professor Anna Ferro-Luzzi
Head, National Research Institute for Food and Nutrition, WHO Collaborating Centre for Nutrition, Rome, Italy

Professor W.P.T. James
Chairman, International Obesity TaskForce, London, United Kingdom

Dr Jørgen H. Jensen
Director, Regional Office for Food Control, Copenhagen, Denmark

Dr Marco Jermini
Head, Food Microbiology Department, Cantonal Laboratory, Public Health Division, Department of Social Affairs, Lugano, Switzerland

Ms Cecile Knai
Consultant, Nutrition and Food Security, WHO Regional Office for Europe

Dr Tim Lobstein
Director, The Food Commission, London, United Kingdom

Dr Aileen Robertson
Regional Adviser, Nutrition and Food Security, WHO Regional Office for Europe

Dr Cristina Tirado
Regional Adviser, Food Safety, WHO European Centre for Environment and Health, Rome, WHO Regional Office for Europe

Abbreviations

Organizations, studies, programmes and projects

cCASHh	Climate Change and Adaptation Strategies for Human Health (WHO project)
CINDI	WHO countrywide integrated noncommunicable disease intervention (programme)
DAFNE	Data Food Networking (study)
DASH	dietary approaches to stop hypertension (trial)
EC	European Commission
ECRHS	European Community Respiratory Health Survey
EFCOSUM	European Food Consumption Survey Method (project)
EPIC	European prospective investigation into cancer
FINE	Finland, Italy and the Netherlands (study)
EU	European Union
FAO	Food and Agriculture Organization of the United Nations
GEMS/Food	Food Contamination Monitoring and Assessment Programme of the Global Environment Monitoring System
GEMS/Food Europe	WHO European Programme for Monitoring and Assessment of Dietary Exposure to Potentially Hazardous Substances
IFOAM	International Federation of Organic Agriculture Movements
MISTRA	Foundation for Strategic Environmental Research
SCOOP	Scientific Co-operation within the European Community
SENECA	Survey Europe on Nutrition in the Elderly: a Concerted Action
UNICEF	United Nations Children's Fund
WTO	World Trade Organization

Technical and other terms

ANGELO	analysis grid for environments linked to obesity (framework)
BMI	body mass index
BSE	bovine spongiform encephalopathy
CAP	(EU) Common Agricultural Policy
CCEE	countries of central and eastern Europe
CHD	coronary heart disease
CO_2	carbon dioxide
CVD	cardiovascular diseases
DALYs	disability-adjusted life-years
DDT	dichlorodiphenyltrichloroethane
DMFT	decayed, missing and filled permanent teeth
GATT	General Agreement on Trade and Tariffs
GMO	genetically modified organism
HACCP	hazard analysis and critical control points
HDL	high-density lipoprotein (cholesterol)
IUD	intrauterine device
LDL	low-density lipoprotein (cholesterol)
NIS	newly independent states
N_2O	nitrous oxide
RDA	recommended daily allowance
PCBs	polychlorinated biphenyls
PCDDs	dibenzo-p-dioxins
PCDFs	polychlorinated dibenzofurans
SD	standard deviation
STEFANI	strategies for effective food and nutrition initiatives (model)
vCJD	variant Creutzfeldt-Jacob disease

Foreword

In 2000, the WHO Regional Committee for Europe requested the Regional Director, in resolution EUR/RC50/R8, to take action to help fulfil WHO's role in implementing its first food and nutrition action plan for the WHO European Region. This included presenting Member States with a review of the scientific evidence needed to develop integrated and comprehensive national food and nutrition policies. This book fills that need, providing a comprehensive, in-depth analysis of the data on nutritional health, foodborne disease, and food safety and public health concerns about the supply and security of food in Europe.

First, this book looks at the burden of diet-related disease in the European Region, discusses the costs to society and asks whether the incidence of these diseases could be reduced. It presents policy options and solutions, along with dietary guidelines and case studies from different countries.

Just like clean air and water, a variety of high-quality, nutritious, safe food is crucial to human health. Many sectors – the health sector and others, such as agriculture and food retailing and catering – influence health. Ensuring the availability of such food is one of the best ways to promote good business while protecting and promoting health. WHO has developed global strategies for nutrition and food safety, and this book makes specific recommendations for the countries in the European Region to ensure consumer confidence while protecting and promoting the population's health.

Efficient agricultural policies have ensured that most populations in Europe have a secure food supply, so much so that many public health experts no longer understand the concept of food security. This book explains what food security means to the health of Europeans today; it also:

- *spells out the health aspects of food production;*
- *examines the forces that shape food consumption patterns; and*
- *explores the opportunities for influencing food policies so that health experts can better understand what evidence exists and what methods can be used to ensure that health receives due priority.*

Fortunately, the solutions for the ethical concerns surrounding food and health are in line with solutions for protecting the environment and promoting sustainable rural development. In addition, the book shows how poverty increases food inequalities in every country in Europe, and suggests policy options to reduce them.

Policy on food and nutrition may be a relatively new concept for some public health experts in Europe. This book presents case studies: examples of policies that promote public health (policy concordance) and of those that ignore it (policy discordance). They show why comprehensive food and nutrition policies can only be successful if the policies on food production and distribution are developed along with those on food safety and nutrition.

Food and its central role in improving health should be perceived as an integral part of a primary health service. While health professionals usually lack a sufficient understanding of this role, the general public is becoming very concerned about it. This publication provides correct and consistent information for use by health professionals. This approach follows the initiatives of WHO and other international bodies to bring human and environmental health and sustainable development into a coherent whole.

Experts working all over Europe contributed technical input to this book. We at the WHO Regional Office for Europe sincerely thank all these people, who are committed to encouraging WHO to develop and promote the scientific evidence that helps governments to implement food and nutrition policies.

The WHO Regional Office for Europe encourages and supports countries in developing and implementing their food and nutrition action plans. The contribution of this publication is to strengthen the capacity of health professionals as an efficient investment in improving public health in Europe. Written to provide the scientific evidence for national action plans and the First Action Plan for Food and Nutrition Policy, WHO European Region 2000–2005, this book is one of the first to give a comprehensive review of the effects of the food we eat on the health we have the right to enjoy.

Marc Danzon
WHO Regional Director for Europe

Introduction: the need for action on food and nutrition in Europe

In the 1950s, Europe was recovering from a devastating war. Food policies were devoted to establishing secure, adequate supplies of food for the population. Refugees and food rationing were still huge problems, and the European Region relied heavily on countries such as Australia, Canada and the United States to provide its bread, cheese and meat.

By the mid-1970s, strong national and regional measures to support agriculture had helped ensure better agricultural supplies within the WHO European Region, in both the western and eastern countries. In general, there was plenty to eat, and a huge food processing industry had become well established.

Yet all was not well. By the 1980s, policies in western Europe had been too successful, creating problems of overproduction and what to do with the huge amounts of food that were not being eaten. In eastern Europe, the political changes of the late 1980s and early 1990s led to increasing problems with food supply and distribution. In addition, the movement of food increased in the 1990s, in terms of both the quantity transported and the distances travelled. Across the Region, there was evidence of increasing rates of disease related to the food being eaten: rising rates of foodborne infectious disease, rising rates of deficiency diseases in pockets of the Region and high rates of chronic, degenerative diseases in which diet plays a key role.

The impact of these diseases – the burden on health services and the costs to economies, societies and families – is beginning to be seen. In particular, health services are becoming conscious of the share of their budgets consumed by food-related ill health. In response, health policy-makers are turning their attention upstream, looking at the early causes of ill health, rather than its diagnosis and treatment. This enables policy-makers to explore possibilities for reducing the burden of disease on the health services and improving the health of the population at large.

This book supports these health policy initiatives. It reviews the current burden of food-related disease in the European Region, examines the links between disease and food, and looks upstream at the nature of food supplies. It

1

shows that policies on food supply and a range of related topics – such as sustainable agriculture and rural development, transport and food retailing and planning – are all linked to the problems of nutrition, food safety and food quality.

In doing this, the book recognizes the very uneven patterns of food production, food safety problems and diet currently prevailing in the European Region. These patterns vary widely between the Nordic, central and Mediterranean countries in the European Union (EU), and even more among the countries of central and eastern Europe (CCEE) and the newly independent states (NIS) of the former USSR. In addition, agricultural policies and support measures differ; food distribution and consumption patterns differ; dietary disease incidence and prevalence differ. These differences can help to reveal the causes of ill health, and point towards their solution.

This book gives data where the figures are available, and points to areas where they are lacking.[1] It shows that knowledge about the links between food production, distribution and consumption and subsequent health patterns is now sufficient to enable these elements to be seen as parts of a greater whole. This whole is influenced by past and present food policies, and can influence future policy-making.

Overview of the book

This book lays out the available data that show the links between health, nutrition, food and food supplies, as outlined in the First Action Plan for Food and Nutrition Policy, WHO European Region, 2000–2005 (Annex 1). Rising concern about health and consumer issues has led EU countries explicitly to include assessments of the effects on health of other sectors' policies, in accordance with the Amsterdam Treaty. The Action Plan recommends that WHO Member States within and outside the EU develop cross-sectoral mechanisms to ensure that health policies are integral to non-health sectors. The WHO Regional Office for Europe has expressed its commitment to supporting Member States in this task.

Diet and disease

Care needs to be taken to distinguish the share of disease attributable to poor diets and that avoidable through better diets. Two assumptions underpin the analysis of the costs and burdens of diet-related ill health: that diet can be a primary cause of disease or cause a reduction in disease, and that the extent of

---

[1] *Food and health in Europe: a new basis for action. Summary* (http://www.euro.who.int/Information-Sources/Publications/Catalogue/20030224_1). Copenhagen, WHO Regional Office for Europe, 2002 (accessed 3 September 2003).

this causation can be measured. Arriving at agreed figures for the extent of causation is not simple. In many diseases, diet is only one of many contributory factors (such as smoking or lack of physical activity), and even the dietary component may vary in different circumstances. Attempts need to be made to tease out the relationships. Chapter 1 looks at patterns of disease and their links to diet.

Fundamental to examining patterns of disease is the notion that they vary between places or over time. These differences allow the suggestion of reasons, which imply causative links, and of remedies, so that people with higher rates of disease may experience the lower rates enjoyed by others.

Chapter 1 reviews chronic noninfectious diseases with links to diet, including the major causes of death in the European Region (cardiovascular diseases and cancer) and those that may not kill but nevertheless are costly to health services, such as dental disease and hypertension. The role of physical activity as an independent and complementary factor reducing the risk of dietary diseases is highlighted.

Chapter 1 also discusses deficiency diseases, such as those related to iodine and iron deficiency, which are still widespread in parts of Europe, including subpopulations in western European countries, and Chapter 4 considers their implications for food and nutrition policies. Chapter 1 presents nutrition data during key stages in the human life cycle, and considers the possibilities that fetal, infant and childhood nutrition may have long-term implications for chronic diseases in adulthood.

Economic status – expressed as household income, earnings or employment category – appears to be a major determinant of many diseases that are known to have dietary links. As illustrated at the end of Chapter 1, poverty is associated with a higher level of risk for these diseases. Various policy implications can be derived from this, and Chapter 4 highlights such issues as access to healthier foods, their cost, the need to store and prepare them, planning and transport policies, education policies and priorities, advertising policies and the social provision of foods through schools and hospitals.

Food safety

Chapter 2 presents short reviews of the links between food safety, health and foodborne diseases. It also looks at toxicological and food safety issues, and considers concerns about the contamination of food with toxic chemicals (such as dioxins), potent microbial agents (such as *Escherichia coli* 0157) and bioactive proteins (such as protease-resistant prions), as well as longer-standing concerns about the impact on health of agrochemicals and veterinary drugs used to enhance agricultural productivity.

Good evidence links these aspects of food and health – principally food safety and nutrition – in certain circumstances. Each affects the other. On the one hand, nutritional status can determine the risk of infectious disease, and dietary patterns can lower the risk of infection. On the other, foodborne disease can reduce nutrient intake.

Food security and sustainable development

The role of food production in generating food-related ill health forms an integral part of this book. Chapter 3 discusses methods of agriculture and food processing, the types of food produced and the increasingly long distances that food commodities travel.

Although production is frequently asserted to follow the patterns of food demanded on the market, there are good reasons to suggest that food production has become dissociated from market demand and that many factors distort the market. The forms of food production determine not only food products' safety but also their nutritional and dietary value. Food production methods – and the factors that influence them – thus form an integral part of the patterns of food-related ill health.

Environmental issues, especially the need to develop farming methods that are sustainable in the long term, have a bearing on food production. A broad degree of concurrence can be foreseen between the production of food for human health and the production of food for environmental protection. Nutrition and environmental policies can thus be developed in parallel, as outlined in the WHO Action Plan.

Food production affects human health in other ways than through food consumption. The nature and sustainable development of the rural economy have implications for rural employment, social cohesion and leisure facilities. These in turn foster improved mental and physical health.

These issues are not mere by-products of sustainable development; they are central to the retention of rural social structures. The wider costs of conventional intensive agriculture have been described, and Chapter 3 gives some figures on their economic impact. Any health impact assessments of rural environmental policies and agricultural policies need to consider these largely hidden costs of different farming methods. Chapter 3 explores a model of social capital and social dividends, and different food production methods can be shown to help increase or deplete them.

Hidden costs or externalities (costs that are not directly borne by the production process) affect both agriculture and food processing, packaging and distribution. Transport, for example, has relatively low direct costs, but can have much higher true costs when externalities are taken into account. These hidden costs include pollution and traffic accidents. They not only indicate that the activity is not sustainable in the long term but also directly affect health, and hence place a burden on society and the health services.

Policies and strategies

Ensuring the safety of food is regulators' and legislators' first priority; its health promoting features and its sustainable supply come second. Breaches in food safety can lead to immediate and often fatal outbreaks of food poisoning, and the main thrust of food inspection and control procedures is to ensure that food is safe to be eaten.

Changes in food production methods, discussed in Chapter 3, have led to the changes in food control strategies discussed in Chapter 4, such as the adoption of hazard analysis and critical control points (HACCP) procedures. In addition, as discussed earlier, it is useful to look upstream and ask why contaminants and hazards find their way into the food supply, rather than relying on minimizing the risks from those that are already present.

Looking upstream at food production is one valuable step, but others also need to be taken. With increasing long-distance distribution of primary and processed products, across national boundaries and around the globe, national regulations are coming under scrutiny, and international agencies (such as the Codex Alimentarius Commission) are increasingly involved in setting safety standards. International standards for the food trade need to be set to protect health, and the health impact of trading policies needs to be assessed.

Chapter 4 discusses nutrition policies from the perspective of improving nutrition at key points during the life-course to maximize opportunities for health in later life. The examples given include exclusive breastfeeding in early infancy to prevent ill health in childhood, and the improvement of women's nutrition before and during pregnancy to ensure optimum growth of the fetus and infant and the prevention of disease in adulthood.

Chapter 4 also discusses the setting of population targets for healthy eating. These targets have become increasingly specific in the last 20 years, moving from general statements about the need to eat a healthy diet to numerical recommendations for certain nutrients and foods. Such targets as increasing fruit and vegetable consumption and reducing fat, salt and sugar intake have implications beyond the orbit of health educators and public advice, and are of direct concern to agricultural production and the food processing and retailing industries.

Population-based nutrition programmes are required to translate population targets into practice. Such programmes include various measures, ranging from specific initiatives advising on healthy lifestyles to controls over food labelling, health claims and advertising. Messages on healthy eating need to be consistent, and widely accepted and promoted by all stakeholders.

Nutrition, food safety and food standards are the policy areas that directly affect food-related ill health. As suggested, many other human activities and the policies that govern them have an influence. These activities include the growing, transport, processing, distribution and marketing of food. Policies on these activities can be presumed to have a bearing on subsequent food safety and nutrition, and hence influence health.

Health impact assessment of such policies is being developed in various forms across Europe and elsewhere, and the procedures have many common threads. The methods involve iterative processes, so that initial conclusions can be re-examined and refined and additional material added to the analysis. They have the advantage of providing the basis for a democratic form of decision-making, and can increase the transparency of the processes and of the interests involved in policy-making.

Different forms of intervention need greater analysis to examine their cost–effectiveness and – efficiency. Surveillance, including monitoring and evaluation, is discussed in Chapter 4.

WHO activities

Discordant agricultural, industrial and food policies can harm health, the environment and the economy, but harmful effects can be reduced and health can be promoted if all sectors are aware of the policy options. National policies on food and nutrition should address three overlapping areas: nutrition, food safety and a sustainable food supply (food security). The First Action Plan for Food and Nutrition Policy calls for interrelated strategies on all three (See Chapter 4, Fig. 4.1, p. 222).

WHO's traditional roles – supporting the health sector in the provision of services and training of health professionals, advising it on planning and assisting in health programmes – can be extended and developed. The Action Plan outlines a series of support measures for national and regional authorities. This book provides a basis for these actions, founded on scientific evidence on the causes of food-related ill health.

1. Diet and disease

The burden of disease varies widely within the WHO European Region and has changed dramatically in many countries over the last 20 years. Patterns of disease and changes in these patterns have environmental determinants, with diet and physical activity playing major roles.

This chapter assesses the range of major health issues confronting European countries and some of the principal determinants of diseases leading to death and disability. Differences and changes in diet explain much of the different patterns of ill health observed in children and adults.

Appropriate public health policies can help prevent the nutrition-related diseases discussed here. Chapter 4 presents recommendations on policy, and cross-references are made where applicable throughout Chapter 1.

Diet-related diseases: the principal health burden in Europe

The burden of disease has been assessed in terms of disability-adjusted life-years (DALYs). These incorporate an assessment of the years of life lost to different diseases before the age of 82.5 years for females and 80 for males *(1)* and the years spent in a disabled state *(2)*. Non-fatal health states are assigned values (disability weights) for estimating years lost to disability based on surveys. Years lost (severity adjusted) to disability are then added to years lost to premature mortality to yield an integrated unit of health: the DALY; one DALY represents the loss of one year of healthy life.

Fig. 1.1 shows the contribution of nutrition to the burden of disease in Europe *(3)*, displaying the share of DALYs lost to diseases that have a substantial dietary basis (such as cardiovascular diseases (CVD) and cancer) separately from that to which dietary factors contribute less substantially but still importantly. In 2000, 136 million years of healthy life were lost; major nutritional risk factors caused the loss of over 56 million and other nutrition-related factors played a role in the loss of a further 52 million. CVD are the leading cause of death, causing over 4 million deaths per year in Europe. Dietary factors explain much of the differences in these diseases in Europe. *The world health report (4)* includes an estimate of the quantitative contribution of dietary risk factors such as high blood pressure, serum cholesterol, overweight,

7

obesity and a low intake of fruits and vegetables. European policy-makers will need to make their own assessments of the relative burden of dietary risk factors in relation to disease prevalence in their own country.

Fig. 1.1. Lost years of healthy life in the European Region, 2000

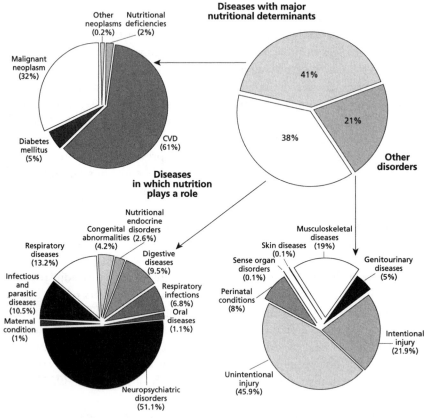

Source: adapted from *The world health report 2000. Health systems: improving performance (3)*.

Diet as a determinant of health

The dietary contributions to CVD, cancer, type 2 diabetes mellitus and obesity have many common components, and physical inactivity is also relevant to all four. The overall effect of each dietary component and of physical inactivity should be calculated and their relative quantitative significance estimated. Unfortunately, only one such assessment of the burden of disease attributable to nutrition in Europe has yet been published (5).

The National Institute of Public Health in Sweden attempted to estimate the burden of disease that could be attributed to various causal factors, including dietary factors, in the EU *(6)*, and ranked the leading risk factors contributing to the burden of disease (Table 1.1). Analyses suggest that poor nutrition accounts for 4.6% of the total DALYs lost in the EU, with overweight and physical inactivity accounting for an additional 3.7% and 1.4%, respectively *(6)*. This analysis does not, however, capture the complexity of the situation and is thus likely to underestimate the importance of nutrition. For example, dietary factors interact with other risk factors. Substantial fruit and vegetable consumption seems to reduce the risk of lung cancer among smokers, although smoking is associated with a large increase in the probability of developing lung cancer even among those with the highest consumption. Other dietary components may moderate the impact of alcohol consumption. Taken together, this evidence suggests that improving nutrition could be the single most important contributor to reducing the burden of disease in the WHO European Region.

Table 1.1. Contribution of selected factors
to the overall burden of disease in the EU

Causal factor	Contribution (%)
Tobacco smoking	9.0
Alcohol consumption	8.4
Overweight	3.7
Occupational risks	3.6
Low fruit and vegetable consumption	3.5
Relative poverty	3.1
Unemployment	2.9
Illicit drugs	2.4
Physical inactivity	1.4
Diet high in saturated fat	1.1
Outdoor air pollution	0.2

Source: Determinants of the burden of disease in the European Union (6).

Studies from Australia and New Zealand *(7–9)* support this finding. In these countries, about 3% of the burden of disease (2.8% in Australia and 2–4% in New Zealand) could be attributed to low consumption of fruits and vegetables. The Australian studies also reported that about 10% of all cancer cases could be attributable to insufficient intake *(8,9)*.

The contribution of various factors to the total burden of disease has been estimated in Australia *(8)* (Fig. 1.2). The multiple interacting processes by which different dietary factors contribute to the disease burden make these analyses more difficult, and there is no agreement on the extent of synergism or on the relative quantitative importance of the main contributors to different diseases or to public health in general.

Fig. 1.2. Proportion of the total burden of disease (in DALYs lost)
attributable to selected risk factors, by sex, Australia, 1996

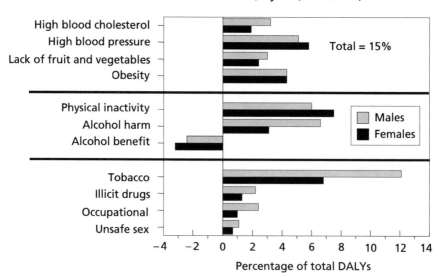

Source: adapted from Mathers et al. *(8)*.

CVD and cancer cause almost two thirds of the overall burden of disease in Europe. Conservative estimates suggest that about one third of CVD is related to inappropriate nutrition, although the need for more research is widely acknowledged. Cancer kills about 1 million adults each year in the WHO European Region. As with CVD, inappropriate diet causes about one third of all cancer deaths worldwide. A report by the World Cancer Research Fund and the American Institute for Cancer Research *(10)* estimated that improved diet, along with maintenance of physical activity and appropriate body mass, could reduce cancer incidence by 30–40% over time. Doll & Peto *(11)* made a widely cited estimate of the diet-related burden of cancer, attributing about 35% of all cancer deaths in the United States to diet (excluding alcohol) and a further 3% to alcohol. They qualified this, however, by also suggesting a range of plausible estimates of between 10% and 70% attributable to diet and a further 2.4% to alcohol. Doll *(12)* later proposed that the evidence available up to the early 1990s associating diet with cancer had become stronger, and gave a narrower range of 20–60%.

Numerous studies have aimed to identify the components of diet that have the greatest influence on CVD and cancer. Many earlier clinical and epidemiological investigations focused on fat intake. In the early 1990s, a study in the United States suggested that reducing fat consumption from 37% of energy intake to 30% would prevent 2% of deaths from CVD and cancer, primarily among people older than 65 years *(13)*. More recently,

Willett *(14)* suggested that replacing saturated and *trans*-fatty acids in the diet could be more important for preventing CVD than reducing the total amount of fat consumed. For example, replacing 6% of energy intake from predominantly animal fat with monounsaturated fat could potentially reduce CVD by 6–8% *(15)*. Growing evidence also indicates that other dietary factors are associated with CVD and cancer risk. There is an international consensus that an excess of energy (more energy consumed in the diet than is expended) and alcohol are risk factors for certain types of cancer (mouth, pharynx, larynx, oesophagus and liver) and that a high intake of fruits and vegetables protects in part against the agents causing cancers of the mouth, pharynx, oesophagus, stomach and lung *(10,16,17)*. Deficiencies of substances such as vitamin A, other antioxidant vitamins and non-nutrient components of fruits and vegetables have also been linked to an increased risk of both CVD and cancer, although this area remains inadequately researched *(10,18)*.

Joffe & Robertson *(19)* investigated the potential health gain if vegetable and fruit intake increased substantially within the EU and three countries in the process of joining it. They estimated that about 23 000 deaths from coronary heart disease (CHD) and major types of cancer before age 65 could be prevented annually if low intake of fruits and vegetables were increased to that of the groups consuming the most.

The importance of nutrition in determining or modulating so many major causes of disability and premature death implies that dietary patterns should differ remarkably across Europe and change over time. Fig. 1.3 displays the remarkable variation in estimated national intake of fruits and vegetables in the EU countries, the Czech Republic, Hungary and Poland. There is a general north–south gradient, with higher intake in the south.

The WHO goal for vegetable and fruit intake is at least 400 g per person per day as a national average throughout the year *(21)*. The intake is less than this in most countries in the European Region, although climate and agricultural conditions in southern and central Europe are ideal for producing sufficient fruits and vegetables to feed the whole Region throughout the year. The mean consumption of fruits and vegetables is a poor measure of the distribution of intake within a population. Fruit and vegetable intake is not normally distributed evenly, but highly skewed. Thus, the mean intake values conceal a large proportion of the population within each country with very low consumption. Despite a relatively high mean consumption of 500 g per day in Greece, for example, 37% of the population is below the recommended level *(22)*.

The availability of fruits and vegetables differs vastly at different times of year. Powles et al. *(23)* found evidence for the importance of seasonality in the role of fresh fruits and vegetables in reducing CVD mortality. This has been

suggested as one explanation for the seasonal cycling and severity of CHD in
the affected countries *(23)*.

Fig. 1.3. Vegetable and fruit intake (mean g/day)
in selected European countries

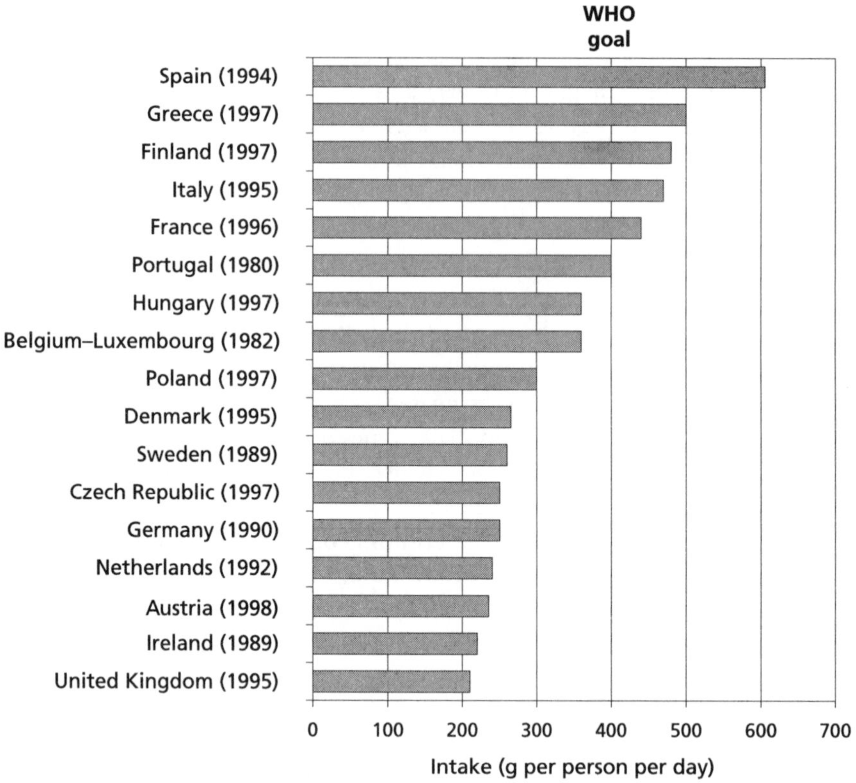

Source: Comparative analysis of food and nutrition policies in the WHO European Region 1994–1999. Full report (20).

Not only does fruit and vegetable intake differ surprisingly across Europe,
but both the total quantity eaten and the variety and choice have changed remarkably over the last 50 years.

Similar changes and differences apply to the availability of milk fat and
fish (according to food balance sheets of the Food and Agriculture
Organization of the United Nations (FAO) – Fig. 1.4 and 1.5). Consumption
of milk fat is very substantial in north-western Europe and especially in the
non-Mediterranean countries. Given its major contribution in inducing high
serum cholesterol levels and CVD, it is not surprising that milk-fat
consumption predicts the prevalence of CVD across Europe *(24)*.

Fig. 1.4. Availability of milk fat, selected countries in the WHO European Region, 1998

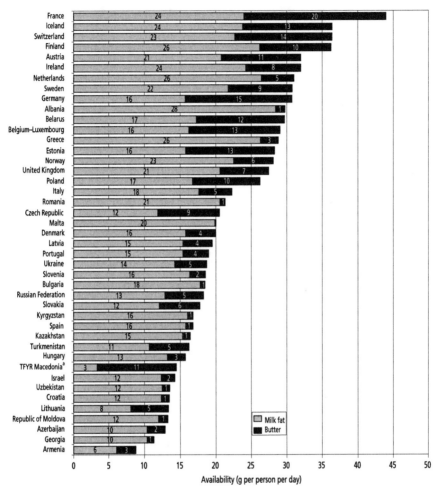

[a] The former Yugoslav Republic of Macedonia.

Source: Food and Agriculture Organization of the United Nations (http://apps.fao.org/lim500/wrap.pl?FoodBalanceSheet&Domain=FoodBalanceSheet&Language=english, accessed 25 September 2003).

The pattern of fish supply shown in Fig. 1.5 may result from the availability of fish in the locality unless a country is affluent enough to import substantial quantities. If an intake of at least 200 g fish per person per week is considered reasonable, consumption reaches this level in only about 10% of countries.

Fig. 1.5. Availability of fish, selected countries in the WHO European Region, 1998

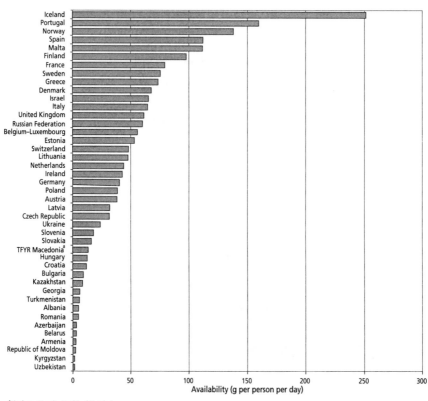

ª The former Yugoslav Republic of Macedonia.

Source: Food and Agriculture Organization of the United Nations (http://apps. fao.org/lim500/wrap.pl?FoodBalanceSheet&Domain=FoodBalanceSheet&Language=english, accessed 25 September 2003).

Government policies and industry initiatives can substantially affect the national consumption of all three categories of food considered here. For instance, when eastern Finland and the province of North Karelia were especially affected by CVD, a major comprehensive prevention project was started in 1972, and developed from a demonstration project into national action. Legislative and other policy decisions included the development of low-fat spreads, fat and salt labelling for many food groups and improving the quality of meals at schools and in the army. The food industry became involved by developing a cholesterol-lowering rapeseed oil from a new type of rape plant that grows well in the northern climate of Finland. This was in effect a domestic, heart-healthy alternative to butter. As a result, from 1972 to 1997, vegetable intake nearly tripled; fish consumption doubled; the use of full-fat milk fell dramatically (Fig. 1.6) and vegetable oil increasingly replaced butter (Fig. 1.7).

Fig. 1.6. Percentage of men and women aged 35–59 years in North Karelia, Finland drinking fat-containing milk and skim milk, 1972 and 1997

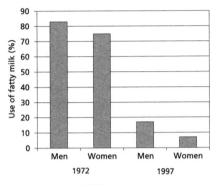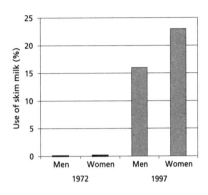

Source: Puska *(25)*.

Fig. 1.7. Percentage of men and women aged 35–59 years in North Karelia, Finland using butter and vegetable oil, 1972 and 1997

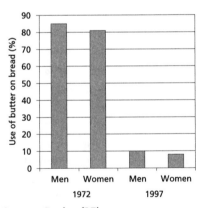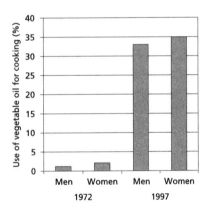

Source: Puska *(25)*.

These comprehensive actions were associated with a remarkable fall in CVD mortality, especially CHD mortality, in eastern Finland (Fig. 1.8).

These differences in intake of fruits and vegetables, fish and milk fat can be linked to other nutritional problems. Thus, pregnant women eating more fruits and vegetables have a higher intake of folic acid; this has been linked to fewer small and premature babies and to the prevention of neural tube defects (see p. 47). Women's consumption of fruits and vegetables limits the likelihood of iron deficiency before pregnancy and of developing anaemia in pregnancy.

In addition, the fruits and vegetables eaten by a nursing mother induce higher blood levels of water-soluble vitamins, which readily pass to the breastfed baby.

Fig. 1.8. Predicted and observed mortality from CHD in females aged 35–64, north-eastern Finland

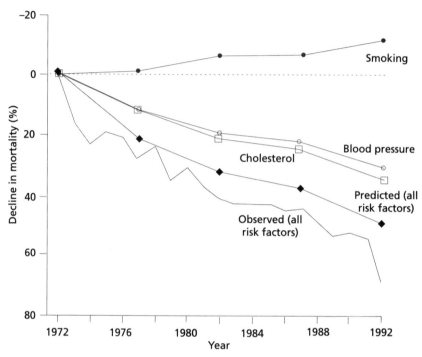

Source: Vartiainen et al. (26).

The consumption of vegetables and fish by young women before and during pregnancy is also crucial to storing omega-3 essential fatty acids in their fat depots, which are called on selectively during pregnancy for channelling to the uterus and the developing fetus. The growth of the fetus and especially the brain of both the fetus and young child crucially depend on having adequate amounts of omega-3 essential fatty acids, which happens only if the mother has been eating an appropriate diet and breastfeeding her child. WHO advocates the gradual introduction of a variety of puréed fruits and vegetables and fish and meats at about 6 months (see Chapter 4, pp. 245–248) (27). Unmodified cow's milk should not be given as a drink before the age of 9 months but can be used in small quantities in preparing complementary foods for babies aged 6–9 months (see Chapter 4, pp. 245–248).

Fish not only is a good source of omega-3 fatty acids but also modulates immune responsiveness, limits disturbances of fat metabolism and stabilizes the excitability of the heart, thereby limiting the risk of sudden cardiac death. Moreover, fish provides an excellent source of zinc, iron and animal proteins that are conducive to the longitudinal growth of the child and the prevention of anaemia.

Given this remarkable interplay between different foods and health, why is the European population not consuming enough of these vital foods at every stage of the life-course? What are the main impediments to their availability and consumption? The precise reasons for poor intake need to be assessed in each country and for each age group, but this book discusses general possibilities in the section on social inequality in this chapter (see pp. 66–73) and gives policy options in Chapter 4.

The widely varying dietary patterns across Europe are governed by not only geographical, climatic and agricultural factors described in Chapter 3 (see Fig. 3.5, p. 166) but also societal conditions, including income levels, civil strife, the status of women, urbanization, exposure to marketing and the changing of family and community structures.

The nutrition transition and its effects on health

National consumption figures for fruits and vegetables and other dietary ingredients (Fig. 1.3–1.5) and breastfeeding rates (see Fig. 1.23, p. 51) differ remarkably. Consumption levels can change over relatively short periods, as shown by the decline in milk-fat consumption in parts of Finland.

Comparison of dietary patterns with other national statistics, such as gross national product, suggests that consumption patterns for dietary components such as meat, fat and vegetables are linked to national wealth, but these patterns change over time and, at the level of households, may depend on income and food security. At a global level, good evidence indicates a transition in nutrition, in which rising national wealth is accompanied by changes in diet, with an increase in consumption of animal-derived products, fat and oil and a reduction in cereal foods and vegetables. The WHO publication *Globalization, diets and noncommunicable diseases (28)* describes this transition:

> Rapid changes in diets and lifestyles resulting from industrialization, urbanization, economic development and market globalization are having a significant impact on the nutritional status of populations. The processes of modernization and economic transition have led to industrialization in many countries and the development of economies that are dependent on trade in the global market. While results include improved standards of living and greater access to services, there have also been significant negative consequences in terms of inappropriate dietary patterns and decreased physical activities, and a corresponding increase in nutritional and diet-related diseases.

Food and food products have become commodities produced and traded in a market that has expanded from an essentially local base to an increasingly global one. Changes in the world food economy have contributed to shifting dietary patterns, for example increased consumption of an energy-dense diet high in fat, particularly saturated fat, and low in carbohydrates. This combines with a decline in energy expenditure that is associated with a sedentary lifestyle, with motorized transport, and labour-saving devices at home and at work largely replacing physically demanding manual tasks, and leisure time often being dominated by physically undemanding pastimes.

Because of these changes in dietary and lifestyle patterns, diet-related diseases – including obesity, type II diabetes mellitus, cardiovascular disease, hypertension and stroke, and various forms of cancer – are increasingly significant causes of disability and premature death in both developing and newly developed countries. They are taking over from more traditional public health concerns like undernutrition and infectious disease, and placing additional burdens on already overtaxed national health budgets.

Dietary patterns, based on food supply data, can be estimated for national populations, using the FAO database, from 1960 onwards. A pattern of nutrition transition can be detected in, for example, southern European countries, which traditionally had diets dominated by plant foods, fish, olive oil and wine. Countries such as Greece, Portugal and Spain show some evidence of moving from Mediterranean-type diets to ones more like those eaten in northern Europe, rich in meat and dairy products.

Simopoulos & Visioli *(29)* suggest that there is not one type of Mediterranean diet, although countries of the Mediterranean region traditionally all have high intakes of fruits and vegetables and low intakes of saturated animal fat. The region includes varied cultures, traditions, incomes and dietary habits and patterns, all of which are evolving with the impact of economic development and globalization. The food supplies and therefore the diets of Europeans seem to be changing rapidly.

The demographic transition – from rural societies with low life expectancy at birth and families with many children to urban societies with higher life expectancy at birth and fewer children – is well known. The epidemiological transition that follows the demographic transition is also fairly well understood: a shift from endemic deficiency and infectious diseases, mostly in early life, to chronic diseases in later life.

Evidence is now sufficient to propose a general theory for these causally and chronologically linked demographic, nutrition and epidemiological transitions. When populations undergo massive social and technological change – as in the NIS, where the level of urbanization is predicted to reach 90% by 2015 – their food supplies and thus disease patterns also change. This pattern can be traced in more economically developed countries, such as the United Kingdom, between the sixteenth and eighteenth centuries following the agrarian and industrial revolutions. In the CCEE and NIS, such transitions are taking place very much faster and in some cases extremely rapidly. This has immense implications for policy-making in public health.

The nutrition transition is marked by a shift away from diets based on indigenous staple foods, such as grains, starchy roots and locally grown legumes, fruits and vegetables, towards more varied diets that include more processed food, more foods of animal origin, more added sugar, salt and fat, and often more alcohol. This shift is accompanied by reduced physical activity in work and leisure. Combined, these changes leading to a rapid increase in obesity and its associated health problems.

Consequently, in most countries of the European Region, diet-related diseases are gaining in magnitude and effects compared with the effects of specific dietary deficiencies, even though certain micronutrient deficiencies (in, for example, iodine and iron) are still prevalent. If appropriate public policies are not implemented to change the transition patterns, these public health problems are likely to continue into future generations.

Costs to the health care system

Information is needed on the cost of diseases attributable to diet and the burden they place on society. It can be valuable in risk management (evaluating the benefits and costs of adopting certain risk control measures or health interventions) and in assessing the impact of ill health on national economies and health service budgets.

In the early 1990s, the Federal Ministry of Health estimated the total costs of diet-related diseases to the health service in Germany at about DM 83.5 billion (Table 1.2), equivalent to 30% of the total cost of health care. The costs include both direct costs (medical and health service expenditure) and indirect costs (from workers' reduced productivity or lost family income). The highest costs resulted from CVD (12% of the total national health care costs), followed by dental caries (7%) and diet-dependent cancer (3%) (30).

In the United Kingdom, Liu et al. (31) estimated that CHD cost £1.65 billion to the health care system, £2.42 billion in informal care and £4.02 billion in productivity loss: a total annual cost of £8.08 billion. This made CHD the most expensive disease in the United Kingdom for which comparable analyses have been done, including back pain, rheumatoid arthritis and Alzheimer's disease.

Liu et al. (31) also noted considerable variation in both the direct health care costs and the productivity and informal care costs per 100 000 CHD patients in different countries. Unsurprisingly, given the different levels of provision and of unit costs, they observed that the direct health and social care costs of CHD were considerably lower in the United Kingdom than in other countries for which data were available. The direct costs were about 1.2 times higher in the Netherlands, 5.5 times higher in Sweden and 6 times higher in Germany. In contrast, the employment and informal care costs in the United Kingdom were higher than those in Switzerland and were very similar to those in Sweden or Germany.

Table 1.2. Costs of diet-dependent conditions in Germany, 1990s

Conditions	Estimated costs (DM billion)		
	Total	Direct	Indirect
CVD	32.9	15.4	17.6
Dental caries	20.2	20.2	<0.1
Cancer	9.6	1.6	8.1
Diabetes	3.8	2.3	1.5
Alcoholism	3.5	0.7	2.8
Diseases of the liver	3.1	0.4	2.6
Other conditions	2.6	1.4	0.5
Diseases of the pancreas	2.6	1.9	0.6
Lipid metabolism	1.4	1.2	0.9
Food poisoning	1.4	0.3	1.1
Goitre	1.3	1.1	0.2
Diseases of the gallbladder	1.1	0.8	0.3
All diet-related conditions	83.5	47.3	36.2

Source: adapted from Kohlmeier et al. (30).

Kenkel & Manning (32) summarized studies by the National Institutes of Health and by Wolf & Colditz (33) of the costs of illnesses associated with dietary factors and physical activity patterns in the United States. The illnesses included CHD, diabetes, stroke, osteoporosis, gall bladder disease and cancers of the breast, colon/rectum and prostate. The estimates are based on the assumption that dietary factors and sedentary lifestyles contribute to 60% of diabetes cases; 35% of breast, colon/rectum and prostate cancer cases; 30% of gall bladder disease; 25% of arthritis; and 20% of CHD and stroke. The total economic cost of all these diet- and exercise-related illnesses was estimated at US $137 billion (32): more than the economic costs of alcohol abuse and dependence (US $118 billion) or smoking (US $90 billion). The direct costs of diet- and exercise-related illnesses – health care expenditure attributable to these conditions – reached US $67 billion, or about 7% of total personal health care expenditure in the United States.

Also in the United States, Oster et al. (34) suggested that a sustained 10% weight loss among obese people would lead to a lifetime saving of US $2200–

5300 per person, depending on age, gender and starting body mass index and an increase in life expectancy of 2–7 months. It would cut lifetime incidence of CHD from 12 cases to 1 case per 1000, and the incidence of stroke from 38 to 13 cases per 1000 *(34)*. In Europe, obesity is estimated to account for about 7% of health care costs *(35)*. Obesity has been estimated to account for substantial direct costs to the health budgets in France *(36,37)*, Germany *(38)*, the Netherlands *(39)* and Sweden *(40)*. The indirect health care costs attributable to obesity are also estimated to be substantial: 3–4% of total health care costs in Germany, for example *(38)*.

Obesity is a highly stigmatized condition in several countries and has been associated with underachievement in education, reduced social activity and discrimination at work *(41)*. Indeed, obese people are often reported to earn less than their lean counterparts because of discrimination or diseases and disabilities caused by obesity *(39)*.

The avoidance of childhood diseases as a result of breastfeeding has been estimated to reduce the economic costs of care to society (http://www.visi.com/ ~artmama/kaiser.htm, accessed 19 September 2003) *(42)*. A study in the United States assessed the potential reduction in costs to society that could be attributed to an increase in breastfeeding from current levels (64% in hospital and 29% at 6 months of age) to those recommended by the Surgeon General of the United States (75% and 50%, respectively). Based on information related to three childhood illnesses (otitis media, gastroenteritis and necrotizing enterocolitis), it was estimated that about US $3.1 billion could be saved by preventing premature death from necrotizing enterocolitis and an additional US $0.5 billion through annual savings associated with reducing traditional expenditure on, for example, visits to physicians or hospitals and laboratory tests. The total estimated savings (US $3.6 billion) probably underestimates the true savings, as the figures reflect savings associated with treating only three illnesses and exclude the cost of over-the-counter medication for otitis media and gastroenteritis symptoms, physician charges for treating necrotizing enterocolitis and savings from reduced long-term morbidity.

In Norway, the National Council on Nutrition and Physical Activity assessed the cost–effectiveness of policies to increase the consumption of fruits and vegetables as a means to reduce cancer *(43)*. It calculated the cost of treating each patient with cancer as NKr 250 000 and estimated that preventing cancer cases could result in savings of NKr 3 million and a delay in cases of 10 years, NKr 1.5 million (using 1997 prices). A similar study in Denmark *(44)* investigated the economic consequences of an increased intake of fruits and vegetables. In 2000, the average daily intake in Denmark was about 250 g per person per day. Using recent estimates *(45)*, the study showed through modelling that, if the population doubled its intake of fruits and vegetables from 250 g to 500 g, life expectancy would increase by 0.9 years and 22% of all cancer incidence could be prevented *(44)*. The lower number of cancer cases, however, seemed not to affect the aggregate health care costs (a 0.1% change), based on data from 1997. This was the outcome of several offsetting effects. Because there were substantial changes across age groups, the disease-specific mean costs were held constant for each group, but the number of people with cancer, as well as the distribution, changes as the intake of fruits and vegetables increases *(44)*.

Early death or ill health creates not only financial costs to the health care system but also personal costs to the people concerned and their families and friends. For example, many people in Europe provide informal care for relatives suffering from diet-related diseases. In the United Kingdom, about 423 000 people have been estimated to give informal care to people with CHD alone, amounting to about 430 million hours of care in 1996 *(46)*. In addition to limiting their personal freedom, this work forces caregivers to leave paid jobs, which creates financial difficulties.

Although a better understanding of the burden of disease attributable to diet is long overdue, more information is needed on its cost to society. Such information can be valuable when evaluating the costs and benefits of adopting certain risk control measures or health interventions (risk management) and in assessing the effects of ill health on national economies and health service budgets.

Cost analysis is an important instrument for the health services in evaluating resources used or lost, and estimates of the direct and indirect costs of diseases are often used to support the argument that prevention can save money. For most programmes, however, the primary gains from a preventive activity or a change in health habits are increased longevity and improved quality of life rather than reduced lifetime medical expenditures. Only in some cases does an intervention improve health and save money at the same time. This is because paying more is usually necessary to receive better, more valued outcomes in health status, morbidity and mortality. The implications of a particular disease for health policy should not be evaluated solely on the basis of financial cost. Value judgements about health gain and the quality of life remain the principal criteria in deciding about investing in health.

Mortality from diet-related diseases

As discussed, CVD and cancer dominate as causes of premature death throughout the Region (Fig. 1.9), and about one third of CVD cases are related to eating a poor diet. CHD is the most common cause of premature death, accounting for nearly 900 000 deaths per year: 16% of all premature deaths in men and 12% in women. Up to the mid-1990s, mortality rates varied widely between the eastern and western countries of the Region. For example, the EU showed a steady fall in deaths from CHD, but most eastern countries exhibited

Fig. 1.9. Main causes of death in groups of countries
in the European Region

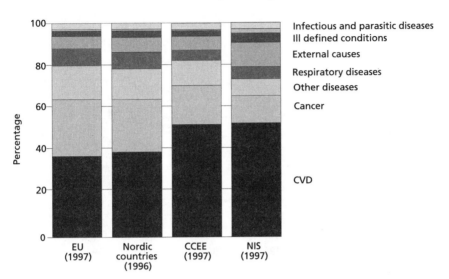

Source: European health for all database, WHO Regional Office for Europe, 2001.

increased rates. In the CCEE and NIS, CHD mortality is almost double that in the EU and still rising in many countries. Fig. 1.10 illustrates the wide range of death rates from cerebrovascular disease.

In the 1990s, however, mortality rates from diet-related diseases started evolving differently in some countries, especially those moving from a centralized to a market economy. The east–west divide is no longer a universally applicable image; significant differences are emerging between the NIS and CCEE.

For example, deaths from CVD decreased dramatically in the Baltic countries – and in the Czech Republic, Poland and Slovakia *(47)* – during the 1990s, while deaths from ischaemic heart disease have continued to increase in Belarus and the Russian Federation (Fig. 1.11). Cancer mortality rates are declining in the CCEE and NIS, falling by 25% in the central Asian republics in only a decade.

Variations in CVD: the fundamental role of diet

Countries in the European Region show marked discrepancies in rates of CVD. Fig. 1.12 shows the huge range in death rates from CHD in Europe, and stroke shows a similar pattern. Some of the poorest countries in the Region clearly have the highest CVD mortality. CVD are not a manifestation

Fig. 1.10. Average age-standardized mortality from cerebrovascular disease in men and women aged 25–64 years, European Region

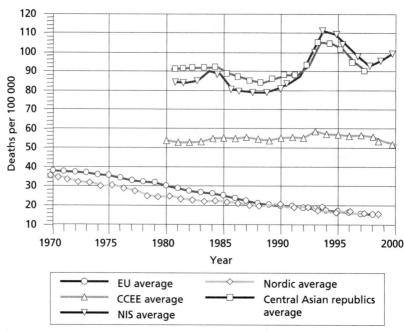

Source: Mortality indicators by cause, age and sex (database), WHO Regional Office for Europe, 2002.

of affluence; the wide differences in death rates are remarkably dependent on social inequalities and poverty (see pp. 69–71 and Chapter 3).

Diet-induced increases in serum cholesterol

For the last 50 years, a strong relationship has been recognized between the level of total cholesterol in the blood and the risk of CHD. This relationship is seen at all levels of CHD mortality – from the lowest, such as those observed in Japan in the 1950s or rural China in the 1970s, to the highest, observed in north-eastern Finland *(48)* – and clearly observed in all major prospective studies of CHD. Men are at much greater risk of CHD than women until women have passed the menopause, when their risk increases markedly.

The measurement of total serum cholesterol has been refined with the recognition that one component of the total cholesterol level, low-density lipoprotein (LDL) cholesterol, is the principal factor contributing to atherosclerosis and that high-density lipoprotein (HDL) cholesterol is protective. HDL is involved in clearing cholesterol from the tissues for disposal and oxidation by the liver. The most effective predictor of risk is the ratio of LDL to HDL

Fig. 1.11. Age-standardized premature mortality from ischaemic heart
disease in men and women aged 0–64 years,
Belarus and the Baltic countries

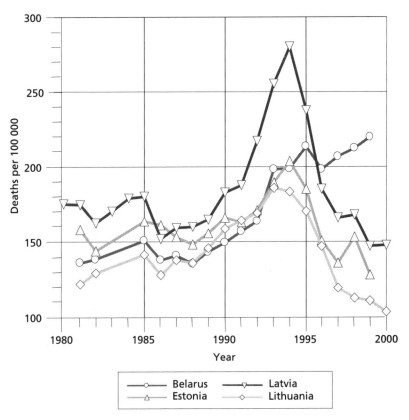

Source: Mortality indicators by cause, age and sex (database), WHO Regional
Office for Europe, 2002.

cholesterol, and smoking, diabetes and high blood pressure amplify the interaction of the two, especially in middle age.

Several hundred carefully controlled studies have illustrated how diet alters
serum cholesterol. The saturated fatty acids in the diet – not dietary
cholesterol – are the primary inducers of increases in LDL cholesterol in the
blood. These saturated fatty acids vary markedly in their effects. Myristic acid,
largely derived from milk fat, is the major stimulus to increased serum levels
of LDL. Lauric acid, present in fat and oil from tropical plants and in milk in
modest amounts, and palmitic acid, present in animal fat and tropical-plant
fat and oil, are also strong stimulators for raising LDL levels, as are some *trans-*
fatty acids *(49)*. A major saturated fat, stearic acid, present in beef fat and lard,

Fig. 1.12. Age-standardized mortality from CHD in men and women aged 25–64 years, European Region, latest available year

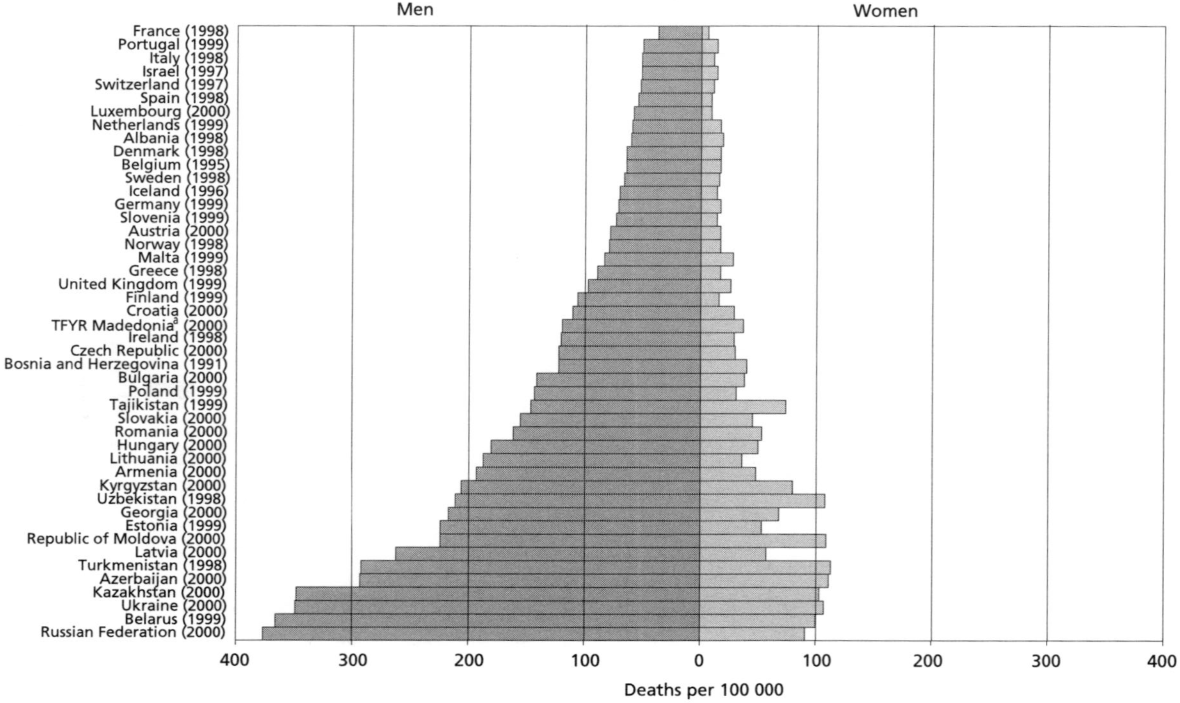

Men

Women

Deaths per 100 000

aThe former Yugoslav Republic of Macedonia.

Source: Mortality indicators by cause, age and sex (database), WHO Regional Office for Europe.

does not increase serum LDL cholesterol levels *(50)*, but all the saturated fatty acids have usually been grouped in one category in an attempt to simplify policy-making and educational messages.

Keys originally showed in the 1950s that the intake of saturated fat crudely predicted the rate of CHD in a population. About 40 years ago, this led the Nordic countries and the American Heart Association to call for a reduction in saturated fat intake. A relationship between intake of milk fat and the prevalence of CHD in European countries has been shown repeatedly; this is understandable, given the powerful effect of the myristic acid in milk fat *(24)*. As mentioned earlier, analyses of major public health programmes, such as those in Finland and Norway, have shown that the substantial fall in CHD rates (see Fig. 1.12) is predominantly explained by a 15% fall in average serum cholesterol levels as the consumption of milk fat – in milk, butter and milk products – drops.

Trans-fatty acids

Trans-fatty acids are unusually structured fatty acids naturally induced by the bacteria within the rumen, and cattle and sheep therefore have appreciable quantities of these fatty acids in their tissues. In addition, over the last 50 years the food industry has increasingly used a hydrogenation process with liquid vegetable and fish oils to produce hardened margarine and oils with a high concentration of *trans*-fatty acids. These are especially valuable in producing crisp or firm products that have a long shelf life before becoming rancid.

The *trans*-fatty acids in such products markedly reduce the intake of polyunsaturated fatty acids and particularly of the valuable omega-3 polyunsaturated fatty acids found in nuts, some vegetables and especially fish. The new chemical species of *trans*-fatty acids produced by hydrogenation have multiple, unusual structures and have been shown to induce deleterious increases in LDL cholesterol levels and decreases in HDL cholesterol levels.

The epidemic of CHD over the last 70–80 years can be attributed to increased intakes of both saturated and *trans*-fatty acids, so WHO recommends that this fatty acid constitute less than 1% of total energy *(21)*. Polyunsaturated fatty acids in a non-hydrogenated form can reduce LDL cholesterol and therefore limit the effect of saturated fat. Monounsaturated fatty acids, such as those found in olive and rapeseed oils, have a neutral effect on serum cholesterol levels.

The quality of the fatty acids in the diet – not total fat intake – determines the incidence of CHD.

Essential fatty acids and sudden cardiac death

The omega-3 polyunsaturated fatty acids are now recognized to have marked effects not only on brain development in infants and children and on immune system function but also on the risk factors for CHD. An increased intake of these fatty acids raises the level of the beneficial HDL cholesterol and reduces the circulating fatty acids in the form of triglycerides, which are an independent risk factor for CHD. In addition, omega-3 polyunsaturated fat reduces the clotting tendency of the blood and further minimize the thrombotic processes that are part of the mechanisms underlying the development of CHD. Perhaps one of their most dramatic effects is in stabilizing the reactivity of the neuronal control of the integrated processes governing the heart's functioning.

Low intake of polyunsaturated fat is linked to a much higher rate of sudden cardiac death. Various careful, placebo-controlled randomized trials have shown a major reduction (45–70%) in the likelihood of sudden death from CHD when intakes of these fatty acids are increased, either by the consumption of fatty fish twice weekly, the provision of fish oils or the inclusion of a Mediterranean-type diet rich in nuts and fish (51). On this basis, the intake of omega-3 fatty acids is a key determinant of CHD rates, acting to reduce the likelihood of sudden death from cardiac arrhythmia in Europe. An analysis of the fatty acids contained in the body fat of patients suffering myocardial infarction showed lower levels of very long-chain omega-3 fatty acids than in controls (51).

Fruits and vegetables and preventing CVD

The more that people consume a variety of fruits and vegetables, the stronger the protection against CVD (52,53). Estimates show that a mean increase in intake of 150 g per day could reduce the risk of mortality from CHD by 20–40%, from stroke by up to 25% and from CVD by 6–22%; the lowest estimates account for the impact of smoking and/or heavy drinking (53).

The precise mechanisms of this protective role are still uncertain. Nevertheless, raising fruit and vegetable intake is known to reduce blood pressure and serum cholesterol levels, the increased plasma antioxidants possibly preventing lipid peroxidation of LDL cholesterol. Fruits and vegetables are rich in dietary fibre and contain over 100 compounds that may be responsible for their protective effects. These include antioxidants, such as vitamins C and E, carotenoids, flavonoids, folic acid, potassium, magnesium and non-nutritive bioactive constituents, such as phytoestrogens and other phytochemicals.

Zatonski et al. (47) investigated the reasons for the decline in CHD deaths in Poland since 1991, after two decades of rising rates. Having considered the potential role of changes in food availability, smoking, alcohol consumption, stress and medical care, the authors attribute the substantial decline in premature mortality to falls in consumption of saturated fat and to an increased supply of fresh fruits and vegetables (47). Similar dietary changes have taken place in the Czech Republic (54).

Gjonca & Bobak *(55)* draw attention to the paradox of high adult life expectancy in Albania, despite its position as the poorest country in the European Region. In 1990, age-standardized mortality for CHD in males aged 0–64 was only 41 per 100 000 in Albania, less than half of the rate in the United Kingdom and similar to that in Italy. A detailed analysis of the geographical distribution of mortality within Albania showed that it was lowest in the south-west, where most of the olive oil, fruits and vegetables are produced and consumed. Albania provided unique opportunities to study this relationship because of the almost complete absence of motorized transport, which limits interregional food distribution, combined with the availability of high-quality mortality data. The authors argue that diet is the most plausible explanation for this paradox of high life expectancy in a poor country: low consumption of total energy, meat and milk products but high consumption of fruit, vegetables and complex carbohydrates. This was the diet eaten in Crete in the 1950s, when Keys showed that it was associated with low rates of CHD.

Trials have shown that mimicking a high intake of fruits and vegetables by using dietary supplements containing vitamins C and E, beta-carotene and flavonol is largely ineffective and sometimes even harmful. One exception is folate: new evidence suggests that folate deficiency may lead to an increased risk of CVD *(56)*. Specifically, inadequate levels of folates raise levels of plasma homocysteine (an essential intermediate in folate metabolism), and elevated plasma homocysteine has been associated with an increased risk of CVD. These high levels can be reduced by extra folic acid intake through dietary folates from vegetables; these are only 50% bioavailable, however, and supplements in people at risk are recommended.

CVD and salt

Dietary salt intake plays a critical role in regulating blood pressure, and populations with low salt intake, all other things being equal, have a lower average blood pressure level. In addition, accumulating evidence shows that a high salt intake could independently predict left ventricular hypertrophy, although this remains controversial *(57,58)*.

The DASH (dietary approaches to stop hypertension) trial *(59)* was conducted in people with "high-normal" blood pressure and stage-one hypertension. They were randomly assigned to a control group or one of two groups with a "normal" diet: one rich in fresh fruits and vegetables and the other containing fresh fruits and vegetables and low-fat dairy products. Estimates of sodium intake indicated a modest reduction to an average of about 130 mmol per day. The group receiving the diet with fresh fruits and vegetables and low-fat dairy products had the lowest blood pressure levels, followed by the group assigned to fresh fruits and vegetables and then the controls. These findings support the concept that a high dietary intake of potassium, magnesium and calcium contributes to reducing blood pressure.

A second version of the DASH trial assigned people with blood pressure of 120/80–159/95 mmHg to a control diet or the DASH combination diet, randomized to one of three dietary sodium levels: high (150 mmol per day), intermediate (100 mmol) or low (50 mmol) *(60)*. People on both the control and DASH combination diets showed a stepwise reduction in blood pressure with each level of reduced salt intake. The difference in blood pressure between those on the DASH diet with the highest and lowest sodium intakes averaged 12 mmHg, a response equal to that of potent antihypertensive drugs. The DASH diet had a greater effect in reducing blood pressure on the two higher levels of salt intake than the control diet. As in the earlier DASH trial, no adverse effects of dietary salt reduction were observed.

Little information is available on salt intake in Europe. In Romania, the daily salt consumption per head is estimated to be 14 g *(61)*. On average, about 12% of adults in Romania have hypertension (blood pressure over 140/90 mmHg), including 32% of men aged 41–65 years. As in all other

Fig. 1.13. Age-adjusted prevalence of high blood pressure (160/95 mmHg) in men aged 35–64, selected countries and regions in the European Region

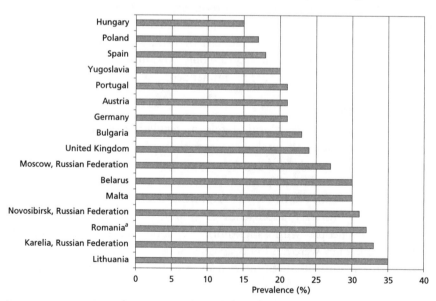

[a] In Romania, the data are for men aged 41–65 years with blood pressure over 140/90 mmHg *(61)*.

Source: data from a risk factor population survey conducted in demonstration centres of the WHO countrywide integrated noncommunicable disease intervention (CINDI) programme, 1999.

European countries, CVD mortality occupies the first place; cerebrovascular accidents caused about 40% of deaths from CVD in 1996, one of the highest rates in the European Region. Fig. 1.13 shows the prevalence of high blood pressure in adult men in some regions and countries in the European Region. The fact that, in countries such as Lithuania, over 40% of adult men in rural areas are hypertensive warrants further studies on salt intake in the Region and renewed emphasis on controlling hypertension by lowering salt intake to less than 5 g per day *(18)*.

The impact of interventions to reduce the daily intake of salt in Norway by 6 g per day was simulated *(62)*. The results suggested that, assuming that the interventions would lead to a reduction of 2 mmHg on average, life expectancy could be increased by 1.8 months in men and 1.4 months in women.

Smoking, stress and CVD

Detailed analyses have shown that eliminating smoking and dramatically improving diet and levels of physical activity could prevent at least 75% of CHD *(63,64)*.

The three classic major risk factors for heart disease are smoking, high blood pressure and high serum cholesterol. The lay press has constantly cited stress as an important cause, but this has been the subject of relatively little research. Nevertheless, four types of psychosocial factors related to stress have been found to be consistently associated with an increased risk of CHD: work stress, lack of social support, depression (including anxiety) and personality traits (especially hostility) *(65,66)*.

In western countries, smoking has usually been considered to be the dominant risk factor, even though Keys, in the original seven countries study *(48)*, highlighted the fact that smoking had far greater impact in northern Europe than in the Mediterranean area, where serum cholesterol levels were so much lower. The smoking rates in Greece are among the highest in Europe. Keys' studies also showed that, in Japan, with the lowest documented CHD rates in the world, men were heavy smokers and had the highest recorded blood pressure but the lowest serum cholesterol levels. Thus, the dietary factors that lead to high total serum cholesterol are fundamental to allowing the impact of smoking and high blood pressure on CHD to become apparent. This is now understandable on a cellular, mechanistic basis *(67)*, because smoking and high blood pressure amplify the effects of abnormalities in cholesterol and fat metabolism, operating by inducing arterial changes.

More recent European analyses than Keys' have re-emphasized the fundamental importance of serum cholesterol levels. Vartiainen et al. *(26)* showed a dramatic 75% fall in CHD rates in women in Finland, despite their increased rates of smoking (see Fig. 1.8). The biggest contributor to the fall was the major decline in serum cholesterol levels, with falling blood pressure also contributing substantially. The implications are that serum cholesterol seems to be the defining risk factor in CHD, and not smoking, as popular understanding has it.

The combined impact of high serum cholesterol, high blood pressure and smoking on CHD is so marked that, even in an affluent western society such as the United States, life expectancy is greater for the groups at lowest risk: 5.8 years more for middle-aged women and 9.5 years for men aged 18–39 years. These differences within one country are analogous to those displayed within the European Region in Fig. 1.9.

Recent analyses have suggested that stress is linked with a greater propensity to CHD in some European societies (68). This stress may not relate simply to crude income inequality or even indices of general distrust but to the insecure situations of people with lower-income jobs. Their livelihood may be prejudiced at any time by actions taken by strangers over whom they have no influence or control. Plausible mechanisms have been suggested, including increased secretions of the stress hormone cortisol and the induction of abdominal obesity with insulin resistance (25).

Diet's role in limiting the development of cancer

As discussed above, 30–40% of all cases of cancer is estimated to be causally related to nutritional factors. The scientific evidence suggests that diet is most convincingly linked to cancer of the lung, stomach, colon/rectum, nasopharynx, oesophagus, mouth and pharynx. A link to cancer of the breast is probable, and diet is possibly associated with cancer of the liver and cervix (10).

Preventive effects of high intake of fruits and vegetables

Diet and physical inactivity are the most important modifiable determinants of cancer risk for the great majority of the population who do not smoke. Apart from the effect of overweight and obesity, the most abundant evidence for an effect of diet on cancer incidence has been related to a lower risk with greater intake of fruits and vegetables (69). Specifically, the evidence shows a statistically significant risk reduction for cancer of the oesophagus, lung, stomach and colon/rectum associated with both fruits and vegetables, for breast cancer associated with vegetables but not with fruits, and for bladder cancer risk associated with fruits but not with vegetables (17).

The role of vitamins and minerals

The potential protective effect of specific vitamins, mainly carotenoids and vitamins A, E and C, has generated considerable interest and research. The carotenoids include beta-carotene (the most common) and xanthophylls, lycopene and cryptoxanthin. High intake of carotenoids from food sources probably decreases the risk of lung cancer *(10)*. Weaker evidence of protective effects of carotenoids has been reported for cancer of the oesophagus, stomach, colon/rectum, breast and cervix. High intake of vitamin C has been reported to decrease the risk of cancer of the stomach, mouth, pharynx, oesophagus and, less consistently, the lung, pancreas and cervix. Studies have shown that high vitamin E intake decreases the risk of cancer of the lung, cervix and colon/rectum *(10)*.

Although clinical trials with antioxidant vitamins have had disappointing results, this is not thought to undermine the epidemiological evidence that points to the protective effect of fruit and vegetable consumption. This is because the doses included in many of the trials result in blood levels of, for example, carotenoids that are 10–20 times higher than could ever be achieved by eating fruits and vegetables. Further, the trials tended to test one or two compounds of the complex mixture of hundreds available *(10)*.

Recent studies have investigated the possible protective effect of folic acid, particularly against colorectal cancer *(70)*. Folates and vitamin B_6 are involved in methionine and choline metabolism, and folate deficiency leads to an accumulation of homocysteine, which may be linked to an increase in cancer mortality. This area, however, requires further investigation.

Harmful effect of meat consumption

Considerable evidence shows a positive association between meat consumption and colorectal cancer. (In this context, *meat* means red meat and meat products, and includes beef, lamb and pork but excludes poultry.) The World Cancer Research Fund considered the evidence for an increased risk of cancer of the colon/rectum from diets high in red meat to be "probable" *(10)*. Meat was first identified as a possible risk factor for cancer in the mid-1970s, when studies identified strong correlations between the worldwide incidence of colorectal cancer and meat consumption.

A consistently positive association has been found between the consumption of preserved and red meat and the risk of colorectal cancer *(71)*. This is supported by results from the European prospective investigation into cancer (EPIC) (Fig. 1.14).

Processed and red meat consumption might help to increase risk in several ways. Constituents of meat, such as fat, protein and iron, are possible risk factors. There is also experimental evidence that meat increases the production of some potentially cancer-causing substances in the large bowel: *N*-nitroso compounds, which may be caused by interactions between bacteria in the bowel and the components of meat. Meat almost always undergoes some type of processing – either cooking or preserving – before it is eaten.

This may complicate the picture, because some processing methods may contribute to the increased risk.

Fig. 1.14. Dose–response relationship between the consumption of red and processed meat and the risk of colorectal cancer

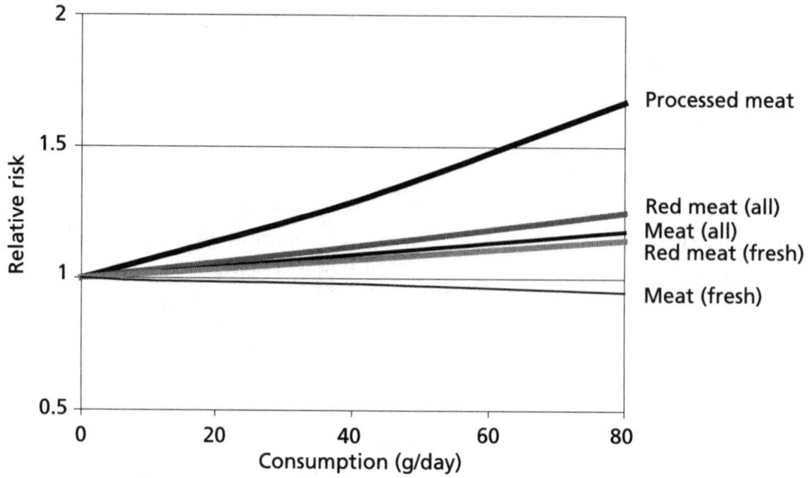

Source: Norat et al. *(72)*. Reprinted by permission of Wiley-Liss, Inc, a subsidiary of John Wiley & Sons, Inc.

Some evidence indicates that diets containing substantial amounts of meat may increase the risk of cancer of the pancreas, breast, prostate and kidney. This evidence is weaker than that linking meat to colorectal cancer and was classified by the World Cancer Research Fund as "possible" *(10)*. Average meat intakes do not vary as much across the European Region as vegetable intakes. Nevertheless, countries show considerable variation in the types of meat consumed and the method of processing used, so national policy-makers should assess their own country's trends.

Overweight and increased risk

A WHO review of the literature linking body weight to the risk of cancer at various sites *(35)* suggests that convincing evidence links excess weight to an elevated risk of endometrial cancer. Good evidence links excess weight to kidney cancer and breast cancer in post-menopausal women *(10)*. The review *(35)* also noted possible links between raised body weight and an elevated risk of colorectal cancer and between high energy intake and pancreatic cancer.

A recent meta-analysis connected overweight with increased risk of cancer of the kidney, endometrium, colon/rectum, prostate, gall bladder and (in post-menopausal women) breast *(73)*. This study also estimated the proportion of cancer in the EU attributable to excess weight. Overall, it accounts for 5% of all cancer cases in the EU: 3% in men and 6% in women, corresponding to cases in over 25 000 males and 44 000 females each year. This included over 21 600 cases of colorectal cancer, 14 200 cases of endometrial cancer and 12 800 cases of breast cancer. On this basis, halving the numbers of people in the EU who are overweight and obese might prevent some 36 000 cases of cancer each year (73).

Epidemic of overweight and obesity

The problem of overweight and obesity has only recently come to the forefront of public health, as public health nutritionists were primarily concerned with the problems of undernutrition, especially in vulnerable groups in society. WHO, however, calls overweight (a body mass index – BMI[2] – of 25–29.9) and obesity (BMI of 30 or more) the biggest unrecognized public health problem in the world; they contribute substantially to both ill health and death in populations (1). Excess weight is calculated to be responsible for nearly 300 000 deaths annually in the EU – nearly 1 in 12 of all deaths recorded – by contributing to CVD and cancer (74).

The major complications of excess weight are type 2 diabetes, high blood pressure, CHD, stroke, a range of cancer types and arthritis. A series of disabilities and psychological problems are linked directly to excess weight. Evidence is accumulating that the emerging epidemic of overweight and obesity in children is markedly amplifying the early onset of other health problems, especially type 2 diabetes. In addition, the risk of gestational diabetes increases in obese pregnant women; this increases the risk of subsequent fetal defects, childhood obesity and diabetes (see pp. 37–38). Recent data sets suggest that many European countries have some of the highest national rates of overweight and obesity among children (75) and adults in the world.

The prevalence of obesity is increasing in all age groups in most European countries. Obesity is a rapidly growing epidemic, now affecting about 30% of the population of the WHO European Region (76).

Published and unpublished data from studies and surveys by WHO and others (73,76–91) show that a considerable proportion of the adult population in many European countries is overweight or obese; Fig. 1.15 and 1.16 arrange these data for groups of countries in the Region. Overweight levels range from 9% to 41% of women and 10% to 50% of men. Further, the trend of overweight is consistently rising, although the rate of increase

---

[2] BMI is one's weight in kg divided by (height in metres)^2.

varies. Even the Scandinavian countries, with historically more active populations relative to many other countries, have been affected.

Fig. 1.15. Overweight adults (BMI 25–29.9), European Region (%)

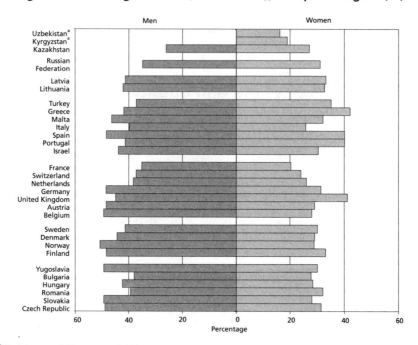

^a No data are available on overweight in men.

Special risks of abdominal obesity

The distribution of excess fat in the body has been recognized as an important predictor of ill health. Excess intra-abdominal fat is linked to a range of health hazards, including diabetes, a greater propensity to hypertension and dyslipidaemia and an increased risk of CHD and stroke. This array of problems is specified as the metabolic syndrome or syndrome X, which is also associated with excessive kidney albumin excretion. This condition is especially seen in men, is amplified by drinking and smoking and has also been linked to mental stress and a programming of fat distribution and disease by poor early fetal and childhood development *(92)*. In women, abdominal obesity is associated with polycystic ovarian syndrome, infertility, menstrual abnormality and hirsutism.

Abdominal obesity can be simply assessed by measuring the waist circumference, and WHO has proposed limits (see Chapter 4, p. 240) for the waist circumference of men and women based on the risk of blood pressure, diabetes and blood lipid abnormalities derived from a population study in the Netherlands *(93)*. There is a new emphasis on highlighting the significance of

Fig. 1.16. Obese adults (BMI ≥30), European Region (%)

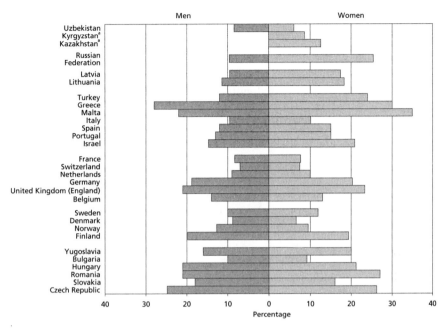

a No data are available on obesity in men.

waist measurements because this can be used in campaigns to alert adults to the problems of weight gain and the particular risk of abdominal obesity. It could also give an early warning to physicians of the likelihood of disease developing in their patients.

Implications of childhood obesity

It is now recognized that large infants (those weighing more than 4 kg at birth) are more likely to develop obesity in later childhood and that low-birth-weight infants who grow very rapidly after the age of 1 year and become overweight are more likely to develop CVD in adult life. Subsequent studies have not borne out the original concern about fat infants being doomed to become overweight and obese adults. The risk of a child persisting with overweight and obesity, however, increases progressively from the age of about 6 years. The prevalence of overweight and obesity among children in Europe is rising significantly, with up to 27% affected in some regions (75).

In examining overweight in preschool children from over 90 countries, de Onis & Blossner (94) used the standard WHO procedure of defining overweight as a BMI exceeding 2 standard deviations (SD) above the median for the WHO international growth charts. They found overweight children in all the 11 countries in the European Region examined: Armenia,

Azerbaijan, Croatia, the Czech Republic, Hungary, Italy, Kazakhstan, Turkey, the United Kingdom, Uzbekistan and Yugoslavia. The prevalence in eastern countries was, for example, 6% overweight young children in Armenia and about 15% in Uzbekistan (94). In addition, about 20% of preschool children in the Russian Federation were overweight in 1997 (http://www.who.int/ nutgrowthdb/intro_text.htm, accessed 19 September 2003).

The major problem associated with childhood and adolescent obesity is its persistence into adult life and its association with diabetes and CVD risk in later life (95). Thus, the problem of obesity in children is arousing intense concern and increasing political attention.

Type 2 diabetes and excessive weight gain

Type 2 diabetes occurs when insulin secretion is insufficient to overcome resistance to its action, leading to inadequate regulation of blood glucose levels. This is the underlying abnormality in most cases with this condition. It was previously a disease of middle-aged and elderly people, but its frequency has escalated in all age groups and the condition is now seen in adolescence and childhood.

The prevalence of type 2 diabetes is expected to increase to more than 10% in all EU and Nordic countries. In addition, the rate of increase is projected to rise dramatically by 2025 (76).

Diabetes rates have risen in parallel with those of overweight and obesity. Powerful evidence indicates that excess weight, especially when centrally distributed, and physical inactivity increase insulin resistance and are independent determinants of diabetes risk. This risk increases even with modest weight increases within the normal range (BMI under 25). A high intake of saturated fatty acids increases insulin resistance and the risk of type 2 diabetes. Weight loss in overweight and obese people, increased physical activity and reduced saturated fat intake have been convincingly shown to reduce the risk of insulin resistance and diabetes.

Impact of physical inactivity on health

Evidence is increasing that regular physical activity has considerable health benefits, such as reducing the risk of CVD, diabetes and osteoporosis (96). In comparison with sedentary people, physically active people (96):

- run 50% less risk of dying from CHD and stroke;
- are at lower risk of hip fracture (30–50%), hypertension (30%), colorectal cancer (40–50%) and type 2 diabetes (20–60%);
- are 50% less likely to become obese;

- have a 25–50% lower risk of developing functional limitations in later life; and
- show a 50% slower decrease of aerobic capacity (which occurs with age), thereby gaining 10–20 years of independent living.

Physical activity plays a role in avoiding overweight and obesity: people with low levels of physical activity have higher body fat and abdominal fat and are more likely to gain body fat than those with high levels of physical activity *(97)*. Physical activity also contributes to maintaining a lower blood pressure throughout life and to lowering the ratio of LDL to HDL cholesterol in the blood. The benefits of physical activity explain its substantial importance in limiting death and illness from CVD.

Assessing physical activity levels, Currie et al. *(98)* found that children exercise progressively less as they grow older. The proportion of 15-year-olds who reported taking part in sports outside school at least twice a week ranged from 37% to 66% in girls and from 60% and 90% in boys (Fig. 1.17).

Fig. 1.17. Proportion of 15-year-olds who report exercising vigorously twice a week or more, European Region

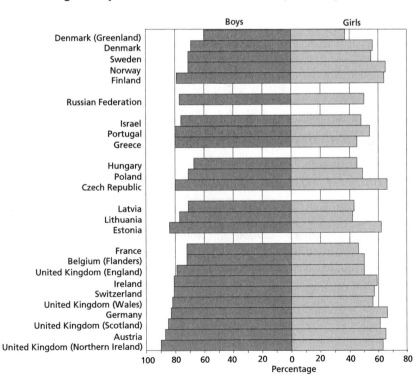

Source: Currie et al. *(98)*.

Associations between physical activity and socioeconomic status have been observed in schoolchildren, with children from lower-status families taking less exercise on average than those from higher-status families, and, in Germany and the United Kingdom at least, undertaking less physical activity outside school *(99,100)*. The survey in Germany involved 3400 children aged 5–7 years and showed that lower physical activity was associated with lower educational status of the family and with unhealthy eating patterns *(100)*. It also found that children watching more than 1 hour of television per day ate significantly more confectionery and fast food than children watching less *(100)*. A later section in this chapter deals with physical activity and inequalities (see pp. 71–72).

The data on physical activity among European adults are poor. A survey of adults in the EU shows that levels of activity are low; on average 32% of adults carry out no leisure-time physical activity in a typical week *(101)*. In general, southern EU countries have lower levels of physical activity than northern and western countries *(101)*.

Physical activity contributes to physical, mental and social health and improves the quality of life of people of all ages. These benefits also help to reduce social and health care costs *(102)*. Physical activity should be considered an essential element of preventing chronic disease, as well as a central part of a healthy lifestyle. Policy-makers' recommendations must address physical activity in children, adolescents, adults and older people and particularly must involve employers and schools, as this is instrumental to making successful policies (see Chapter 4, pp. 238–239).

Impaired infant and child development from micronutrient deficiency

Iodine deficiency

Iodine deficiency leads to what are collectively called iodine deficiency disorders, and is the primary cause of avoidable mental deficiency in childhood. The most severe forms of these disorders can result in cretinism or severe brain damage. In children and adolescents, iodine deficiency leads to overt or subclinical hypothyroidism, impaired mental and physical development, and goitre. A comprehensive WHO report on iodine deficiency disorders and their control *(103)* presents an overview of the situation in the European Region.

Mild and moderate forms of iodine deficiency are still common in Europe *(104)*, with neurological defects and minor impairments of brain functioning evident. According to the WHO global database on iodine deficiency disorders, they are estimated to affect about 130 million people in the Region.

Iodine deficiency disorders are considered unlikely in a number of European countries: Austria, Finland, Ireland, Monaco, the Netherlands,

Norway, San Marino, Sweden, Switzerland and the United Kingdom *(105)*. Nevertheless, recent surveys of the prevalence of goitre show that many people in the European Region still suffer from moderate iodine deficiency. (The prevalence of goitre only reveals a proportion of the iodine deficiency problem, however, and insufficiency of iodine is likely to be much higher.) For example, the prevalence of goitre was 11% for adults in Azerbaijan in 1996 and 37% for the population of Uzbekistan in 1998. Fig. 1.18 shows the prevalence in school-age children *(105)*. In addition, iodine deficiency disorders are still a public health problem in some western European countries, such as Belgium *(105)* and Italy *(106)*.

Fig. 1.18. Prevalence of goitre in school-age children in selected countries in the European Region

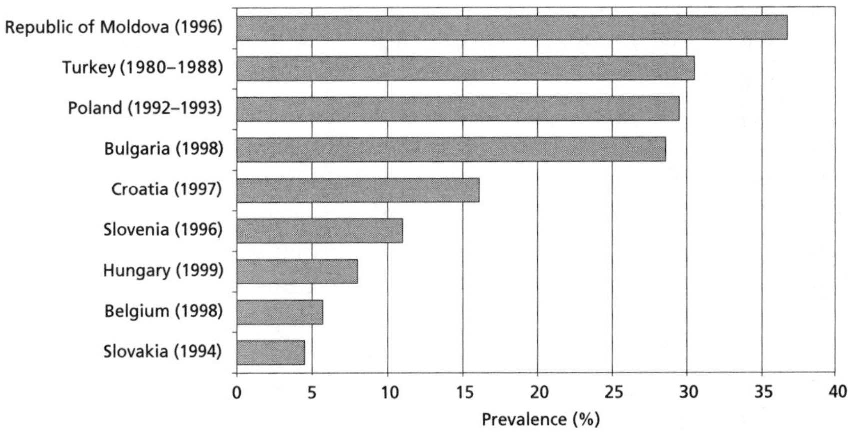

Note: The data for the Republic of Moldova, Slovakia, Slovenia and Turkey are taken from the country responses to a 1998 WHO questionnaire on iodine deficiency disorders, not official survey reports, so they should be treated as preliminary.

Source: WHO global database on iodine deficiency disorders, Geneva, World Health Organization and de Benoist & Allen *(105)*.

Iodine deficiency is easy to eradicate, but this has not yet happened in Europe. Policy-makers should implement the universal iodization of salt in their countries (see Chapter 4, p. 250).

Iron deficiency
Iron deficiency can result in impaired brain development in children and poor mental concentration and cognitive performance in both children and adults. In addition, iron deficiency anaemia compromises adults' work capacity.

The body needs iron as a component of a variety of enzyme systems in all tissues and for the production of blood haemoglobin, crucial for the transport of oxygen. Dietary iron in its normal inorganic form is poorly absorbed by the intestine because of the interaction of a variety of dietary inhibitors, which bind the iron and reduce its bioavailability to 3–15% (see Chapter 4, pp. 251–252). Bioavailability is much improved when iron is consumed with vitamin C from fruits and vegetables or when dietary iron is eaten in the organic form, for example, as part of the haem iron protein found in meat and fish. Important compounds in vegetable foods interfere with iron bioavailability: the phytates found, for example, in unrefined grains; the albumin from eggs; and the polyphenols and other compounds found in tea. Fruits and vegetables rich in vitamin C limit the impact of phytates. Calcium and zinc intake may also modify iron bioavailability.

A variety of factors can cause iron deficiency and anaemia: insufficient dietary iron, dietary anti-nutrients (such as phytates and polyphenols), blood loss and intestinal parasites, especially helminths such as hookworm, and gastrointestinal infections. Pica – the craving for non-food items such as soil and chalk – is still claimed to be quite prevalent in certain parts of Europe. Pica can occur during pregnancy, and the unusual items eaten amplify the malabsorption of iron (107), leading to iron deficiency anaemia.

In the European Region, infants and children may develop iron deficiency anaemia from poor feeding practices, such as giving tea to infants and children, or when weaning off breast-milk does not coincide with the introduction of fruits and vegetables, along with meat and fish. Prematurity exacerbates the problem of anaemia because iron stores are limited in a small newborn baby; any infestation with parasites or helminths, as a result of poor hygiene and impure water, markedly exacerbates the problem by amplifying malabsorption and stimulating excessive intestinal blood loss.

In addition to poor feeding practices, low breastfeeding rates can be considered a major cause of iron deficiency anaemia in infants and young children. Very high prevalence has been reported from the central Asian republics (80,82,108,109), Bosnia and Herzegovina (110) and parts of western Europe (111). Even in affluent countries, such as the United Kingdom, the prevalence in children of Asian background has been observed to be 12% in those aged 1–2 years and 6% in those aged 2–4 years (111). Children in other countries in western Europe also show high levels of iron store depletion (112).

In addition, many adolescents in Europe have either iron deficiency anaemia or depleted iron stores (112). The latter is a precursor to the development of anaemia. Adolescent girls tend to have higher rates of iron deficiency and anaemia than boys; these are due not only to the onset of puberty, with its increased iron requirements, but also the iron loss with menstruation (113,114).

The high rates of anaemia and iron depletion among women of reproductive age in the European Region are of great concern. They can have a number of causes.

Although women throughout the Region are affected, Fig. 1.19 shows that the prevalence of anaemia is highest in central Asian countries *(80,82,108, 109,111,114)*. Evidence from Kazakhstan *(115)* shows that women had a relatively low mean iron intake (13.2 mg/day) and about 35% of Kazakh women of reproductive age were suffering from anaemia (haemoglobin under 12 g/dl blood) in 1999. In Sweden, over 30% of women of reproductive age have low iron stores.

Fig. 1.19. Prevalence of anaemia and depleted iron stores[a] in women of reproductive age, selected European countries

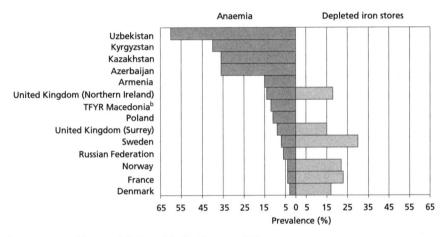

[a] Investigators used their own definitions of depleted iron stores *(112)*.
[b] The former Yugoslav Republic of Macedonia.

Sources: Kazakhstan demographic and health survey (DHS), 1999 (80), Kyrgyzstan demographic and health survey (DHS), 1997 (82), Uzbekistan demographic and health survey, 1996 (109), Branca et al. (personal communication, 1996), Hercberg et al. *(112)* and Branca et al. *(116)*.

Significant socioeconomic deprivation can in part explain some of these high rates, although probably not those in Sweden. For example, a cohort study of 15 000 people in the United Kingdom found that women in the lowest social class were 1.5 times more likely to be anaemic that those in the highest social class *(117)*.

In pregnancy, substantial iron stores are mobilized because of the need not only to supply extra maternal tissues (such as the placenta) and the growing fetus but also to expand the woman's blood volume. In some countries of the

Region, pregnant women have a high prevalence of anaemia, especially those with successive pregnancies. In such cases, the women's bodies cannot meet the repeated high demands for haemoglobin production from their already depleted iron stores; the depletion is exacerbated by the normal iron demands of the growing fetus and the loss of blood in childbirth.

The severity and prevalence of anaemia during pregnancy depend on the prevalence of pre-existing iron deficiency and anaemia. In Armenia, 50% of the women in the third trimester of pregnancy have mild or moderate anaemia *(116)*. In Uzbekistan, 27% of pregnant women have moderate anaemia; children born to these women are also likely to be anaemic *(109)*.

Multiple pregnancies and repeated abortions worsen anaemia in women of reproductive age. In some countries, abortion is an important cause of iron depletion through blood loss, especially where rates are high and abortion is still practised as a method of birth control *(118)*. In certain central Asian republics, the prevalence of moderate-to-severe anaemia among women with two or more births can be twice as high as that among women with fewer than two births or no pregnancies *(80)*.

Wide use of the intrauterine device (IUD) provides a further explanation for high rates of anaemia. Contraceptive pills reduce menstrual losses by half *(119)*, while an IUD doubles menstrual iron losses *(120)*. Data on the contraceptive methods used in central Asian republics show that the IUD is used far more often than the contraceptive pill: almost 10, 5 and 4 times more often in Uzbekistan, Kyrgyzstan and Kazakhstan, respectively *(80,82,108,109)*.

Helminth infestation, especially by hookworms, is also a major cause of anaemia. Hookworms cause chronic intestinal blood loss, leading in turn to severe anaemia. The degree of anaemia they produce is linked to their number. There is some evidence *(121,122)* that the burden of intestinal parasitism is high in the central Asian republics, in keeping with the lack of satisfactory sanitation and clean water supplies. A dramatic increase in

Table 1.3. Incidence of worm infestation in school-age adolescents in Armenia, 1993–1997

Worm type	Cases per 100 000 population				
	1993	1994	1995	1996	1997
Pinworm	297.6	373.0	361.7	1140.1	613.6
Roundworm	106.5	120.0	110.6	519.3	284.2
Trichuris spp.	12.0	9.3	7.0	22.1	17.4
Echinococcus spp.	1.7	0.8	1.5	3.15	1.6

Source: adapted from *Health and health care (123)*.

intestinal worm infestation among school-age adolescents in Armenia probably resulted from the difficult socioeconomic conditions (123) (Table 1.3). Evidence suggests that women benefit more from parasite elimination than from iron supplementation, since the parasites induce intestinal blood losses and double iron requirements (124). Information is urgently needed on the severity and prevalence of parasitic conditions in the European Region, especially in the central Asian republics.

A consultation organized by WHO and the United Nations Children's Fund (UNICEF) reviewed iron deficiency in the central Asian republics (125). Contributory factors appear to include high intakes of wheat, with its well recognized iron-inhibitory phytate content. Further, substantial tea drinking and relatively low meat intake by women – for example, a mean meat intake of 50 g per day in Kazakhstan (115) – are likely to amplify the iron absorption problem. The relative importance of all these issues, however, needs to be assessed. It seems clear that dietary practices can harm women and their children and that intestinal parasitism and abortions and the use of IUDs exacerbate these problems.

Pregnancy and fetal development

A poor diet not only deprives the developing fetus of nutrients but can also increase the loss of nutrients from the mother's body.

Several risk factors can harm a woman's health during pregnancy. For example, teenage pregnancy puts a double nutritional burden on the body. While the adolescent has to meet increasing needs for nutrients for her own growth and development, the extra needs of the fetus jeopardize the nutritional health of both.

Teenage pregnancy is a serious issue, especially in the CCEE and NIS; Fig. 1.20 shows that rates vary more than fivefold between countries in the Region (126,127). Adolescent pregnancy exposes both mother and child to adverse health and socioeconomic consequences, especially if the mother is not tall and has only modest reserves of nutrients. These conditions are especially likely to occur in the central Asian republics and Turkey (114). Pregnancy among teenagers warrants special attention, as young mothers and their children are at a higher risk of food insecurity and social and health problems. Children born to young mothers in the Region tend to have higher levels of illness, and their children, higher rates of death (80).

Another important aspect of pregnancy is the need for a sufficient intake of micronutrients, especially iron, folates and iodine. Micronutrient malnutrition may begin in utero and depends largely on the mother's nutritional status. Deficiencies retard intrauterine development and growth, which may persist through the first 2 years and permanently impair the child's cognitive development and other functions later in life. Even if micronutrient deficiencies are corrected in later childhood, the early consequences cannot be corrected, and may perpetuate the problem of stunted growth from one generation to the next.

Fig. 1.20. Adolescent pregnancy rates per 1000 women aged 15–19 years
in groups of European countries, 1990s

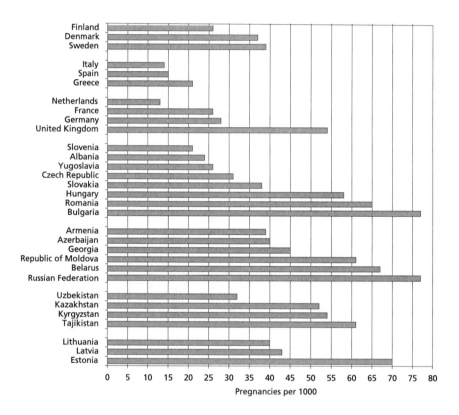

Note: Data on live births and abortions are taken together to represent pregnancy rates. The unweighted average teenage birth rate in the EU dropped from 16.1 to 12.3 per 1000 women aged 15–19 years between 1990 and 1995. Birth and abortion data for the EU refer to 1990, however, since no more recent abortion data are available for some countries. No abortion data are published for several EU countries, usually because abortion is legal only in particular circumstances. For Albania, data on births refer to 1997, and data on abortions to 1995. Data for Tajikistan come from 1995; for Yugoslavia, data on abortions refer to 1996.

Source: Young people in changing societies (126) and Micklewright & Stewart *(127).*

Folates and neural tube defects

Adequate intakes of folic acid are important in preventing birth defects such as spina bifida. Folate supplementation prior to and during the early weeks of pregnancy prevents up to 75% of neural tube defects occurring in the developing fetus *(128)*. Further, growing evidence indicates that maternal folic acid may reduce the child's likelihood of CVD in later life *(128)*. The most vulnerable stages of life are during the early weeks of pregnancy, when a woman may not know she is pregnant. Thus, women's folate status should always be adequate because many pregnancies are not planned.

A supplement of 400 µg folic acid has been shown to reduce the incidence of neural tube defects. Such high levels can be achieved through supplementation or fortification, but with difficulty through an unfortified diet. Possible causal factors in folate deficiency are dietary insufficiency from, for example, a low intake of vegetables and from the low bioavailability of some dietary folates.

Within the EU, the prevalence of neural tube defects varies widely between countries. Fig. 1.21 shows that it ranged from about 35 cases per 10 000 in certain parts of the United Kingdom and Ireland to just under 11 in Paris, France in the late 1980s *(129)*.

Fig. 1.21. Total reported prevalence of neural tube defects in 14 EUROCAT registries, 1980–1986

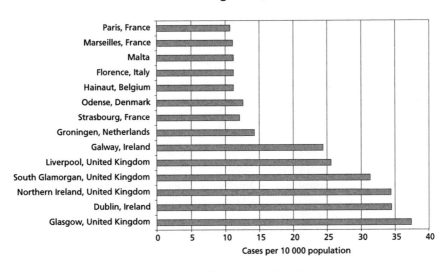

Source: adapted from EUROCAT Working Group *(129)*.

Fetal programming

Fetal programming, or the fetal origins hypothesis, suggests that alterations in fetal nutrition and endocrine status result in developmental adaptations that predispose an individual to CVD and metabolic and endocrine disease in later life *(92,130)*. Growing evidence links conditions in the intrauterine environment to the later likelihood of adult chronic diseases such as CVD, type 2 diabetes and hypertension *(92,130–134)*. The relevant factors in fetal life include:

• intrauterine growth retardation, which can result in low birth weight
• premature delivery of a fetus with normal growth for gestational age
• intergenerational factors.

Effect of maternal weight
The incidence of maternal complications increases with increasing body weight. Several studies *(135–137)* suggest an increased risk of gestational hypertension, gestational diabetes and/or Caesarean delivery among overweight or obese women *(138)*. In contrast, the fetuses of women whose weight is low before conception and/or inadequate during gestation are at increased risk of growth restriction.

There is some evidence that low rates of weight gain may be associated with preterm delivery *(139,140)*. Finally, recent studies suggest that overweight and obese women are less successful at initiating and continuing breastfeeding than women of normal weight *(141,142)*.

Low birth weight
Low weight at birth (less than 2500 g) is the result of either preterm delivery or intrauterine growth retardation, which can be related to the poor nutritional status of the mother. Fig. 1.22 shows the prevalence of low birth weight in groups of countries across the European Region. Rather surprisingly, of the CCEE, only The former Yugoslav Republic of Macedonia shows a significantly higher prevalence than western European countries. Within the EU, the proportion of low-birth-weight children has remained relatively constant over the past 20 years; only the Nordic countries have seen a fall.

In contrast, the prevalence of low birth weight appears to have increased in the NIS. In Armenia, for example, preterm delivery was recorded in 5.6% of live births in 1991 and 6.6% in 1996 *(123)*. Births do not always take place in hospital, however, so country information on the prevalence of low birth weight can be incomplete. Further, differences in reporting and the definition of low birth weight may bias figures from the CCEE. In some countries, infants born weighing less than 1000 g are not included because their risk of dying is so high. As a result, the extent to which the present data reflect the real situation is difficult to determine. The definition and collection of data clearly need to be standardized to improve comparisons between countries.

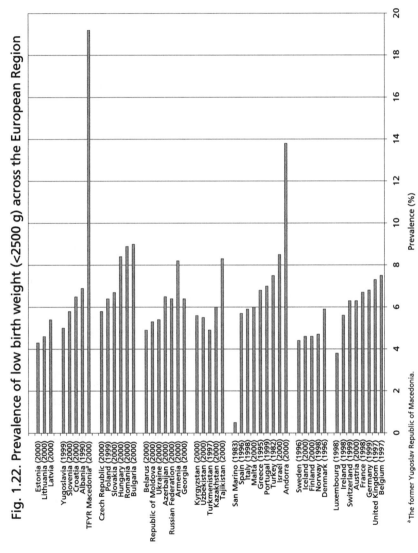

Fig. 1.22. Prevalence of low birth weight (<2500 g) across the European Region

a The former Yugoslav Republic of Macedonia.

Source: European health for all database, WHO Regional Office for Europe, 2002.

The high incidence of low birth weight in babies may be one indication of the nutritional inadequacy of the maternal diet. A study of social variation in birth outcome in the Czech Republic noted that mean birth weight fell between 1989 and 1991 and then rose again. The gap in mean birth weight between the babies of mothers with primary education and those of mothers with university education widened by about 40% from 1989 to 1996. The implications are that the relatively poorer birth outcome for less educated mothers may be linked to their nutritional intake before and during pregnancy and that social differences in birth outcome may have increased in the European Region.

Having smaller nutrient reserves not only handicaps small infants but also may compromise development of their immune systems and brains. The greater propensity of low-birth-weight infants to infantile anaemia further handicaps cognitive development because of the effects of marked iron deficiency with anaemia on the iron-dependent process of brain development in infancy.

Intergenerational factors
As mentioned above, young girls who grow poorly become stunted women. They are more likely to give birth to low-birth-weight babies, who are in turn likely to continue the cycle by being stunted in adulthood, and so on. Low maternal birth weight is associated with higher blood pressure levels in a child, independent of the relation between the child's own birth weight and blood pressure. There are clear intergenerational factors in obesity, such as parental obesity, maternal gestational diabetes and maternal birth weight.

Feeding of infants and young children
Breastfeeding is the most beneficial way of feeding an infant, as breast-milk provides not only the appropriate amounts of nutrients but a range of other factors that contribute to growth and the development of the immune system and intestines and other organs. For example, the iron in breast-milk is highly bioavailable and is normally sufficient for the needs of a fully breastfed infant up to 6 months of age (http://www.who.int/child-adolescent-health/NUTRITION/global_strategy.htm, accessed 25 September 2003) (26).

Breastfeeding practice varies remarkably between European countries. As Fig. 1.23 shows, at 3 months, over 90% of infants in Uzbekistan are at least partially breastfed, compared with about 25% in the United Kingdom (143).

Nevertheless, breastfeeding rates seem to be increasing across the Region. Nordic countries especially have very high rates compared with those 20 years ago. In Norway, for instance, the prevalence of breastfeeding at 3 months rose from only 25–30% in 1969 to about 80% in 1985 (144). Bottle-feeding with

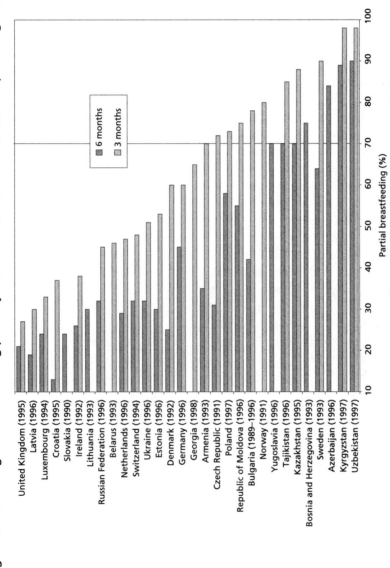

Fig. 1.23. Percentage of infants being partially breastfed at 3 and 6 months, European Region, 1990s

Source: Comparative analysis of implementation of the Innocenti Declaration in WHO European Member States (143).

cow's milk, however, is still common throughout the Region, leading to possible gastrointestinal blood loss, micronutrient deficiency and anaemia *(27)*. For example, a survey in Uzbekistan found that 35% of children under 3 months of age were fed using a bottle, 12% with infant formula and 23% with evaporated milk *(109)*.

The exclusive breastfeeding of infants is essential for proper growth and development. The weight of current evidence indicates that breastfeeding helps reduce the risk of developing CVD in later life.

HIV and breastfeeding

About one third to one half of overall mother-to-child transmission of HIV occurs during the period of breastfeeding *(145)*. This overall rate is roughly twice as high in populations where breastfeeding is the norm as in those where it is uncommon *(146,147)*. Several studies have shown that the rate of transmission can be further increased if HIV-positive mothers combine breastfeeding regimes with formula feeding *(148,149)*. The reason may be that feeding with formula introduces foreign bacteria into the infant's intestinal tract, which alters the mucosal lining's functioning and its ability to act as a barrier against ingested HIV *(150)*. Clinical risk factors, such as bleeding nipples, mastitis and breast abscesses *(151–153)*, have been associated with mother-to-child transmission of HIV, as has the viral load of the breast-milk.

Despite the declining trends in HIV/AIDS in the European Region, HIV continues to spread among injecting drug users in the CCEE and central Asian republics. Until the mid-1990s, this part of the Region appeared to have been spared the worst of the epidemic. It now holds an estimated 270 000 people living with HIV, and AIDS incidence is expected to increase in the near future (http://www.euro.who.int/eprise/main/WHO/Progs/SHA/ Home, accessed 25 September 2003) (see Chapter 4, pp. 244–245, for WHO recommendations).

Complementary feeding

After 6 months of exclusive breastfeeding, infants should receive other appropriate foods (see Chapter 4, pp. 245–248). As shown in Fig. 1.24, however, this does not always happen in the Region; infants are given water (boiled or not), tea with sugar and cereals as early as 2 weeks in most central Asian republics *(80,82,108,109,154–162)*. These feeding practices can lead to diarrhoeal diseases (Fig. 1.25) and anaemia in both infants and young children (see above) *(80–82,108, 109)*.

Growth retardation

Poor feeding practices can be considered a major cause of undernutrition. The main manifestation of undernutrition in the Region is stunting: chronic reduction in height for age to 2 SD below the median. The highest incidence of stunting occurs in and soon after the weaning period. Early childhood stunting is not reversible, although improved diets can achieve some catch-up growth.

Fig. 1.24. When liquids and complementary foods are introduced into the infant's diet according to surveys, selected European countries

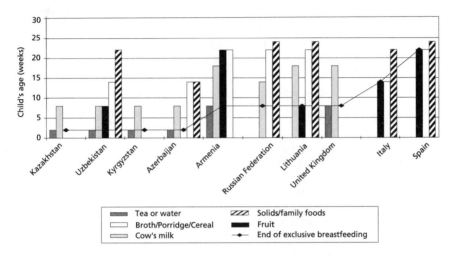

Fig. 1.25. Prevalence of diarrhoeal diseases in children aged 0–59 months, four European countries

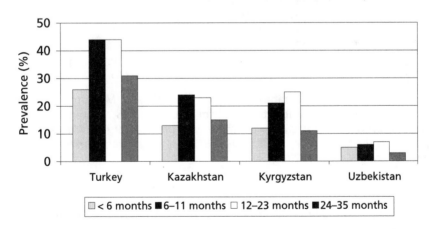

Note: Information was obtained from the vaccination card or the mother in the absence of written records.

Sources: *Kazakhstan demographic and health survey (DHS), 1999 (80), Turkey demographic and health survey (DHS), 1998 (81), Kyrgyzstan demographic and health survey (DHS), 1997 (82), Kazakhstan demographic and health survey (DHS), 1995 (108) and Uzbekistan demographic and health survey, 1996 (109).*

A sign of deprivation, stunting increases the risk of morbidity, impaired cognitive development and poor school performance in childhood and reduced work productivity in later life *(163,164)*. Stunting is a sensitive measure of poverty and is clearly linked with low birth weight *(165)*.

In the European Region, levels of stunting in young children are low in western countries but high in eastern ones, especially the central Asian republics. Fig. 1.26 shows that in Tajikistan, for example, over half the children under 5 years of age are stunted (http://www.who.int/nutgrowthdb/intro_text.htm, accessed 25 September 2003) *(80–82,109)*. In Uzbekistan, 31% of preschool children are stunted and 14% of these are severely stunted *(166)*.

Fig. 1.26. Prevalence of stunting
in preschool children, selected European countries, 1990s

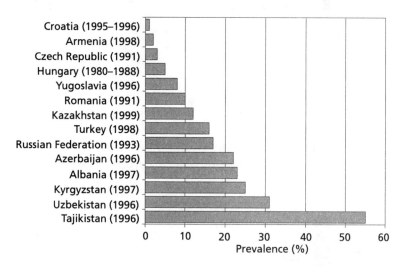

Sources: WHO Global Database on Child Growth and Malnutrition (http://www.who.int/nutgrowthdb/intro_text.htm, accessed 25 September 2003), *Kazakhstan demographic and health survey (DHS), 1999 (80)*, *Turkey demographic and health survey (DHS), 1998 (81)* and *Kyrgyzstan demographic and health survey (DHS), 1997 (82)*.

Stunting is usually more pronounced in rural than in urban areas. This suggests that hygiene and environmental conditions partly determine stunting *(166)*. Kazakhstan *(80)*, Kyrgyzstan *(82)* and Yugoslavia (http://www.who.int/nutgrowthdb/intro_text.htm, accessed 25 September 2003) all report about twice the rate of stunting in rural as in urban areas. The exception to the pattern is Uzbekistan, where stunting was reported to be slightly higher in urban areas *(109)*.

While stunting is most common in the central Asian republics, less than optimal growth patterns may be found among poorer groups in relatively wealthy countries, such as the United Kingdom. Gregory & Lowe *(167)* have shown that the average height of children from the wealthiest households (with over £600 weekly income) is 10 cm over that of children from the poorest households.

Dental health

Dental caries is a process of enamel and dentine demineralization caused by various acids formed from bacteria in dental plaque. The DMFT (decayed, missing and filled permanent teeth) index is a universally accepted measure of dental health. The score for any individual can range from 0 to 32 and represents the number of teeth affected *(168)*.

Caries is caused by acids produced mainly from the interaction of specific bacteria with dietary sugar: the bacteria do not produce enough acid to demineralize enamel without sugar. Fluoride is the main factor altering the resistance of teeth to acid attack. Fluoride reduces caries by reducing demineralization of enamel, by remineralizing enamel and by altering the ecology of dental plaque to reduce bacterial acid production *(168)*.

Fig. 1.27 shows DMFT scores in children in Europe *(169)*. Even in the countries with relatively low DMFT scores, 65% of children have had dental caries in their permanent teeth *(170)*. The CCEE and NIS continue to have significantly higher caries levels than other European countries; these levels are well above the European average and the WHO target of a population average of 3 or fewer DMFT *(169)*. In addition, caries affects the vast majority of people in eastern countries from an early age; in most of western Europe, it is concentrated in certain groups. Further, the percentage of untreated caries lesions in 12-year-olds has been reported to be 11% in the Czech Republic, 29% in France, 45% in the United Kingdom, 46% in Hungary and 53% in Poland *(169)*.

Dental care is expensive. Table 1.2 shows how dental caries accounted for the largest proportion of all direct costs to the health care service in Germany in the 1990s and the second-largest share of total costs.

In older people, oral health status is especially important and influences nutritional status. Dental caries, traditionally considered a problem of childhood, progresses throughout life and may accelerate with old age *(168)*. Periodontal disease increases with age. As a result, older people have fewer natural teeth, are more likely to be toothless (edentulous) and are also vulnerable to dietary restrictions for other reasons such as disability and medical or social conditions.

Chewing problems are relatively common in older people. They can cause dietary restrictions and thus compromise nutritional status and wellbeing

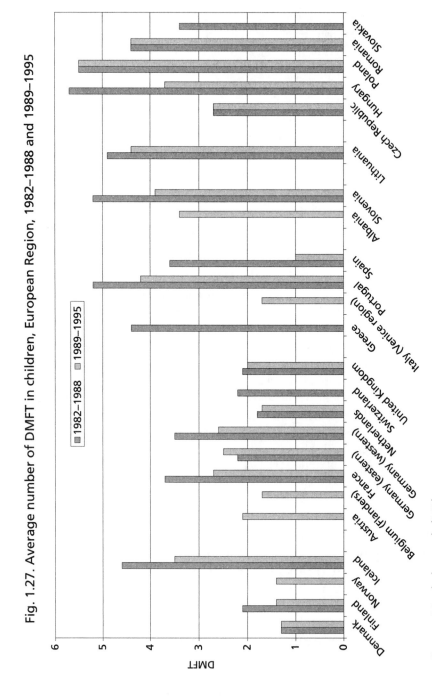

Fig. 1.27. Average number of DMFT in children, European Region, 1982–1988 and 1989–1995

Source: Marthaler et al. (169).

(171,172). Wearing dentures limits dietary intake and nutritional status, as it may alter food choices, which may result in lower intakes for key nutrients such as iron and fibre *(173–176)*.

Tooth loss is associated with a lower intake of hard-to-chew foods such as apples and carrots, and edentulous people consume fewer fruits and vegetables, less fibre and carotene, and more cholesterol, saturated fat and energy than people who have retained their teeth *(175)*. In older people living in their own homes, intakes of most nutrients, fruits and vegetables were significantly lower in the edentulous. In the United Kingdom, raw carrots, apples, well done steak or nuts were difficult for many edentulous older people to eat: for about 20% of those living in their own homes and over 50% of those in institutions. The daily intake of fruits and vegetables, non-starch polysaccharides, protein, calcium, non-haem iron, niacin, vitamin C, intrinsic and milk sugars and plasma ascorbate and retinol were significantly lower in edentulous people. Plasma ascorbate was significantly related to the number of pairs of teeth at the back of the mouth that are capable of chewing fruits and vegetables *(177)*.

The health of the ageing population of Europe

The population of Europe is ageing, and within the EU alone, the number of people aged over 80 years is estimated to increase by about 30% over the next 50 years *(178)*. Because life expectancy is increasing across the European Region, despite the differences (see Fig. 1.28), an increasing proportion of the population is older. This means that the overall disease burden can be expected to rise sharply, which will tend to offset the benefits of good preventive measures.

For a variety of physical, social and psychological reasons, older adults are considered to be at risk of nutritional problems, either as a result of impaired food intake or reduced nutrient utilization. Both cross-sectional and longitudinal studies in older people show a decline in energy intake with age *(179,180)*. Several of the health problems and bodily changes they experience have long been attributed to the normal ageing process but are increasingly being linked to lifestyle, socioeconomic or environmental factors *(181)*. For example, four fifths of pensioners in Romania have incomes below the official subsistence limits *(67)*.

Diet and morbidity and mortality among older people

The FINE (Finland, Italy and the Netherlands) study investigated the association of dietary patterns and mortality in more than 3000 men aged 50–70 years in the three countries. Of the 59% of men who died during the twenty-year follow-up, mortality was highest in eastern Finland and lowest in Italy. The national differences were striking in that Finnish men with healthier diets had higher mortality rates than Italian men with more unhealthy diets *(182)*.

Other detailed studies on older people in Europe have emphasized the importance of an appropriate diet in determining mortality and morbidity rates as well as mental functioning *(183)*. From 1988 to 1999, the Survey Europe on Nutrition in the Elderly: a Concerted Action (SENECA) found evidence of deficiency in 47% for vitamin D, 23.3% for vitamin B_6, 2.7% for vitamin B_{12} and 1.1% for vitamin E *(184)*.

There is evidence that plasma homocysteine levels in many older people are related to inadequate intake of folic acid *(185–187)*. Homocysteine levels relate not only to lower levels of plasma folate but also to estimates of folate intake, and have been associated with an increased propensity to CVD and especially thrombosis. The association of high homocysteine levels with poor mental functioning may therefore reflect the impact of a series of small cerebral thromboses. Detailed studies in Italy have revealed that low folate levels are especially evident among older people living at home, with higher rates among men and among those who drink more alcohol and take a variety of drugs, which reduce the bioavailability of dietary folate. Thus, those taking drugs for a variety of medical conditions have 2–3 times the prevalence of low folate deficiency. Other European studies have shown that about 75% of older

Fig. 1.28. Trends in the proportion of the population 65 years or older in the WHO European Region, 1970–1998

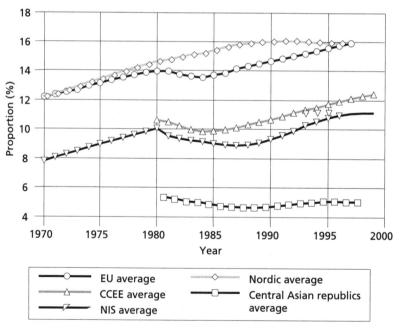

Source: European health for all database, WHO Regional Office for Europe.

people have abnormally high homocysteine levels, which are correlated inversely with both plasma and dietary folate *(188)*.

Fat-soluble vitamins, such as vitamins A, E and D, are important for older people. Studies in Italy show a clear decline in vitamin A status with age as food intake falls *(189)*, and a higher level of vitamin E in the plasma lowers the likelihood of marked atherosclerosis among older people *(190)*. It is therefore not surprising that vitamin E status, as well as the adequacy of intake of B vitamins, has been linked to a higher survival rate and lower mortality. The SENECA study shows a high prevalence of vitamin E and B_6 deficiency among older people in Europe. An appreciable proportion of the poor mental functioning of older people in Europe may therefore prove to be preventable.

As older people reduce their food intake in response to decreasing physical activity, iron intake falls. Any difficulty in chewing food because of dental loss reduces the intake of iron-enhancing vegetables and meat *(173–176)*. In a follow-up to the SENECA study, Martins et al. *(191)* reported that, of people in Portugal aged 81–86 years, 49% of men and 73% of women consumed less than the lowest European recommended dietary intake. Anaemia rates, however, are not unusually elevated, except in the central Asian republics, where iron availability is severely compromised or intestinal parasitism or other intestinal disease limits iron absorption. The modest prevalence of frank anaemia among older people needs to be distinguished from the much higher prevalence of anaemia among people who are ill and depend on nursing and other help with food, either at home or in institutions. Many well recognized techniques identify older people at risk, such as those living on their own, having difficulty in moving and shopping or displaying poor appetite and poor dental health *(192,193)*.

The importance of a healthy lifestyle in later life

The decline of the vitamin status of older people in Europe is of serious public health concern and is related not only to the marked decline in physical activity but also to the often poor quality of the diet among very old people, many of whom are either edentulous or have serious dental problems *(168)*. This suggests that the quality of the diet needs to be improved. The general importance of adequate vitamin status in older people was assessed in a double-blind placebo-controlled trial. Giving the equivalent of the recommended daily allowances of vitamins and some minerals to apparently healthy older people not only markedly improved their immune status but also led to a halving of intercurrent illnesses in the subsequent year.

How much the health of older people can be generally improved – by either improving the quality of the diet or simply increasing their physical activity so that they increase their intake – is uncertain. Nevertheless, the importance of increasing physical activity in older people has certainly been underestimated. Detailed studies in the Netherlands have shown that the greater the physical activity of older men, the lower the subsequent mortality rate. Thus, the rate among the most active third of older people was more than halved *(194)*. This surprisingly strong effect of physical activity may reflect not only improved nutrition but the well recognized impact of even modest physical activity in reducing CVD mortality *(195)*. In older people, physical activity is also likely not only to maintain better bone structure and greater power in better maintained muscle mass but also to limit the adverse metabolic effects of obesity. Intervention studies encouraging older people to take up even modest physical activity markedly improved their flexibility and sense of wellbeing *(196)*. This is a neglected area of public health in Europe.

Fig. 1.29. Adjusted hazard ratios of the individual and combined effects of diet, nonsmoking and physical activity on mortality in a sample of European men and women born between 1913 and 1918

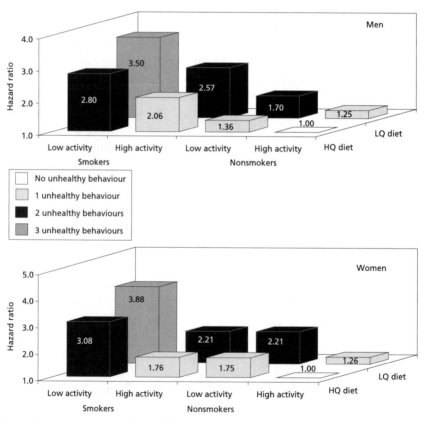

Note: The ratios were adjusted for age at baseline, region and the number of chronic diseases. HQ diet = high-quality diet; LQ diet = low-quality diet.
Source: Haveman-Nies et al. *(197)*.

The SENECA study highlighted the interaction between a good diet and physical activity by investigating their effects on the survival of older people individually and in combination with nonsmoking. The study population, aged 70–75 years, consisted of 631 men and 650 women from cities in Belgium, Denmark, Italy, the Netherlands, Portugal, Spain and Switzerland. A lifestyle score was calculated by adding the scores of the three lifestyle factors. Each factor and the total lifestyle score were related to survival in these European populations (Fig. 1.29). Combining types of unhealthy behaviour increased the risk of death: men and women with three unhealthy types of behaviour had a three- to fourfold increase in mortality. These results *(197)* emphasize the importance of a healthy lifestyle, including multiple lifestyle factors, and maintaining it with advancing age.

Healthy behaviour is related not only to a higher chance of survival but also to a delay in the deterioration of health status. Ideal healthy ageing is described as a situation in which people survive to an advanced age with their vigour and functional independence maintained and with morbidity and disability compressed into a relatively short period before death *(198)*.

Fig. 1.30 shows the effect of healthy behaviour on life expectancy and health status. The health status of survivors of the SENECA birth cohorts with healthy and unhealthy lifestyles is presented, with hypothetical extrapolations from the age of 82.5 years. During the ten-year follow-up period, the health status of the survivors with healthy lifestyles declined less quickly.

Fig. 1.30. Effect of healthy lifestyles on healthy ageing in a sample of Europeans born between 1913 and 1918, including hypothesized effects after 2000

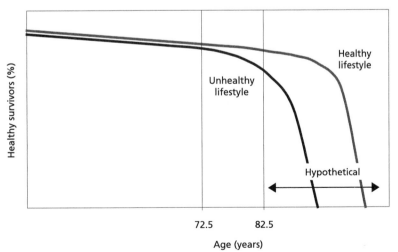

Source: adapted from Haveman-Nies et al. *(197)*.

In conclusion, healthy behaviour increases the chance of survival and delays the onset of illnesses. Although the SENECA study could not determine the net effect of these two relationships on the process of healthy ageing, postponing the onset of major morbidity is likely to compress morbidity into a shorter period.

The burden of osteoporosis

Osteoporosis means that the amount of bone per unit volume decreases but the composition remains unchanged. It occurs progressively after people reach peak bone mass as young adults. The two nutrients essential for bone health are vitamin D and calcium. Vitamin D deficiency is common among elderly people, often caused by poor nutrition and/or inadequate exposure to sunlight *(199)*. Subclinical deficiency of vitamin D, known as vitamin D insufficiency, may increase the risk of bone fractures if osteoporosis is already present. The yearly incidence of osteoporotic hip fractures in the EU is projected to more than double, from over 400 000 (80% in women) to almost 1 million, by 2050 (Fig. 1.31).

Fig. 1.31. Projected numbers of yearly incident hip fractures in EU countries, 1995–2050

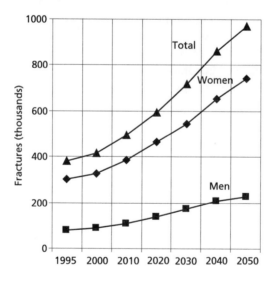

Source: adapted from *Report on osteoporosis in the European Community – action on prevention (200).*

Osteoporotic fractures have an overall mortality of 15–30% *(201,202)*. They are associated with considerable morbidity and often require hospitalization, rehabilitation and home care. The economic burden of osteoporosis is considerable. For example, the total cost of hospitalization for hip fractures in the EU was ECU 3.6 billion in 1995, and is expected to rise with the number of fractures *(203)*. Fig. 1.32 shows the direct estimated costs; these include surgery and postoperative stay, but not longer rehabilitation. For Sweden and the United Kingdom, for which data are available for the indirect costs of hip fracture (such as primary care, outpatient care and institutional care), the total amount is 2.5 times the direct hospital costs.

Fig. 1.32. Estimated total direct hospital costs arising from hip fractures in 13 EU countries, 1996

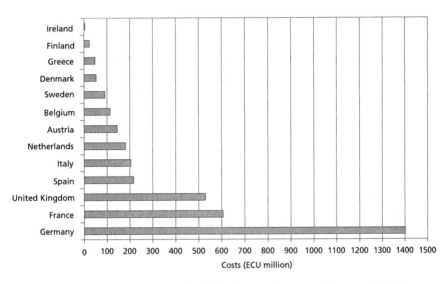

Note: No national data were available for Luxembourg or Portugal. The figures for Austria are based on the costs in Germany.

Source: adapted from *Report on osteoporosis in the European Community – action on prevention (200).*

Physical activity plays a well established role throughout the lifespan in maintaining the normal structure and functional strength of bone. Specifically, physical activity can prevent or slow down the bone loss that begins occurring in women as a normal process after menopause *(204).*

In summary, while most chronic diseases manifest in later life, the quality of life needs to be maximized until death. Adopting health promoting behaviour, such as physical activity and healthy diets, provides clear benefits to ageing individuals and populations. As the proportion of older European increases, interventions will influence an even greater number of people. In turn, improved health results in less dependence and reduces the cost of health care and institutional care (see Chapter 4, pp. 237–239, for policy recommendations).

Nutritional health of vulnerable groups
Refugees and internally displaced people
In the midst of major socioeconomic and political transition, and in part as a result of the severance from traditional trade and financial links with the former USSR, many of the NIS and CCEE are not maximizing their industrial and agricultural potential and some are further crippled by natural disaster and political strife. These conditions continue to damage food security and the nutritional status of the affected populations.

For instance, the three-year conflict in Bosnia and Herzegovina jeopardized the health and nutritional status of older people. By January 1994, 15% had a BMI below 18.5. Because the vegetable supply was poor, so were plasma carotenoid levels and plasma 25-hydroxyvitamin D_3 levels in 65% of older people, most likely because of poor exposure to sunlight after months of siege (205). Protein and energy undernutrition was not a widespread public health problem, however (110).

In 1999 in Kosovo, 11 000 children older than 5 years were estimated to be acutely malnourished and about 17 000 would be affected by stunting. Over 5% of the surveyed mothers had a BMI below 18.5 and more than 10% were obese (206). Other examples are Tajikistan and Uzbekistan, where both drought and civil conflict have increased the frequency of both wasting and stunting.

Migrant groups, refugees and travellers constitute minorities residing – sometimes temporarily – within populations. Surveys of dietary patterns and nutritional status among these groups are sparse. As of 1 January 2002, the United Nations High Commission for Refugees classified nearly 5 million people in Europe as persons of concern, including refugees and asylum seekers (http://www.unhcr.ch/cgi-bin/texis/vtx/home?page=statistics, accessed 25 September 2003).

Transient populations such as the Roma, an ethnic minority group of northern Indian origin that is especially numerous in the CCEE and western NIS, suffer additional strains on their health, as they are often stigmatized. More than 5 million Roma live in the CCEE. They are estimated to account for more than 5% of the population in Bulgaria, Hungary, Romania and Slovakia (207). With few exceptions, members of groups such as the Roma have low socioeconomic status. A study of Romany children aged 9–13 years in the Czech Republic found inadequate consumption of vegetables (19% of the recommended daily allowances (RDAs)), fruit (20% of RDA), milk and milk products (32% of RDA), cereal foods (63% of RDA) and fish, meat, poultry and eggs (on average, 78% of RDA) *(208)*. The children were consuming more than four times the recommended amounts of various snack foods containing fat and sugar. Compared with Czech children, Romany children typically consumed half the amounts of fruit, vegetables, milk and milk products. Yet when asked what foods they liked, 90% of Romany children mentioned fruit of various types. Their low consumption may reflect the constraints on choice arising from low income *(209)* and lack of access to fruits and vegetables because of high seasonality in rural areas *(210,211)*. This highlights the need to address availability and expense rather than concentrating only on education and information campaigns. These results may also help explain the reports of elevated obesity rates in Romany children *(211)*.

Children who are especially vulnerable to food insecurity and poor diet tend to grow and develop more slowly than others of their age *(208)*. In Azerbaijan, anaemia rates were consistently higher among internally displaced populations (http://web.azerweb.com/NGO_and_International_Organiza-tion_Reports/1996/CDCsurvey.html, accessed 25 September 2003). In Kazakhstan, the Kazakh ethnic group has a higher rate of anaemia than the Russian ethnic group *(212)*.

People in hospital

Evidence shows that some patients in European hospitals are undernourished and that undernutrition may increase during hospital stay. The prevalence of underweight (BMI < 20) among hospital patients is 20–30%. This problem has been described in Denmark *(213)*, Germany, Italy *(214)*, Norway *(215)*, Sweden *(216)*, Switzerland *(217,218)* and the United Kingdom *(219)*.

Good nutritional care for patients provides clear benefits, but several factors have prevented its adequate provision in Europe (see Chapter 4, pp. 242–243, for recommendations on nutrition in hospitals):

- unclear responsibilities in planning and managing nutritional care;
- insufficient education on nutrition for some staff groups;
- patients' lack of influence and knowledge;
- insufficient cooperation between staff groups; and
- inadequate involvement of hospital managers.

Some patients who have little fat-free mass could be undernourished despite having a normal BMI *(218)*. Most of the studies assessing the nutritional status of patients have excluded those who are most ill and hence most likely to be undernourished *(213,220)*. Finally, obese patients could become undernourished while losing weight *(221)*.

The prevalence of undernutrition is much higher among some patient groups, such as gastrointestinal patients, than among others, such as people admitted for obstetric services or elective surgery. In addition, undernutrition is higher among old patients (213,219,222–224). The prevalence has been suggested to be slightly higher among medical than surgical patients (219), among women (225,226) and among patients in teaching hospitals than those in district general hospitals (220,227).

A survey of hospitalized children under 5 years in Kosovo found that 44% were fed vegetables and 84% fruit; 58% of the children were anaemic (18% severely and 40% moderately), possibly in part because tea was given to 80% of infants. The average age at which tea was introduced into their diet was 5 months. In 68% of hospital cases, children had not been breastfed for 6 full months, and 63% of the children had been given cow's milk before reaching 6 months of age.

Many studies have shown that the risk of undernutrition increases during hospital stay (228–232). For example, of 112 patients with all kinds of diagnoses hospitalized for more than 1 week, 64% had lost weight when discharged (mean weight loss: 5.4%), including 75% of those initially most undernourished. In contrast, 20% gained weight, including only 12.5% originally classified as undernourished. None gained sufficient weight to allow them to be reclassified as having normal weight (219).

A reduced length of stay in hospital and decreased complication rates benefit both the patient and the health services. Improving hospital nutrition may bring the services substantial savings: at least £330 per surgical patient according to one estimate (233).

A study in Denmark suggested that nutritional support could save the health services €133 million for every 100 000 patients (221). A study in the United Kingdom estimated that the National Health Service could save £266 million per year through nutritional support, based on the assumption that 10% of patients would benefit (234). A study in the United States (235) suggested that appropriate and timely nutritional support could save a typical large hospital over US $1 million per year.

Social inequalities and poverty

Various studies have surveyed the dietary patterns of different socioeconomic groups in Europe using a variety of indicators, such as household income, occupational class or the educational level of the head of the household (see Chapter 3, pp. 158–168).

The DAFNE (Data Food Networking) study looked at household food purchases made by different socioeconomic groups based on educational attainment levels in Belgium, Greece, Hungary and Poland in 1990 (236).

The study found that dietary patterns differ considerably between countries, possibly reflecting different phases of the nutrition transition. These differences were generally greater than the differences found between socioeconomic groups, although the latter showed certain patterns. In general, lower socioeconomic groups tend to consume more meat, fat and sugar, although not necessarily the lowest socioeconomic groups, who may be partly excluded from more commercialized food supplies. The groups with the highest educational level appeared to consume more fruits and vegetables, although in some countries the groups with the lowest educational level, who may be growing their own produce, consumed a great deal.

De Irala-Estevez et al. *(237)* and Roos et al. *(238)* support these findings; they examined dietary survey data for several western European countries and showed large socioeconomic differences in fruit and vegetable intake, with the higher socioeconomic groups usually consuming more fruits and vegetables (Table 1.4).

Table 1.4. Difference in fruit and vegetable consumption among groups with high and low education in selected European countries and regions, 1980s and 1990s

| Country or region | Difference (g per 10 MJ consumed per day) | |
	Fruits	Vegetables
Finland	+55	+30
Sweden	+18	+23
Norway	+26	− 3
Denmark	+46	+43
United Kingdom	+31	+33
Germany	+16	+14
Netherlands	+52	+19
Spain		
Navarra	+14	+ 9
Catalonia	+ 6	−19
Basque Country	−97	+31

Source: Roos et al. *(238)*.

These figures are based on surveys made in the 1980s and 1990s. A more recent examination of fruit and vegetable consumption in Spain *(239)* suggested that the patterns of fruit and vegetable consumption now reflect those of northern Europe, with people in higher educational groups having higher intakes than those in lower educational groups.

Among over 3000 Norwegian adults, those with higher educational and occupational status ate more fruits and vegetables and more dietary fibre and less fat *(240)*. People living in cities also had healthier diets than those living in rural areas, although other data indicated that farmers in Norway tended to have a lower-fat diet, lower serum cholesterol and less CHD than people in urban areas (Gunn-Elin Bjørnboe, National Council on Nutrition and Physical Activity, Oslo, Norway, personal communication, 2000).

The United Kingdom has a long history of monitoring dietary patterns related to income levels, and annual food purchasing surveys have shown that household income is consistently related to certain dietary patterns. Families living on low incomes tend to consume less fruit and vegetables (Fig. 1.33) *(241)*, fish and whole-grain cereal foods and more refined cereal foods, sweet foods, fat and oil *(242)*. As a result, the intake of essential nutrients shows a marked social gradient from poorer to richer households (Table 1.5).

Fig. 1.33. Relationship of income to consumption of fresh fruits and vegetables and the share of income spent on food in the United Kingdom

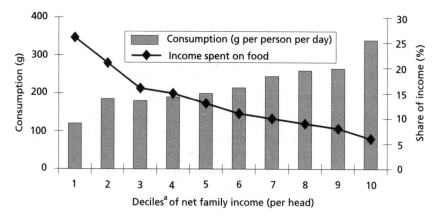

ᵃ 1 = lowest incomes; 10 = highest incomes.

Source: Department for Food, Environment and Rural Affairs *(241)*.

Further surveys in the United Kingdom have shown that vulnerable groups – including older people, children from manual social classes, families claiming state benefits and children from lone-parent families – have lower intake and lower blood levels of many vitamins and minerals than others in the population *(111,167,243)*. Intakes of vitamin C, folate, iron, zinc and magnesium are well below reference levels in households with incomes below £180 a week (the lowest income cut-off) or in households with more than three children or headed by a lone parent *(241)*. Among the poorest fifth of families, the intake of some nutrients declined over a period of 15 years: vitamin C by 23% and beta-carotene by 47% *(244)*.

Table 1.5. Household income and average levels of consumption
of several essential nutrients in the United Kingdom

Income decile (%)	Beta-carotene (µg/day)	Folate (µg/day)	Vitamin C (mg/day)	Iron (mg/day)	Zinc (mg/day)
0–10	1.175	204	43.2	8.3	6.6
10–20	1.601	231	50.8	9.5	7.3
20–30	1.631	245	54.7	10.0	7.8
30–40	1.742	250	56.7	10.2	7.8
40–50	1.773	253	60.7	10.3	7.9
50–60	1.914	257	63.2	10.5	8.1
60–70	1.921	256	62.3	10.5	8.0
70–80	1.984	266	69.4	10.8	8.2
80–90	1.937	269	73.4	11.0	8.3
90–100	2.075	273	80.8	11.2	8.3

Source: Ministry of Agriculture, Fisheries and Food *(241).*

Studies of socioeconomic status and breastfeeding suggest that, in more af-fluent countries, the frequency and duration of breastfeeding are greatest among higher-income groups. In the United Kingdom, for example, mothers in the highest-income group are twice as likely to be breastfeeding during the first week after a baby's birth than mothers in the lowest group, and the social-class differences grow over subsequent weeks (Table 1.6).

Table 1.6. Breastfeeding rates in high and low socioeconomic groups
in the United Kingdom, 1999

Time	Breastfeeding rates (%)	
	Social class I	Social class V
At 1 week	84	40
At 6 weeks	73	23
At 4 months	56	13

Source: Nelson *(245).*

Inequality and diet-related diseases

The dietary patterns described above may go some way in explaining the dif-ferent disease patterns experienced by different social groups. A survey of more than 15 000 adults in the United Kingdom found significant differences in the prevalence of disease factors across different social classes defined by occupation (Table 1.7).

The short-term effects on disease of inequality between social classes can be illustrated among individuals who change social class during their adult lives. A study in Oslo found that people who moved from lower to higher income or vice versa showed mortality rates that approached but did not equal those of the class to which they had moved *(246).*

Table 1.7. Social class and ill health: prevalence of diseases
and risk factors in adults in the United Kingdom, 1994

Diseases and risk factors	Social class					
	Highest		Intermediate non-manual		Lowest	
	Men	Women	Men	Women	Men	Women
Ischaemic heart disease (%)	5.1	1.8	6.0	5.2	6.4	7.2
Stroke (%)	1.3	0.5	1.7	2.3	2.1	2.5
Mean blood pressure (mm/Hg)	136/76	130/72	138/76	136/73	139/77	141/75
Cholesterol > 6.5 mmol/l (%)	26	26	27	35	26	36
Haemoglobin < 13 g/dl (%)	3	9	5	12	5	13
Obesity (BMI > 30) (%)	9.9	11.8	13.7	15.0	14.0	22.6
Physically inactive (%)	14	15	15	17	21	22

Source: Colhoun & Prescott-Clarke (117).

Cancer rates can show a similar change in pattern: after Turkish migrants move to Germany, their disease rates rise towards the levels prevailing there (247). This implies that changing lifestyle – including food and diet – can affect the health experience of the groups being assimilated and can therefore explain some of the inequality in disease rates among these populations.

As shown in Table 1.7, lower-income groups in the United Kingdom tend to have higher heart disease rates, and many countries in Europe show a similar relationship. The cause is likely to be multifactorial, including smoking, physical activity, stress, occupational factors and other psychosocial factors (248), as well as nutrition.

Nevertheless, the same pattern may not be found among populations adhering to diets more like those traditionally eaten in southern Europe. Kunst et al. (249) examined data on socioeconomic status and heart disease mortality in several European countries. Although data sources were not perfectly compatible, and data for some groups were unobtainable, the figures fairly consistently show that lower socioeconomic status and heart disease are most strongly associated in northern Europe and among younger populations. In contrast, the association tended to be reversed among older populations in southern Europe (Table 1.8). The analysis was based on data from longitudinal and cross-sectional studies using national population censuses of 1981. For most of the longitudinal studies, follow-up covered the period from 1980 to 1989.

The trends shown in Table 1.8 may result from several factors, but diet will play a part. A transition from the heart-protecting diets (rich in fruits, vegetables and fish) eaten traditionally in southern Europe to diets rich in animal products and refined carbohydrates will increase the risk of heart disease.

The fact that such a transition in diet has occurred to a greater degree among poorer populations and has affected younger more than older members of a population needs further investigation.

Table 1.8. Relative risk[a] of heart disease for men in manual versus non-manual occupations in selected countries in western Europe

Country	Relative risk in men aged:		
	30–44 years	45–59 years	60–64 years
Sweden	1.80	1.38	Not available
United Kingdom (England and Wales)	1.68	1.50	1.26
France	1.18	0.96	Not available
Italy	1.35	1.08	0.85
Portugal	0.82	0.76	Not available
Norway	1.77	1.35	1.26

[a] >1 = elevated risk; <1 = lower risk.

Source: adapted from Kunst et al. (249).

Obesity, physical activity and inequality

Inequality in disease experience may also be related to energy expenditure and physical activity (see Chapter 3, pp. 165–167). A fitness survey in England found that people who had more education or owned their homes tended to engage in more physical activity (250). Unemployed men, and to some extent unemployed women, tended to be more sedentary than those in employment (251). Professional people were twice as likely as unskilled manual workers or economically inactive people to take part in sports or other leisure physical activity. In addition, a survey of over 15 000 adults in the United Kingdom found that physical inactivity in both men and women increased as social class decreased.

Socioeconomic status and obesity have often been found to be inversely related among women in Europe (Fig. 1.34) (252). The relationship among men, although less clear in earlier reviews (253), seems to be similar to that among women. In the consumer survey of the entire EU, in which BMI was calculated from subjects' self-reported height and weight, levels of obesity and social class were strongly associated, with social class being defined variously by household income, occupation or educational level (252). The survey involved over 15 000 people aged over 15 years in the member states of the EU.

In 1997–1998, the WHO Health Behaviour in School-aged Children study found consistent links between greater family affluence and more self-reported exercise among 15-year-olds surveyed in several European countries (98). Exercise was more common among more affluent children in Austria,

Fig. 1.34. Prevalence of obesity among adult men and women
according to economic status (measured by household income
or occupation) in the EU

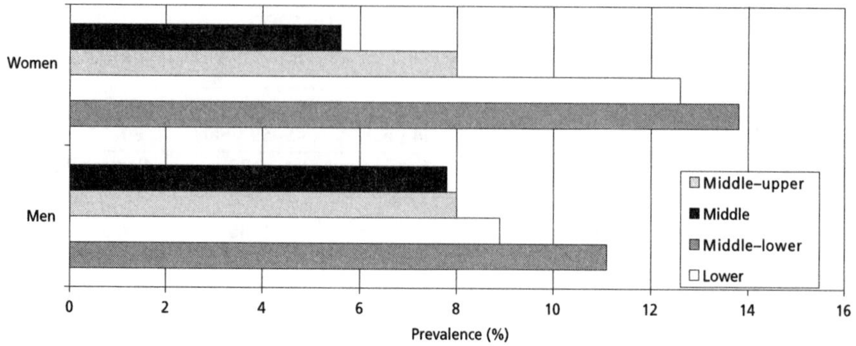

Source: adapted from Martinez et al. *(252).*

Denmark, Germany, Hungary, Latvia, Portugal, the Russian Federation and
the United Kingdom, but not in Norway.

A consumer survey in the EU suggested that adults with less education are
more likely to have physically active jobs and are more likely to spend time in
sedentary leisure when not working *(254).* Those who were older and had
only primary education were the least likely both to take part in physical
exercise and to consider such activity necessary for health.

Lifestyle and choice

In countries where undernutrition and poor child growth are still relatively
common, there is evidence that obesity and underweight may coexist. Studies
carried out in Kyrgyzstan, the Russian Federation and Tajikistan *(255)* show
that 30–60% of households with underweight individuals also had
overweight individuals: typically an underweight child and an overweight
adult. The causes may be complex, but some evidence suggests that, the more
rapid the nutrition transition, the more likely that both under- and
overweight problems will coexist in the same household *(256).*

The data reviewed here show wide variation between countries in the
WHO European Region. More economically advanced countries show a post-
transition pattern, in which people who are poorer in material or social conditions are likely to eat less healthily and take less exercise. These unhealthy lifestyles in turn generate the inequality observed in morbidity and mortality
from CVD and a wide range of other causes.

In countries with limited access to commercialized food supplies, dietary
patterns may be more like a subsistence diet, relying on staple cereal crops,

some vegetable foods and limited amounts of animal products. Health indicators such as infant mortality rates may be high, but rates of CVD and other adult noncommunicable diseases may be low, indicating that such diets may contribute to better adult health.

As discussed elsewhere in this book, factors such as fetal nutrition, birth weight, child growth and subsequent obesity and disease experience are shaped by environmental and material circumstances that may be far beyond the individual's control. In such situations, efforts to improve health by exhorting members of the population to improve their lifestyles may have only limited impact: as Dowler *(257)* points out:

> The implication is that people are able to exert personal choice over what they eat, or whether they walk/cycle or undertake active exercise, rather than leading a sedentary life, and that the role of those implementing health promotion is to encourage or enable them to make "the right" choices …

In practice, choices in relation to food and activity are not solely individual matters, unconstrained by family, neighbourhood or material conditions. The evidence is that structural and social influences – such as the amount of time and money people can devote to pursuit of good food and active living, the cost and accessibility of both, the physical area where households are located and the general social circumstances of the lives of those classified as lower classes by whatever indicators – constrain and govern choice to a considerable extent.

Public health policies are necessary to ensure that the choices required for a healthy lifestyle are available to the population and that a healthy choice is an easy one for all people to make (see Chapter 4).

References

1. MURRAY, C.J.L. & LOPEZ, A.D. *The global burden of disease. A comprehensive assessment of mortality and disability from diseases, injuries, and risk factors in 1990 and projected to 2020.* Cambridge, MA, Harvard School of Public Health, 1996.
2. MURRAY, C.J. & LOPEZ, A.D. Global mortality, disability, and the contribution of risk factors: Global Burden of Disease Study. *Lancet,* **349**: 1436–1442 (1997).
3. *The world health report 2000. Health systems: improving performance.* Geneva, World Health Organization, 2000.
4. *The world health report 2002: reducing risks, promoting healthy life* (http:// whqlibdoc.who.int/publications/2002/9241562072.pdf). Geneva, World Health Organization, 2002 (accessed 3 September 2003).

5. POMERLEAU, J. ET AL The burden of disease attributable to nutrition in Europe. *Public health nutrition,* **6**(5): 453–461 (2003).
6. *Determinants of the burden of disease in the European Union.* Stockholm, National Institute of Public Health, 1997.
7. TOBIAS, M. *The burden of disease and injury in New Zealand* (http://www.moh.govt.nz/moh.nsf/ea6005dc347e7bd44c2566a40079ae6f/a313645fbc60bf02cc2569f400791b9b?OpenDocument). Wellington, New Zealand Ministry of Health, 2001 (Public Health Intelligence Occasional Bulletin No. 1) (accessed 25 September 2003).
8. MATHERS, C. ET AL. *The burden of disease and injury in Australia.* Canberra, Australian Institute of Health and Welfare, 1999.
9. VOS, T. & BEGG, S. *The Victorian burden of disease study: mortality.* Melbourne, Public Health and Development Division, Victorian Government Department of Human Services, 1999.
10. WORLD CANCER RESEARCH FUND & AMERICAN INSTITUTE FOR CANCER RESEARCH. *Food, nutrition and the prevention of cancer: a global perspective.* Washington, DC, American Institute for Cancer Research, 1997.
11. DOLL, R. & PETO, R. *The causes of cancer.* Oxford, Oxford University Press, 1981.
12. DOLL, R. The lessons of life. Keynote address to the nutrition and cancer conference. *Cancer research,* **52**: 2024S–2029S (1992).
13. BROWNER, W.S. ET AL. What if Americans ate less fat? A quantitative estimate of the effect on mortality. *Journal of the American Medical Association,* **265**: 285–291 (1991).
14. WILLETT, W.C. Will high-carbohydrate/low-fat diets reduce the risk of coronary heart disease? *Proceedings of the Society for Experimental Biology and Medicine,* **225**:187–190 (2000).
15. WILLETT, W.C. Diet, nutrition and avoidable cancer. *Environmental health perspectives,* **103**(Suppl. 8): 165–170 (1995).
16. RIBOLI, E. ET AL. *Alimentation et cancer: évaluation des données scientifique?* Paris, Editions Techniques et Documentation, Lavoisier, 1996.
17. COMMITTEE ON MEDICAL ASPECTS OF FOOD POLICY WORKING GROUP ON DIET AND CANCER (COMA). *Nutritional aspects of the development of cancer.* London, H.M. Stationery Office, 1998 (Department of Health Reports on Health and Social Subjects, No. 48).
18. PAPAS, A.M., ED. *Antioxidant status, diet, nutrition, and health.* Boca Raton, FL, CRC Press, 1998.
19. JOFFE, M. & ROBERTSON, A. The potential contribution of increased vegetable and fruit consumption to health gain in the European Union. *Public health nutrition,* **4**: 893–901 (2001).

20. *Comparative analysis of food and nutrition policies in the WHO European Region 1994–1999. Full report.* Copenhagen, WHO Regional Office for Europe (in press).

21. *Diet, nutrition and the prevention of chronic diseases. Report of a joint WHO/FAO expert consultation* (http://whqlibdoc.who.int/trs/WHO_TRS_916.pdf). Geneva, World Health Organization, 2003 (WHO Technical Series, No. 916) (accessed 3 September 2003).

22. TRICHOPOULOU, A. *Nutrition in Europe: nutrition policy and public health in the European Community and models for European eating habits on the threshold of the 21st century.* Brussels, European Parliament Scientific and Technological Options Assessment (STOA), 1997.

23. POWLES, J.W. ET AL. Protective foods in winter and spring: a key to lower vascular mortality? *Lancet,* **348**: 898–899 (1996).

24. RENAUD, S. & LANZMANN-PETITHORY, D. Coronary heart disease: dietary links and pathogenesis. *Public health nutrition,* 4(2B): 459–474 (2001).

25. PUSKA, P. Nutrition and mortality: the Finnish experience. *Acta cardiologica,* **55**: 213–220 (2000).

26. VARTIAINEN, E. ET AL. Changes in risk factors explain changes in mortality from ischaemic heart disease in Finland. *British medical journal,* **309**: 23–27 (1994).

27. MICHAELSEN, K. ET AL. *Feeding and nutrition of infants and young children. Guidelines for the WHO European Region, with emphasis on the former Soviet countries* (http://www.euro.who.int/InformationSources/Publications/Catalogue/20010914_21). Copenhagen, WHO Regional Office for Europe, 2003 (WHO Regional Publications, European Series, No. 87) (accessed 25 September 2003).

28. *Globalization, diets and noncommunicable diseases* (http://whqlibdoc.who.int/publications/9241590416.pdf). Geneva, World Health Organization, 2002 (accessed 3 September 2003).

29. SIMOPOULOS, A.P. & VISIOLI, F., ED. *Mediterranean diets.* Basle, Karger, 2000 (World review of nutrition and dietetics, Vol. 87).

30. KOHLMEIER, L. ET AL. *Ernährungsabhängige Krankheiten und ihre Kosten.* Baden-Baden, Nomos-Verlagsgesellschaft, 1993.

31. LIU, J.L.Y. ET AL. The economic burden of coronary heart disease in the UK. *Heart,* **88**: 597–603 (2002).

32. KENKEL, D.S. & MANNING, W. Economic evaluation of nutrition policy. Or there's no such thing as a free lunch. *Food policy,* 24: 145–162 (1999).

33. WOLF, A.M. & COLDITZ, G.A. Current estimates of the economic cost of obesity in the United States. *Obesity research,* 6: 97–106 (1998).

34. OSTER, G. ET AL. Lifetime health and economic benefits of weight loss among obese persons. *American journal of public health*, **89**: 1536–1542 (1999).

35. *Obesity – preventing and managing the global epidemic. Report of a WHO Consultation*. Geneva, World Health Organization, 1998 (Technical Report Series, No. 894).

36. LEVY, E. ET AL. The economic cost of obesity: the French situation. *International journal of obesity and related metabolic disorders*, **19**: 788–792 (1995).

37. DETOURNAY, B. ET AL. Obesity morbidity and health care costs in France: an analysis of the 1991–1992 Medical Care Household Survey. *International journal of obesity and related metabolic disorders*, **24**: 151–155 (2000).

38. KURSCHEID, T. & LAUTERBACH, K. The cost implications of obesity for health care and society. *International journal of obesity and related metabolic disorders*, **22**(Suppl. 1): S3–S5 (1998).

39. SEIDELL, J.C. & DEERENBERG, I. Obesity in Europe: prevalence and consequences for use of medical care. *Pharmacoeconomics*, **5**(Suppl. 1): 38–44 (1994).

40. SJÖSTRUM, L. ET AL. Costs and benefits when treating obesity. *International journal of obesity and related metabolic disorders*, **19**(Suppl. 6): S9–S12 (1995).

41. GORSTEIN, J. & GROSSE, R.N. The indirect costs of obesity to society. *Pharmacoeconomics*, **5**(Suppl. 1): 58–61 (1994).

42. HOLTERMAN, M. & NOUT, S.M. *The economic benefit of breast feeding in the Netherlands.* Amsterdam, Free University, 1998.

43. *Kostnad-nytte vurderinger av tiltak for å øke forbruket av frukt og grønnsaker, for å redusere forekomsten av kreft* [Cost–benefit evaluations of policies to increase the consumption of fruit and vegetables to reduce cancer]. Oslo, National Council on Nutrition and Physical Activity, 1998 (Report 4/98) (in Norwegian).

44. GUNDGAARD, J. ET AL. [Evaluation of health economic consequences of an increased intake of fruit and vegetables]. Odense, Center for Anvendt Sundhedstjenesteforskning og Teknologivurdering, Syddansk Universitet, 2002 (in Danish).

45. VAN'T VEER, P. ET AL. Fruit and vegetables in the prevention of cancer and cardiovascular disease. *Public health nutrition*, **3**: 103–107 (2000).

46. RAYNER, M. ET AL. *Coronary heart disease statistics. British Heart Foundation statistics database 1998. Annual compendium.* Oxford, British Heart Foundation Health Promotion Research Group, 1998.

47. ZATONSKI, W.A. ET AL. Ecological study of reasons for sharp decline in mortality from ischaemic heart disease in Poland since 1991. *British medical journal,* **316**: 1047–1051 (1998).

48. KEYS, A.B. *Seven countries: a multivariate analysis of death and coronary heart disease.* Cambridge, Harvard University Press, 1980.

49. MULLER, H. ET AL. Serum cholesterol predictive equations with special emphasis on *trans* and saturated fatty acids: an analysis from designed controlled studies. *Lipids,* **36**: 783–791 (2001).

50. YU, S. ET AL. Plasma cholesterol – predictive equations demonstrate that stearic acid is neutral and monounsaturated fatty acids are hypocholesterolemic. *American journal of clinical nutrition,* **61**: 1129–1139 (1995).

51. SCHMIDT, E.B. ET AL. N-3 fatty acids from fish and coronary artery disease: implications for public health. *Public health nutrition,* **3**: 91–98 (2000).

52. PETERSEN, S. & RAYNER, M. *Coronary heart disease statistics, 2000 edition.* Oxford, British Heart Foundation Health Promotion Research Group, 2000.

53. KLERK, M. ET AL. *Fruits and vegetables in chronic disease prevention. Part II: Update and extension (literature up to early 1998).* Wageningen, Wageningen Agricultural University, 1998.

54. DOFKOVA, M. ET AL. The development of food consumption in the Czech Republic after 1989. *Public health nutrition,* **4**: 999–1003 (2001).

55. GJONCA, A. & BOBAK, M. Albanian paradox, another example of protective effect of Mediterranean lifestyle? *Lancet,* **350**: 1815–1817 (1997).

56. WILCKEN, D.E. MTHFR 677CT mutation, folate intake, neural-tube defect, and risk of cardiovascular disease. *Lancet,* **350**: 603–604 (1997).

57. ALDERMAN, M.H. Salt, blood pressure, and human health. *Hypertension,* **36**: 890–893 (2000).

58. PERRY, I.J. Dietary salt intake and cerebrovascular damage. *Nutrition, metabolism and cardiovascular diseases,* **10**: 229–235 (2000).

59. APPEL, L.J. ET AL. A clinical trial of the effects of dietary patterns on blood pressure. DASH Collaborative Research Group. *New England journal of medicine,* **336**: 1117–1124 (1997).

60. SACKS, F.M. ET AL. Effects on blood pressure of reduced dietary sodium and the dietary approaches to stop hypertension (DASH) diet. *New England journal of medicine,* **344**: 3–10 (2001).

61. MINCU, I. *Nutrition, lifestyle and state of health. The alimentation of Romanians.* Bucharest, Editura Enciclopedica, 2001.

62. SELMER, R.M. ET AL. Cost and health consequences of reducing the population intake of salt. *Journal of epidemiology and community health,* **54**: 697–702 (2000).

63. STAMLER, J. ET AL. Low risk-factor profile and long-term cardiovascular and non-cardiovascular mortality and life expectancy: findings for 5 large cohorts of young adult and middle-aged men and women. *Journal of the American Medical Association*, **282**: 2012–2018 (1999).

64. MAGNUS, P. & BEAGLEHOLE, R. The real contribution of the major risk factors to the coronary epidemics: time to end the "only-50%" myth. *Archives of internal medicine*, **161**: 2657–2660 (2001).

65. HEMINGWAY, H. & MARMOT, M. Psychosocial factors in the aetiology and prognosis of coronary heart disease: systematic review of prospective cohort studies. *British medical journal*, **318**: 1460–1467 (1999).

66. THEORELL, T. & KARASEK, R.A. Current issues relating to psychosocial job strain and cardiovascular disease research. *Journal of occupational health psychology*, **1**: 9–26 (1996).

67. ROSS, R. Atherosclerosis – an inflammatory disease. *New England journal of medicine*, **340**: 115–126 (1999).

68. BJORNTORP, P. Heart and soul: stress and the metabolic syndrome. *Scandinavian cardiovascular journal*, **35**: 172–177 (2001).

69. RIBOLI, E. & NORAT, T. Epidemiological evidence of the protective effect of fruits and vegetables on cancer risk. *American journal of clinical nutrition* (in press).

70. KONINGS, E.J. ET AL. Intake of dietary folate vitamers and risk of colorectal carcinoma: results from The Netherlands Cohort Study. *Cancer*, **95**: 1421–1433 (2002).

71. RIBOLI, E. & NORAT, T. Cancer prevention and diet: opportunities in Europe. *Public health nutrition*, 4(2B): 475–484 (2001).

72. NORAT, T. ET AL. Meat consumption and colorectal cancer risk: dose–response meta-analysis of epidemiological studies. *International journal of cancer*, **98**: 241–256 (2002).

73. BERGSTROM, A. ET AL. Overweight as an avoidable cause of cancer in Europe. *International journal of cancer*, **91**: 421–430 (2001).

74. BANEGAS, J.R. ET AL. *A simple estimate of mortality attributable to excess weight in the European Union*. Madrid, Department of Preventive Medicine and Public Health, Autonomous University of Madrid, 2002.

75. LOBSTEIN, T. ET AL. *Childhood obesity: the new crisis in public health*. London, International Obesity Task Force, 2003.

76. ASTRUP, A. Healthy lifestyles in Europe; prevention of obesity and type II diabetes by diet and physical activity. *Public health nutrition*, 4(2B): 499–515 (2001).

77. TRICHOPOULOU, A. ET AL. Body mass index in relation to energy intake and expenditure among adults in Greece. *Epidemiology*, **11**: 333–336 (2000).

78. DJORDJEVIC, P. ET AL. *Screen, treat and prevent*. Belgrade, YASO, 1998.

79. ZAJKAS, G. & BIRO, G. Some data on the prevalence of obesity in Hungarian adult population between 1985-88 and 1992-94. *Zeitschrift für Ernahrungswissenschaft*, 37(Suppl 1): 134–135 (1998).

80. *Kazakhstan demographic and health survey (DHS), 1999.* Calverton, MD, Macro International Inc., 2000.

81. *Turkey demographic and health survey (DHS), 1998.* Calverton, MD, Macro International Inc., 1999.

82. *Kyrgyzstan demographic and health survey (DHS), 1997.* Calverton, MD, Macro International Inc., 1998.

83. PRIOR, G. & PRIMATESTA, P., ED. *Health survey for England 2000.* London, The Stationery Office, 2002.

84. DE BACKER, G. De zwaarlijvige Belgen: met hoeveel zijn ze [Obese Belgians: how many are there]? *RUG nieuwsbrief over gezond en lekker eren*, 70: 3 (2000) (in Flemish).

85. VISSCHER, T.L.S. ET AL. Long-term and recent time trends in the prevalence of obesity among Dutch men and women. *International journal of obesity*, 26: 1218–1224 (2002).

86. EGGER, S. ET AL. [Overweight and obesity in the Zurich canton. A LuftiBus study]. *Schweizerische Rundschau für Medizin Praxis*, 90: 531–538 (2001).

87. *Il sovrappeso e l'obesitá* [Overweight and obesity in Italy] (http://www.ausl.mo.it/pps/salute/download/sovrappe.pdf). Rome, National Institute of Statistics (ISTAT), 2000 (in Italian) (accessed 25 September 2003).

88. ARANCETA, J. ET AL. *Prevalencia de la obesidad en España: estudio SEEDO'97* [Prevalence of obesity in Spain: The SEEDO 97 study] (http://www.seedo.es/prevalencia97.htm). Barcelona, Sociedad Española para el Estudio de la Obesidad, 1998 (in Spanish) (accessed 6 October 2002).

89. MATTHIESSEN, J. ET AL. [The significance of diet and physical activity for the development of obesity in Denmark from 1985 to 1995]. *Ugeskrift for laeger*, 163: 2941–2945 (2001) (in Danish).

90. LAHTI-KOSKI, M. ET AL. Age, education and occupation as determinants of trends in body mass index in Finland from 1982 to 1997. *International journal of obesity and related metabolic disorders*, 24: 1669–1676 (2000).

91. LISSNER, L. ET AL. Social mapping of the obesity epidemic in Sweden. *International journal of obesity and related metabolic disorders*, 24: 801–805 (2000).

92. GODFREY, K.M. & BARKER, D.J. Fetal programming and adult health. *Public health nutrition*, 4(2B): 611–624 (2001).

93. HAN, T.S. ET AL. Waist circumference action levels in the identification of cardiovascular risk factors: prevalence study in a random sample. *British medical journal*, **311**: 1401–1405 (1995).

94. DE ONIS, M. & BLOSSNER, M. Prevalence and trends of overweight among preschool children in developing countries. *American journal of clinical nutrition*, **72**: 1032–1039 (2000).

95. STARK, D. ET AL. Longitudinal study of obesity in the National Survey of Health and Development. *British medical journal*, **283**: 12–17 (1981).

96. VUORI, I.M. Health benefits of physical activity with special reference to interaction with diet. *Public health nutrition*, 4(2B): 517–528 (2001).

97. PRENTICE, A.M. & JEBB, S.A. Obesity in Britain: gluttony or sloth? *British medical journal*, **311**: 437–439 (1995).

98. CURRIE, C. ET AL., ED. *Health and health behaviour among young people: international report* (http://www.euro.who.int/document/e67880.pdf). Copenhagen: WHO Regional Office for Europe, 2000 (Health Policy for Children and Adolescents Series, No. 1) (accessed 25 September 2003).

99. *Tomorrow's young adults: 9–15-year-olds look at alcohol, drugs, exercise and smoking*. London, Health Education Authority, 1991.

100. MÜLLER, M.J. ET AL. Physical activity and diet in 5 to 7 years old children. *Public health nutrition*, 2(3A): 443–444 (1999).

101. *A Pan-EU survey on consumer attitudes to physical activity, body-weight and health*. Dublin, Institute of European Food Studies, Trinity College, 1999.

102. *Active living. Report from the meeting of "The Active Living National Policy Group". Hämeenlinna, Finland, 25–27 August 1997*. Geneva, World Health Organization, 1997 (document HPR 97/9).

103. *Iodine deficiency in Europe: a continuing public health problem*. Geneva, World Health Organization (in press).

104. DELANGE, F. ET AL., ED. *Elimination of iodine deficiency disorders (IDD) in central and eastern Europe, the Commonwealth of Independent States and the Baltic states. Proceedings of a conference held in Munich, Germany, 3–6 September 1997* (http://whqlibdoc.who.int/hq/1998/WHO_EURO_NUT_98.1.pdf). Copenhagen, WHO Regional Office for Europe, 1998 (document WHO/EURO/NUT/98.1) (accessed 25 September 2003).

105. DE BENOIST, B. & ALLEN, H. *IDD situation in Europe*. Geneva, World Health Organization, 2001 (unpublished document).

106. RAPA, A. ET AL. Puberty and urinary iodine excretion. *Journal of pediatric endocrinology and metabolism*, **12**: 583–584 (1999).

107. SUGITA, K. Pica: pathogenesis and therapeutic approach. *Japanese journal of clinical medicine*, **59**: 561–565 (2001).

108. *Kazakstan demographic and health survey (DHS), 1995*. Calverton, MD, Macro International Inc., 1996

109. *Uzbekistan demographic and health survey, 1996.* Calverton, MD, Macro International Inc., 1997.

110. ROBERTSON, A. ET AL. Nutrition and immunization survey of Bosnian women and children during 1993. *International journal of epidemiology,* 24: 1163–1170 (1993).

111. GREGORY, J.R. *National diet and nutrition survey: children aged 1 1/2 to 4 1/2 years. Vol. 1. Report of the diet and nutrition survey.* London, H.M. Stationery Office, 1995.

112. HERCBERG, S. ET AL. Iron deficiency in Europe. *Public health nutrition,* 4(2B): 537–545 (2001).

113. HALLBERG, L. ET AL. Iron balance in menstruating women. *European journal of clinical nutrition,* 49: 200–207 (1995).

114. DELISLE, H. *Nutrition in adolescence: issues and challenges for the health sector.* Geneva, World Health Organization, 1999 (document).

115. SHARMONOV, T.S. & ABUOVA, G.O. *National nutrition survey of 15–80 year olds of the Republic of Kazakhstan, 1996.* Almaty, Institute of Nutrition of the Republic of Kazakhstan, 1996.

116. BRANCA, F. ET AL. *The health and nutritional status of women and children in Armenia.* Rome, National Institute of Nutrition, 1998.

117. COLHOUN, H. & PRESCOTT-CLARKE, P. *Health survey for England 1994.* London, H.M. Stationery Office, 1996.

118. *Sharing responsibilities. Women, society & abortions worldwide.* New York, Alan Guttmacher Institute, 1999.

119. NILSSON, L. & SÖLVELL, L. Clinical studies on oral contraceptives – a randomised, double blind, crossover study of 4 different preparations. *Acta obstetrica et gynaecologica scandinavica,* 46(Suppl. 8): 1–31 (1967).

120. GUILLEBAUD, J. ET AL. Menstrual blood-loss with intrauterine device in the treatment of menorrhagia. *British journal of obstetrics and gynaecology,* 97: 690–694 (1990).

121. ABDIEV, T.A. ET AL. [An evaluation of the economic loss from intestinal helminthiases in the Uzbek SSR]. *Meditsinskaia parazitologiia i parazitarnye bolezni,* 2: 37–39 (1990) (in Russian).

122. KARIMOV, S.I. ET AL. Epidemic aspects of echinococcosis. *Khirurgiia,* 7: 37–39 (1998).

123. *Health and health care.* Yerevan, Ministry of Health of Armenia, 1997.

124. SANTISO, R. Effects of chronic parasitosis on women's health. *International journal of gynaecology and obstetrics,* 58: 129–136 (1997).

125. *Complementary feeding of young children in developing countries. A review of the current scientific knowledge.* Copenhagen, WHO Regional Office for Europe, 1998 (document WHO/NUT/98.1).

126. *Young people in changing societies. The MONEE Project CEE/CIS/Baltics.* Florence, UNICEF Innocenti Research Centre, 2000.

127. MICKLEWRIGHT, J. & STEWART, K. *The welfare of Europe's children: are EU member states converging?* Bristol, The Policy Press, 2000.

128. MOLLOY, A.M. & SCOTT, J. Folates and prevention of disease. *Public health nutrition*, 4(2B): 601–609 (2001).

129. EUROCAT WORKING GROUP. Prevalence of neural tube defects in 20 regions of Europe and the impact of prenatal diagnosis, 1980–1986. *Journal of epidemiology and community health*, 45: 52–58 (1991).

130. BARKER, D.J. *Mothers, babies and health in later life*, 2nd ed. Edinburgh, Churchill-Livingstone, 1998.

131. OSMOND, C. ET AL. Early growth and death from cardiovascular disease in women. *British medical journal*, 307: 1519–1524 (1993).

132. BARKER, D.J. ET AL. The relation of small head circumference and thinness at birth to death from cardiovascular disease in adult life. *British medical journal*, 306: 422–426 (1993).

133. FRANKEL, S. ET AL. Birthweight, body mass index in middle age, and incident coronary heart disease. *Lancet*, 348: 1478–1480 (1996).

134. RICH-EDWARDS, J.W. ET AL. Birth weight and risk of cardiovascular disease in a cohort of women followed up since 1976. *British medical journal*, 315: 396–400 (1997).

135. BAETEN, J. ET AL. Pregnancy complications and outcomes among overweight and obese nulliparous women. *American journal of public health*, 91: 436–440 (2001).

136. CRANE, S.S. ET AL. Association between pre-pregnancy obesity and the risk of Caesarean delivery. *Obstetrics and gynecology*, 89: 213–216 (1997).

137. KAISER, P. & KIRBY, R. Obesity as a risk factor for cesarean in a low-risk population. *Obstetrics and gynecology*, 97: 39–43 (2001).

138. *Nutrition today matters tomorrow. A report from The March of Dimes Task Force on Nutrition and Optimal Human Development*. White Plains, NY, March of Dimes, 2002.

139. KRAMER, M. Socioeconomic determinants of intrauterine growth retardation. *European journal of clinical nutrition*, 52(Suppl. 1): S29–S33 (1998).

140. SIEGA-RIZ, A. ET AL. Maternal underweight status and inadequate rate of weight gain during the third trimester of pregnancy increases the risk of pre-term delivery. *Journal of nutrition*, 126: 146–153 (1996).

141. HILSON, J. ET AL. Maternal obesity and breast-feeding success in rural population of white women. *American journal of clinical nutrition*, 66: 1371–1378 (1997).

142. DAVIS, M., ET AL., ED. *Integrating population outcomes, biological mechanisms and research methods in the study of human milk and lactation*. New York, Kluwer Academic, Plenum, 2001.

143. *Comparative analysis of implementation of the Innocenti Declaration in WHO European Member States. Monitoring Innocenti targets on the protection, promotion and support of breastfeeding* (http://www.euro.who.int/document/e63687.pdf). Copenhagen, WHO Regional Office for Europe, 1999 (document EUR/ICP/LVNG 01 01 02) (accessed 25 September 2003).

144. HEIBERG ENDERSEN, E. & HELSING, E. Changes in breastfeeding practices in Norwegian maternity wards: national surveys 1973, 1982 and 1991. *Acta paediatrica*, **84**: 719–724 (1995).

145. DUNN, D.T. ET AL. Risk of human immunodeficiency type 1 transmission through breastfeeding. *Lancet*, **340**: 585–588 (1992).

146. NICOLL, A. ET AL. Infant feeding and HIV-1 infection – year 2000. *AIDS*, **14**(Suppl. 3): S57–S74 (2000).

147. DE COCK, K.M. ET AL. Prevention of mother-to-child HIV transmission in resource-poor countries. Translating research into policy and practice. *Journal of the American Medical Association*, **283**: 1175–1182 (2000).

148. COUTSOUDIS, A. ET AL. Influence of infant-feeding patterns on early mother-to-child transmission of HIV-1 in Durban, South Africa: a prospective cohort study. *Lancet*, **354**: 471–476 (1999).

149. GOTO, K. ET AL. Epidemiology of altered intestinal permeability to lactulose and mannitol in Guatemalan infants. *Journal of pediatric gastroenterology and nutrition*, **28**: 282–290 (1999).

150. COUTSOUDIS, A. ET AL. Method of feeding and transmission of HIV-1 from mothers to children by 15 months of age: prospective cohort study from Durban, South Africa. *AIDS*, **15**: 379–387 (2001).

151. JOHN, G. ET AL. *Correlates of perinatal HIV-1 transmission in the Kenyan Breastfeeding Study.* Seattle, WA, Department of Biostatistics, Medicine and Epidemiology, University of Washington, p. 16.

152. SEMBA, R.D. ET AL. Human immunodeficiency virus load in breast-milk, mastitis, and mother-to-child transmission of human immunodeficiency virus type 1. *Journal of infectious diseases*, **189**: 93–98 (1999).

153. EKPINI, E.R. ET AL. Late postnatal mother-to-child transmission in Abidjan, Cote d'Ivoire. *Lancet*, **349**: 1054–1059 (1997).

154. *Nutrition survey of children under 5 of Azerbaijan.* Geneva, World Health Organization, 1997.

155. SEMENOVA, G. *Breastfeeding and weaning practices in Uzbekistan: preliminary summary report.* Almaty, Institute of Nutrition, Kazakhstan, 1998.

156. *The adaptation of infant and young child feeding recommendations for IMCI. Report on the household trials of improved feeding practices for the Almaty and Semipalatinsk oblasts, Kazakhstan.* Almaty, National Institute of Nutrition, Kazakhstan in collaboration with BASICS (Basic Support for Institutionalizing Child Survival), 1998.

157. *Protracted relief and recovery operation – Armenia 6120.01. Relief and recovery assistance for refugees and vulnerable groups in Armenia (proposal).* Rome, World Food Programme, 1999.

158. MILLS, A. & TYLER, H. *Food and nutrient intakes of British infants aged 6–12 months.* London, H.M. Stationery Office, 1992.

159. *Breastfeeding in Sweden.* Penang, World Alliance for Breastfeeding Action, 1992.

160. FERRENTE, E. ET AL. [Retrospective study on weaning practice in Rome and its province. Results and critical considerations]. *Minerva pediatrica,* **46**: 275–283 (1994) (in Italian).

161. SAVINO, F. ET AL. [Weaning practice in Torinese area: epidemiological study on practice and age of introduction of complementary food]. *Minerva pediatrica,* **46**: 285–293 (1994) (in Italian).

162. VAN DEN BOOM, S.A.M. ET AL. Weaning practices in children up to 19 months of age in Madrid. *Acta paediatrica,* **84**: 853–858 (1995).

163. MCGUIRE, J. S. *The nutrition pay-off paper.* Washington, DC, Population, Health and Nutrition Division, World Bank, 1996.

164. SAVAGE-KING, F. & BURGESS, A. *Nutrition for developing countries,* 2nd ed. Oxford, Oxford University Press, 1995.

165. JAMES, W.P.T. ET AL. *Ending malnutrition by 2020: an agenda for change in the millennium. Final report to the ACC/SCN by the Commission on the Nutrition Challenges of the 21st Century. Supplement to the Food and Nutrition Bulletin, September/October 2000.* Boston, International Nutrition Foundation, 2000.

166. ROKX, C. ET AL. *Prospects for improving nutrition in eastern Europe and central Asia.* Washington, DC, World Bank, 2001.

167. GREGORY, J.R. *National diet and nutrition survey: young people aged 4–18 years. Vol. 1. Report of the diet and nutrition survey.* London, The Stationery Office, 2000.

168. SHEIHAM, A. Dietary effects on dental diseases. *Public health nutrition,* 4(2B): 569–591 (2001).

169. MARTHALER, T.M. ET AL. The prevalence of dental caries in Europe, 1990–1995. *Caries research,* **30**: 237–255 (1996).

170. PITTS, N.B. ET AL. The total dental caries experience of 12 year old children in the United Kingdom. Surveys coordinated by the British Association for the Study of Community Dentistry in 1996/97. *Community dental health,* **15**: 49–54 (1998).

171. PAPAS, A.S. ET AL. The effects of denture status on nutrition. *Special care in dentistry,* **18**: 17–25 (1998).

172. HOLLISTER, M.C. & WEINTRAUB, J.A. The association of oral status with systemic health, quality of life, and economic productivity. *Journal of dental education,* **57**: 901–911 (1993).

173. BRODEUR, J.M. ET AL. Nutrient intake and gastrointestinal disorders related to masticatory performance in the edentulous elderly. *Journal of prosthetic dentistry,* 70: 468–473 (1993).

174. MOYNIHAN, P.J. ET AL. Intake of non-starch polysaccharide (dietary fibre) in edentulous and dentate persons: an observational study. *British dental journal,* 177: 243–247 (1994).

175. JOSHIPURA, K.J. ET AL. The impact of edentulousness on food and nutrient intake. *Journal of the American Dental Association,* 127: 459–467 (1996).

176. KRALL, E. ET AL. How dentition status and masticatory function affect nutrition intake. *Journal of the American Dental Association,* 129: 1261–1269 (1998).

177. SHEIHAM, A. ET AL. The relationship among dental status, nutrient intake, and nutritional status in older people. *Journal of dental research,* 80: 408–413 (2001).

178. KAFATOS, A.G. & CODRINGTON, C.A., ed. EURODIET reports and proceedings. *Public health nutrition,* 4(2A) (2001).

179. HORWATH, C.C. Dietary intake studies in elderly people. *World review of nutrition and dietetics,* 59: 1–70 (1989).

180. MOREIRAS, O. ET AL. Longitudinal changes in the intake of energy and macronutrients of elderly Europeans. SENECA Investigators. *European journal of clinical nutrition,* 50(Suppl 2): S67–S76 (1996).

181. MANN, J. & TRUSWELL, A.S., ED. *Essentials of human nutrition.* Oxford, Oxford Medical Publications, 1998.

182. HUIJBREGTS, P. ET AL. Dietary pattern and 20 year mortality in elderly men in Finland, Italy and the Netherlands: longitudinal cohort study. *British medical journal,* 315: 13–17 (1997).

183. SELHUB, J. ET AL. B vitamins, homocysteine, and neurocognitive function in the elderly. *American journal of clinical nutrition,* 71(2): 614S–620S (2000).

184. HALLER, J. The vitamin status and its adequacy in the elderly: an international overview. *International journal for vitamin and nutrition research,* 69: 160–168 (1999).

185. ORTEGA, R.M. ET AL. Homocysteine levels in elderly Spanish people: influence of pyridoxine, vitamin B_{12} and folic acid intakes. *Journal of nutrition, health & aging,* 6: 69–71 (2002).

186. SELHUB, J. Folate, vitamin B_{12} and vitamin B_6 and one carbon metabolism. *Journal of nutrition, health & aging,* 6: 39–42 (2002).

187. VENTURA, P. ET AL. Hyperhomocysteinemia and related factors in 600 hospitalized elderly subjects. *Metabolism: clinical & experimental,* 50: 1466–1471 (2001).

188. BATES, C.J. ET AL. Micronutrients: highlights and research challenges from the 1994–5 National Diet and Nutrition Survey of people aged 65 years and over. *British journal of nutrition*, **82**: 7–15 (1999).

189. MAIANI, G. ET AL. Vitamin A. *International journal for vitamin and nutrition research*, **63**: 252–257 (1993).

190. CHERUBINI, A. ET AL. High vitamin E plasma levels and low low-density lipoprotein oxidation are associated with the absence of atherosclerosis in octogenarians. *Journal of the American Geriatrics Society*, **49**: 651–654 (2001).

191. MARTINS, I. ET AL. Vitamin and mineral intakes in elderly. *Journal of nutrition, health & aging*, **6**: 63–5 (2002).

192. KAFATOS, A. ET AL. Nutritional status: serum lipids. Euronut SENECA investigators. *European journal of clinical nutrition*, **45**(Suppl. 3): 53–61 (1991).

193. DE GROOT, L.C. ET AL. Nutrition and health of elderly people in Europe: the EURONUT-SENECA Study. *Nutrition reviews*, **50**: 185–194 (1992).

194. BIJNEN, F.C. ET AL. Baseline and previous physical activity in relation to mortality in elderly men: the Zutphen Elderly Study. *American journal of epidemiology*, **150**: 1289–1296 (1999).

195. BLAIR, S.N. & JACKSON, A.S. Physical fitness and activity as separate heart disease risk factors: a meta-analysis. *Medicine and science in sports and exercise*, **33**: 762–764 (2001).

196. MCMURDO, M.E. & BURNETT, L. Randomised controlled trial of exercise in the elderly. *Gerontology*, **38**: 292–298 (1992).

197. HAVEMAN-NIES, A. ET AL. Evaluation of dietary quality in relationship to nutritional and lifestyle factors in elderly people of the US Framingham Heart Study and the European SENECA study. *European journal of clinical nutrition*, **55**: 870–880 (2001).

198. CAMPION, E.W. Aging better. *New England journal of medicine*, **338**: 1064–1066 (1998).

199. VAN DER WIELEN, R.P. ET AL. Serum vitamin D concentrations among elderly people in Europe. *Lancet*, **346**: 207–210 (1995).

200. *Report on osteoporosis in the European Community – action on prevention*. Luxembourg, Office of Official Publications of the European Communities, 1998.

201. BROWNER, W.S. ET AL. Mortality following fractures in older women. The Study of Oestoporotic Fractures. *Archives of internal medicine*, **156**: 1521–1525 (1996).

202. KEENE, G.S. ET AL. Mortality and morbidity after hip fractures. *British medical journal*, **307**: 1248–1250 (1993).

203. GENNARI, C. Calcium and vitamin D nutrition and bone disease of the elderly. *Public health nutrition*, **4**(2B): 547–559 (2001).

204. *Surgeon General's report on physical activity and health.* Washington, DC, US Department of Health and Human Services, 1996.
205. ROBERTSON, A. & JAMES, W.P.T. War in former Yugoslavia: coping with nutritional issues. *In*: Mann, J. et al., ed. *The essentials of human nutrition.* Oxford, Oxford University Press, 1998.
206. *Nutrition anthropometric report, Kosovo.* London, Action Against Hunger UK, 2000.
207. MCKEE, M. The health of Gypsies. *British medical journal,* 315: 1172–1173 (1997).
208. BRAZDOVA, Z. ET AL. [Dietary habits of Romany children]. *Ceskoslovenska pediatrie,* 53: 419–423 (1998) (in Czech).
209. SOOMAN, A. ET AL. Scotland's health – a more difficult challenge for some? The price and availability of healthy foods in socially contrasting localities in the west of Scotland. *Health bulletin (Edinburgh),* 51: 276–284 (1993).
210. KOUPILOVA, I. & MCKEE, M., ED. *Health needs of the Roma population in the Czech and Slovak republics.* London, European Centre on Health and Societies in Transition, 2000.
211. BRAZDOVA, Z. ET AL. [Serving equivalents of food groups as a tool for evaluation of food consumption of Romany children]. *Hygiena,* 43: 195–206 (1998) (in Czech).
212. SHARMANOV, A. Anaemia in central Asia: demographic and health service experience. *Food and nutrition bulletin,* 19: 307–317 (1998).
213. BECK, A.M. ET AL. [Nutritional status in hospitalized younger and elderly patients]. *Ugeskrift for laeger,* 162: 3193–3196 (2000) (in Danish).
214. INCALZI, R.A. ET AL. Energy intake and in-hospital starvation. *Archives of internal medicine,* 156: 425–429 (1996).
215. MOWÉ, M. ET AL. Reduced nutritional state in an elderly population (> 70 years) is probable before disease and possibly contributes to the development of disease. *American journal of clinical nutrition,* 59: 317–324 (1994).
216. SJÖBERG, M. ET AL. [Hospital meals – what do patients need and what are they given?]. *Scandinavian journal of nutrition,* 36: 138–141 (1992) (in Swedish).
217. MÜHLETHALER, R. ET AL. The prognostic significance of protein-energy malnutrition in geriatric patients. *Age and ageing,* 24: 193–197 (1995).
218. KYLE, U.G. ET AL. Contribution of body composition to nutritional assessment at hospital admission in 995 patients: a controlled population study. *British journal of nutrition,* 86: 725–731 (2001).
219. MCWHIRTER, J.P. & PENNINGTON, C.R. Incidence and recognition of malnutrition in hospital. *British medical journal,* 308: 945–948 (1994).

220. EDINGTON, J. ET AL. Prevalence of malnutrition on admission to four hospitals in England. The Malnutrition Prevalence Group. *Clinical nutrition*, **19**: 191–195 (2000).

221. COUNCIL OF EUROPE. *Food and nutritional care in hospitals: how to prevent undernutrition.* Strasbourg, Council of Europe Publishing, 2003.

222. CEDERHOLM, T. ET AL. Nutritional status and performance capacity in internal medical patients. *Clinical nutrition*, **12**: 8–14 (1993).

223. CIANCIARUSO, B. ET AL. Nutritional status in the elderly patient with uremia. *Nephrology dialysis transplantation*, **10**(Suppl. 6): 65–68 (1995).

224. TAYLOR, S.J. Audit of nasogastric feeding practice at two acute hospitals: is early enteral feeding associated with reduced mortality and hospital stay? *Journal of human nutrition and dietetics*, **6**: 477–489 (1993).

225. CONSTANS, T. ET AL. Protein-energy malnutrition in elderly medical patients. *Journal of the American Geriatric Society*, **40**: 263–268 (1992).

226. PAILLAUD, E. ET AL. Nutritional status and energy expenditure in elderly patients with recent hip fracture during a 2-month follow-up. *British journal of nutrition*, **83**: 97–103 (2000).

227. ELIA, M. & STRATTON, R.J. How much undernutrition is there in hospitals? *British journal of nutrition*, **84**: 257–259 (2000).

228. NABER, T.H. ET AL. Prevalence of malnutrition in nonsurgical hospitalized patients and its association with disease complications. *American journal of clinical nutrition*, **66**: 1232–1239 (1997).

229. BRUUN, L.I. ET AL. Prevalence of malnutrition in surgical patients: evaluation of nutritional support and documentation. *Clinical nutrition*, **18**: 141–147 (1999).

230. GARIBALLA, S.E. ET AL. Nutritional status of hospitalized acute stroke patients. *British journal of nutrition*, **79**: 481–487 (1998).

231. ULANDER, K. ET AL. Postoperative energy intake in patients after colorectal cancer surgery. *Scandinavian journal of caring sciences*, **12**: 131–138 (1998).

232. CORISH, C.A. & KENNEDY, N.P. Protein-energy undernutrition in hospital in-patients. *British journal of nutrition*, **83**: 575–591 (2000).

233. GREEN, C.J. Existence, causes and consequences of disease-related malnutrition in the hospital and the community, and clinical and financial benefits of nutritional intervention. *Clinical nutrition*, **18**(Suppl. 2): 3–28 (1999).

234. DAVIS, A.M. & BRISTOW, A. *Managing nutrition in hospital.* London, Nuffield Trust, 1999, p. 26.

235. TUCKER, H.N. & MIGUEL, S.G. Cost containment through nutrition intervention. *Nutrition reviews*, **54**(4): 111–121 (1996).

236. TRICHOPOULOU, A. & LAGIOU, P. *DAFNE II Data Food Networking Network for the pan-European food data bank based on household budget*

survey (HBS) data. Methodology for the exploitation of HBS food data and results on food availability in six European countries. Luxembourg, Office for Official Publications of the European Communities, 1998.

237. DE IRALA-ESTEVEZ, J. ET AL. A systematic review of socio-economic differences in food habits in Europe: consumption of fruit and vegetables, *European journal of clinical nutrition*, 54: 706–714 (2000).

238. ROOS, G. ET AL. Disparities in vegetable and fruit consumption: European cases from the north to the south, *Public health nutrition*, 4: 35–43 (2000).

239. AGUDO, A. & PERA, G. Vegetable and fruit consumption associated with anthropometric, dietary and lifestyle factors in Spain. EPIC Group of Spain. European Prospective Investigation into Cancer. *Public health nutrition*, 2: 263–271 (1999).

240. JOHANSSON, L. ET AL. Healthy dietary habits in relation to social determinants and lifestyle factors. *British journal of nutrition*, 81: 211–220 (1999).

241. DEPARTMENT FOR FOOD, ENVIRONMENT AND RURAL AFFAIRS. *National food survey 2000.* London, The Stationery Office, 2001.

242. MINISTRY OF AGRICULTURE, FISHERIES AND FOOD. *National food survey, 1998. Annual report on food expenditure, consumption and nutrient intakes.* London, The Stationery Office, 1999.

243. FINCH, S. *National diet and nutrition survey: people aged 65 years and over. Vol. 1. Report of the diet and nutrition survey.* London, The Stationery Office, 1998.

244. DOWLER, E. & LEATHER, S. Intake of micronutrients in Britain's poorest fifth has declined. *British medical journal*, 314: 1412 (1997).

245. NELSON, M. Nutrition and health inequalities. *In*: Gordon, D. et al., ed. *Inequalities in health: studies in poverty, inequality and social exclusion.* Bristol, The Policy Press, 1999.

246. NAESS, O. & CLAUSSEN, B. Social inequalities in mortality in Oslo: is health-related selection the main cause? *In*: *Health inequalities in Europe.* Paris, Société Française de Santé Publique, 2000, p. 188.

247. RAZUM, O. & ZEEB, H. Risk of coronary heart disease among Turkish migrants to Germany: further epidemiological evidence. *Atherosclerosis*, 150: 439–440 (2000).

248. MARMOT, M. & WILKINSON, R.G., ED. *Social determinants of health.* Oxford, Oxford University Press, 1999.

249. KUNST, A.E. ET AL. Occupational class and ischemic heart disease mortality in the United States and 11 European countries. *American journal of public health*, 89: 47–53 (1999).

250. *Allied Dunbar national fitness survey: main findings.* London, Health Education Authority and Sports Council, 1992.

251. *Health update 5: physical activity.* London, Health Education Authority, 1995.

252. MARTINEZ, J.A. ET AL. Variables independently associated with self-reported obesity in the European Union. *Public health nutrition*, 2(1A): 125–133 (1999).

253. SORBAL, J. & STUNKARD, A.J. Socio-economic status and obesity: a review of the literature. *Psychological bulletin*, 105: 260–275 (1989).

254. KAFATOS, A. ET AL. Regional, demographic and national influences on attitude and beliefs with regard to physical activity, body weight and health in a nationally representative sample in the European Union. *Public health nutrition*, 2(1A): 87–95 (1999).

255. POPKIN, B. ET AL. Diet-related conditions that increase the risk of chronic diseases. *Food and nutrition bulletin*, 22(4 Supplement): 26–30 (2001).

256. DOAK, C. ET AL. Overweight and underweight co-exist in Brazil, China and Russia. *Journal of nutrition*, 130: 2965–2980 (2000).

257. DOWLER, E. Inequalities in diet and physical activity in Europe. *Public health nutrition*, 4(2B): 701–709 (2001).

2. Food safety

Food safety and food control

Of the issues discussed in this book, food safety has commanded the most attention from the public, politicians and officials in Europe in recent years. While nutrition patterns may have greater influence on overall population health and food supply policies on rural economic activity, food safety has broad and considerable importance. Foodborne diseases impose substantial health and social burdens, and food safety issues have significant implications for global trade: half the world's food exports are produced in Europe *(1)*.

Concerns over the safety and control of food supplies have arisen from a number of factors, such as:

- rising numbers of incidents of foodborne disease;
- the emergence of new, serious hazards in the food chain;
- the globalization of the food trade;
- demographic changes and an increase in vulnerable groups;
- new opportunities for chemical contamination; and
- the need for appropriate risk assessment procedures for new technology.

These have led to increased advocacy of microbiological and chemical risk assessment techniques and the integration of food safety and food production policies to develop risk-based, farm-to-table approaches to control foodborne hazards.

Food safety is the assurance that food will not cause harm to the consumer when it is prepared and/or eaten.

Food security is sometimes confused with food safety because the words security and safety are synonymous in many languages. Food security means ensuring that all members of a population have access to a supply of food sufficient in quality and quantity, regardless of their social or economic status (see Chapter 3 for food supply concerns).

Food control is a mandatory regulatory activity through which national or local authorities protect consumers and ensure that, during production, handling, storage, processing and distribution, all foods are safe, wholesome and fit for human consumption, meet quality and safety requirements, and are honestly and accurately labelled as prescribed by law.

Causes of foodborne disease

Foodborne disease is defined as any disease of an infectious or toxic nature caused, or thought to be caused, by the consumption of food or water. It can result from contamination with an extrinsic chemical or biological hazard and sometimes from the intrinsic toxicity associated with food (Table 2.1).

Table 2.1. Causes of foodborne disease

Causes	Examples
Extrinsic hazards	
Chemical contaminants	Dioxins, polychlorinated biphenyls, heavy metals, cadmium, mercury, lead, pesticide residues, veterinary drug residues
Biological contaminants	Bacteria causing infection (such as *Salmonella*) or intoxication (such as *Clostridium botulinum*), helminths (such as roundworms), protozoa (such as *Giardia lamblia*), viruses (such as hepatitis A and Norwalk-like human caliciviruses), fungi and mycotoxins (such as aflatoxin), algae (such as dinoflagellates leading to paralytic shellfish poisoning), prions
Intrinsic hazards (natural toxins or antinutritional factors)	Oxalic acid (in rhubarb and spinach), alkaloids, solanine (in potatoes), dioscorine (in yams), cyanide (in cassava and lima beans), haemagglutinin (in red kidney beans), protease inhibitors (in legumes), phytic acid (in bran), amatoxin, psilocybin and others (in toxic mushrooms)

Adverse health effects can result from both acute and chronic exposure to foodborne chemicals and may include kidney and liver damage, fetal developmental disruption, endocrine system disruption, immunotoxicity and cancer *(2)*. Chemical hazards in foods can arise from several sources:

- environmental pollutants such as lead, mercury, polychlorinated biphenyls (PCBs), dioxins and radionuclides;
- agricultural and veterinary practices such as pesticides, fertilizers and veterinary drugs; and
- food-processing and packaging techniques (such as the use of chloropropanols and nitrosamines).

Most foodborne disease is thought to be of microbial origin. Microorganisms cause foodborne illness by one of essentially two mechanisms:

- infection: when viable organisms (bacteria, viruses or parasites) are present in food and enter the body, where their growth and metabolism produce the disease response; and

- intoxication: when the presence and (usually) growth of an organism in the food because of incorrect storage are accompanied by the accumulation of a toxin that is ingested with the food and causes illness.

For example, organisms causing intoxication include the bacteria *Bacillus cereus*, *Clostridium botulinum* and *Staphylococcus aureus*, algae and mycotoxins (mould toxins).

Prions, which are thought to be responsible for bovine spongiform encephalopathy (BSE) in cattle and new variant Creutzfeldt-Jacob disease (vCJD) in humans, are very different. They are proteins rather than complete organisms and recruit or convert proteins on the surface of neurons to an abnormal form that accumulates, which causes symptoms in the nervous system.

Effects of foodborne disease

The effects of foodborne disease on individuals depend on factors such as their age, health and nutritional status and the virulence of the pathogen involved. For otherwise healthy adults, foodborne illness is mostly an unpleasant but not life-threatening condition restricted to a self-limiting gastroenteritis. Typically it is characterized by a combination of nausea, vomiting, stomach pains and diarrhoea, although some foodborne illnesses, such as listeriosis, botulism and paralytic shellfish poisoning, are not restricted to the intestinal tract and present different symptoms or additional, more severe ones.

All types of foodborne illness, however, can be far more serious in vulnerable groups such as infants and children, and people who are elderly, sick, pregnant or immunocompromised. *Listeria monocytogenes* infection, which mainly affects vulnerable groups, has a mortality rate of 20–30%, and an estimated 10% of patients (mainly children) with haemorrhagic colitis caused by verotoxin-producing *Escherichia coli* later develop the life-threatening complication haemolytic uraemic syndrome *(3)*.

Evidence is also growing of the serious long-term health effects of foodborne hazards, including a number of chronic sequelae such as kidney failure, reactive arthritis and brain and nervous system disorders *(4)*. About 1 of 1000 people infected with *Campylobacter jejuni*, the most common cause of foodborne disease in many European countries, develop the nervous system disease Guillain-Barré syndrome *(5)*. In a 1985 outbreak of salmonellosis in Chicago caused by contaminated pasteurized milk, more than 2% of the 170 000–200 000 people infected had reactive arthritis as a result *(6)*.

The numbers of elderly, chronically ill and immunocompromised people are increasing, which means that overall susceptibility to foodborne illness in the European population is likely to increase and its consequences to become more severe.

Dietary exposure to hazardous chemicals among vulnerable populations, such as pregnant women, children and elderly people, is of particular concern. The intake of chemicals differs between groups in the population, and risk assessment is needed for the most susceptible.

For example, infants and children can be more sensitive to some chemicals (such as organophosphate pesticides) than adults. They have greater exposure to chemical residues in their diet in relation to their body weight; their diet is less diverse, and potential sources of exposure are broader. Specific data on prenatal and postnatal developmental toxicity and exposure are lacking for many of the currently used pesticides. Risk assessment to establish acceptable daily intakes and acute reference doses and to evaluate proposed maximum residue limits for pesticides in foods often does not consider these important aspects so as fully to ensure the health and safety of infants and children.

Extent of foodborne disease

European situation

Overall, the incidents of foodborne disease reported to the WHO Surveillance Programme for Control of Foodborne Infections and Intoxication in Europe have increased over the last 20 years. Illness caused by *Salmonella* and *Campylobacter* – the most common agents of foodborne infection – has increased dramatically in many European countries. An epidemic of salmonellosis started in about 1985 and peaked in the mid-1990s in most countries in the WHO European Region. Reported cases of *Campylobacter* infection have increased continually since 1985 (Fig. 2.1), so that it is now the most commonly reported cause of gastrointestinal infection in many countries, including Denmark, Finland, Iceland, the Netherlands, Norway, Sweden, Switzerland and the United Kingdom *(7)*.

The incidence of zoonotic diseases such as brucellosis, trichinosis and hydatidosis is in general rather low, but these diseases are still endemic in some areas. Brucellosis is prevalent in many countries in the Mediterranean and eastern parts of the European Region, although continuously declining in most of them. The reported incidence of hydatidosis is highest in the central Asian republics and that of trichinosis is highest among the non-Muslim populations in the Balkan countries.

Food intoxications such as botulism remain relevant in the eastern part of the Region. These are frequently related to traditional ways of food preparation at home. Most of the cases reported have been associated with the consumption of home-canned meats and vegetables and of home-smoked or -cured fish or meat.

Fig. 2.1. Reported incidence of campylobacteriosis
in selected European countries, 1985–1998

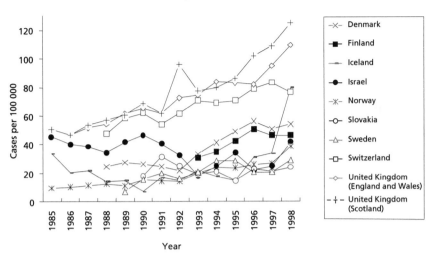

Toxic mushrooms that resemble edible ones are also important causes of ill
health in several areas of the Region. In central Europe, misidentification of
toxic mushrooms is a main cause of outbreaks of foodborne disease.

Few countries report cases of infection with *L. monocytogenes*, and countries in which notification is mandatory, such as France, report higher incidence. In addition, few countries provide information on the numbers of *E.
coli* O157 infections or cases of haemolytic uraemic syndrome. Since the
reporting systems differ greatly among countries, analysing the trends for
these conditions is difficult.

In contrast to the traditional forms of foodborne disease, vCJD has
affected younger patients, has a relatively longer duration of illness and is
strongly linked to exposure to BSE, probably through food. From October
1996 to November 2002, 128 cases of vCJD were reported in the United
Kingdom, 5 in France and 1 in Ireland. Insufficient information is available to
make any well founded prediction about the future number of cases.

Responding to a questionnaire survey in 1999, WHO European Member
States indicated that contaminated food and water was a priority environment
and health issue, especially in the CCEE and NIS. Countries expressed more
concern about microbial contaminants in foods (52% and 70% of EU countries) than about chemical contamination (48.5% and 62.5% of the NIS) *(8).*

Chemicals are a significant source of foodborne diseases although chemical
risks are often uncharacterized and usually difficult to link with a particular

food. Chemical contamination usually results from environmental contamination or agricultural practices.

Several chemical substances may be present in the food supply as a result of environmental contamination. Heavy metals – such as lead, cadmium, arsenic or mercury present in soil, coastal and continental waters – can accumulate in seafood, especially in bottom-feeder and predatory fish, shellfish or crustaceans. For example, data from the Food Contamination Monitoring and Assessment Programme of the Global Environment Monitoring System (GEMS/Food) indicate that dietary intake of lead by adults in some countries in the European Region exceeds the provisional tolerable weekly intake. Similarly, children's lead intake in some countries approaches the provisional tolerable weekly intake. Since human beings are exposed to lead through air, water, soil and food, significantly reducing such exposure requires the coordinated efforts of several government agencies and sectors. The general trend towards decreasing intake in western Europe has mostly resulted from the switch to unleaded petrol, the decreasing use of lead in water pipes and the banning of lead for canning and other contact with food.

Dioxins and PCBs (see also pp. 112–113) are mainly by-products of industrial processes and waste incineration and are among a group of toxic chemicals known as persistent organic pollutants. Their effects on health may be extremely serious and have caused great concern. Although the sources of these compounds are strictly controlled, both dioxins and PCBs are found at low concentrations in nearly all foods, but especially dairy products, meat, fish and shellfish. Data from a WHO-coordinated study of levels of dioxin and related compounds in human breast-milk suggest that dietary exposure is decreasing in most European countries and that source-directed measures have reduced environmental emissions *(9)*.

Pesticides, veterinary drugs and other agricultural chemicals can pose hazards if they are not properly regulated or appropriately used. For example, such pesticides as dichlorodiphenyltrichloroethane (DDT), aldrin, dieldrin and lindane, herbicides and defoliants have been applied heavily on cotton crops in the Aral Sea region for almost 30 years, and this has created hazards to the health of the local population.

The inadequate use of food additives and accidental or intentional adulteration of food by toxic substances have also resulted in serious public health incidents in Europe.

Mycotoxicosis has been a major but unrecognized food safety issue in Europe for several centuries. Animal studies have shown that, besides acute effects, mycotoxins can cause carcinogenic, mutagenic and teratogenic effects. In view of their presence in many foods and their stability during processing, mycotoxins are considered a major public health concern. Aflatoxin-contaminated animal feed can lead to the transfer of toxins through milk and meat to human beings. Other mycotoxins of concern include ergot alkaloids, ochratoxin A, patulin, fumonisin B and the trichothecenes. Continuous regulatory efforts are being made to lower their maximum limits to reduce risk to health.

Reporting systems and underreporting
Surveillance of foodborne diseases
Most countries in the Region periodically report incidence statistics to the WHO Surveillance Programme for Control of Foodborne Infections and Intoxication in Europe. The WHO Regional Office for Europe supervises the Programme, and the FAO/WHO Collaborating Centre for Research and Training in Food Hygiene and Zoonoses at the Federal Institute for Health Protection of Consumers and Veterinary Medicine in Berlin coordinates it.

Although these data may be useful in indicating trends, they are not strictly comparable across countries, as apparent differences in morbidity rates may simply reflect differences in national reporting systems. For example, some countries report the total number of cases, and others, only the cases in larger outbreaks. Some countries consider a disease foodborne only when the causative pathogen is isolated from both the patient and the suspected food, while others count all cases of diarrhoeal disease as foodborne.

Official statistics capture only a small proportion of actual cases. An increase in reported incidence over time may therefore simply reflect improvement in the reporting system. The degree of underreporting varies from country to country, and less severe types of illness are less likely to be reported. Official agencies discover an estimated 1–10% of cases. The infectious intestinal diseases study *(10)*, conducted in 1993–1996 in England, United Kingdom, gave results broadly similar to those from an earlier study in the Netherlands, and indicated that 20% of the population suffered from such diseases each year *(11)*. Not all of this is necessarily foodborne in origin. For every 1000 cases in the community in England, 160 resulted in a visit to a physician, 45 had a stool sample sent for microbiological examination, 10 had a positive result and 7 were reported, going on to appear in the official statistics *(10)*. The degree of underreporting varied according to the pathogen. For *Salmonella* 1 in 3.2 cases was reported, but for *Campylobacter* the ratio was 1:7.6. Underreporting was much greater for the relatively milder pathogen *Clostridium perfringens* (1 in 343) but most severe for Norwalk-like viruses (1 in 1562 cases) *(10)*.

Monitoring of chemical contamination
Information on chemical food contamination in Europe is variable and usually not recorded in monitoring programmes. In 1996, the EU and Norway initiated a monitoring programme that collects common data on pesticide residue levels in fruits, vegetables and cereals. The Scientific Co-operation

within the European Community (SCOOP) projects coordinate studies in the EU on the intake of certain contaminants such as PCBs and dioxins, mycotoxins and lead. In less affluent parts of Europe, the risks posed by chemicals in food are uncharacterized. Most of these countries have no monitoring capabilities, and little information, from total diet studies, for example, is available about the dietary exposure of their populations to chemicals in food.

GEMS/Food is an international source of health-oriented, population-based information on human exposure to potential chemical hazards in food. The WHO European Programme for Monitoring and Assessment of Dietary Exposure to Potentially Hazardous Substances (GEMS/Food Europe) was re-established to support the provision of specific data from the Region. GEMS/Food Europe updated the core, intermediate and comprehensive lists of contaminants and food commodities to be reported (Table 2.2).

Trends in foodborne disease

Over the last 50 years, food safety has presented a continually changing picture as new problems have emerged and established ones either resisted or responded to control measures. The sources of food contamination are no longer local, given increasing international travel and worldwide shipping in a global food market *(13)*:

> The emergence of new pathogens and pathogens not previously associated with food consumption is a major concern. Microorganisms have the ability to adapt and change, and changing modes of food production, preservation and packaging have therefore resulted in altered food safety hazards.
>
> Organisms such as *Listeria monocytogenes*, and to a lesser extent *Clostridium botulinum*, have re-emerged because of changes in the way high-risk foods are packaged and processed. *E. coli* O157:H7 was identified for the first time in 1979 and has subsequently caused illness and death (especially in children) following the consumption of ground beef, unpasteurized apple cider, raw milk, lettuce, alfalfa sprouts and drinking-water in several countries.
>
> *Salmonella typhimurium* DT104 has developed chromosomally encoded resistance to five commonly prescribed antibiotics and is a major concern in several countries because of its rapid national and international spread during the 1990s.

The factors that can influence the emergence of or increase in foodborne disease include *(8)*:

1. changes in the pathogenic organism, increased resistance and new virulence properties;

2. new analytical techniques to detect previously unsuspected hazards;
3. new production systems, including more mass production and longer food chains;
4. new environmental pollutants and changing ecology and climate;
5. new food products, processing techniques, ingredients, additives and packaging;
6. changing social conditions and increasing poverty or pollution;
7. changes in the health status of the population or a subpopulation;
8. changing diets and increasing demand for minimally processed foods;
9. changing food purchasing, more street consumption and eating outside the home;
10. travel and migration and the movement of pathogen hosts; and
11. increased trade in food, animal feed and livestock and exposure to contaminants.

Specific examples of these factors in practice are legion. For example, new diseases can appear following changes in food production practices, as vCJD did after recycled animal protein was used in ruminant feed. Existing diseases can extend their range to new populations or areas, as in the spread of exotic *Salmonella* serotypes through increased trade and tourism or the threat from hepatitis A in areas where it is no longer endemic. Foods previously considered unlikely carriers of illness, such as fruit juices or chocolate, can be implicated in outbreaks of foodborne illness, and previously unrecognized problems can emerge following the introduction of new analytical techniques, as occurred in the 1970s when the first successful isolation media for *Campylobacter* were developed. Changing consumer habits, such as increased consumption of poultry or ready-to-eat chilled foods, can increase concerns over pathogens associated with poultry or those capable of growth at chill temperatures such as *L. monocytogenes*. Food preservation techniques such as vacuum packaging can provide a new niche for *C. botulinum*. Economic difficulty and increasing affluence can affect social behaviour and food safety; the former has been given as a reason for the increased levels of botulism reported in many NIS.

Trends in the chemical contamination of food are difficult to identify. The health effects of foodborne chemical hazards are not easily characterized, as they may be difficult to link to a particular food and may occur long after consumption *(14)*.

New industrial processes may lead to the emission of unknown potentially harmful environmental pollutants (such as endocrine disrupters and carcinogens) that could eventually contaminate water and food. This requires continuous assessment and control. Further research is necessary to understand whether many chemicals are linked to endocrine system disruption, immunotoxicity, neurotoxicity and carcinogenesis.

Table 2.2. GEMS/Food Europe comprehensive list
of contaminants and foods

Contaminants	Foods
Aldrin, dieldrin, DDT (*p,p'*- and *o,p'*-), TDE (*p, p'*-), DDE (*p,p'*- and *p,o'*-) endosulfan hexachlorobenzene, heptachlor, heptachlor epoxide, chlordane, polychlorinated biphenyls (congeners no. 28, 52, 77, 101, 105, 114, 118, 123, 126, 138, 153, 156, 167, 169, 180 and 189), and dioxins (polychlorinated dibenzo-*p*-dioxins (PCDDs) and polychlorinated dibenzofurans (PCDFs))	Whole milk, dried milk, butter, eggs, animal fats and oils, fish, cereals,[a] vegetable fats and oils, human milk, total diet, drinking-water
Lead	Milk, canned/fresh meat, kidney, fish, mollusks, crustaceans, cereals,[a] pulses, legumes, canned/fresh fruit, fruit juice, spices, infant food, total diet, drinking-water
Cadmium	Kidney, molluscs, crustaceans, cereals,[a] flour, vegetables, total diet
Mercury	Fish, fish products, mushrooms, total diet
Aflatoxins	Milk, milk products, maize, cereals,[a] groundnuts, other nuts, spices, dried figs, total diet
Ochratoxin A	Wheat, cereals,[a] wine
Dioxynivalenol	Wheat, cereals[a]
Patulin	Apple juice
Fumonisins	Maize, wheat
Diazinon, fenitrothion, malathion, parathion, methyl parathion, methyl pirimiphos, chlorpyrifos	Cereals,[a] vegetables, fruit, total diet
Aldicarb, captan, dimethoate, folpet, phosalone	Cereals,[a] vegetables, fruit, total diet
Dithiocarbamates	Cereals,[a] vegetables, fruit, total diet, drinking-water
Radionuclides (caesium-137, strontium-90, iodine-131, plutonium-239)	Cereals,[a] vegetables, fruit, total diet, drinking-water
Nitrate/nitrite	Drinking-water
Inorganic arsenic	Drinking-water

[a] Includes other staple foods.

Source: Improved coordination and harmonization of national food safety control services: report on a joint WHO/EURO–FSAI meeting, Dublin, Ireland 19–20 June 2001 (12).

New food technologies, food-processing techniques and packaging materials may lead to the contamination of food. Their potential risks should be rigorously assessed before the food industry introduces them.

Improved risk assessment, analytical methods and developments in food tracing and post-market monitoring allow continuing improvement in the identification of hazardous chemicals in food products. Affluent countries may have well established and well resourced systems for monitoring and managing chemical hazards in food, while less affluent ones may be poorly equipped to manage even basic chemical contamination problems.

Climate change may affect the incidence of foodborne diseases. Surface air temperatures increased by about 0.8 °C in most of Europe during the 20th century. Projections of regional changes over the 21st century suggest that temperature and precipitation changes are likely to be unprecedented, leading to milder winters in much of Europe and thus greater problems with food contamination (15). The replication rates of most bacteria are positively correlated with temperature. Other possible potential effects of global climate change include the spread of contaminants across food crops by flooding and an increase in fungal growth with increased humidity, raising the risk of fungal contamination of food (such as with ochratoxin and aflatoxin).

The effects of global environmental changes on foodborne diseases have not been assessed (see Chapter 3, pp. 180–181 for effects on food security). In response to this need, the WHO European Centre for Environment and Health is coordinating a pan-European project Climate Change and Adaptation Strategies for Human Health (cCASHh). This project includes an assessment of the potential impact of weather and climate on food- and waterborne disease in Europe.

The burden of foodborne disease

The disease burden

Estimating the importance of foodborne diseases in the total disease burden of a population is difficult. The Danish Veterinary and Food Administration (16) listed common food-related problems and their incidence in the general population. Table 2.3 shows some of these and also shows the agency's hazard rating, indicating the need for action. Other factors may also be significant, such as foodborne viruses, heavy metals and possibly food additives. For example, phenylalanine, found in some artificial sweeteners, is a hazard for the estimated one in 10 000 people born with the enzyme disorder phenylketonuria.

More detailed work has been undertaken using a measure of the number of years of healthy life lost due to disease: DALYs (see Chapter 1, pp. 7–8). In the EU, diarrhoeal disease accounts for barely 0.2% of the total DALYs lost, according to estimates made by the Swedish National Institute of Public Health (17). Corresponding figures are just over 0.3% of total DALYs lost in the CCEE and the westernmost NIS but 10% for the area including the central Asian republics (18).

Table 2.3. Comparison of food safety hazards in Denmark

Foodborne hazard	Annual disease burden		Food control effort rating[a]
	Cases per million population	Cancer deaths	
Salmonella	10 000–20 000		2
Campylobacter	6 000–12 000		1
L. monocytogenes	8		2
E. coli O157:H7	2–4		1
Yersinia	1 000–2 000		3
Hepatitis A	2–40		3
Prions	0		2
Parasites	>20		3
Aflatoxins		<0.1	3
Dioxins, PCBs		Unknown	2
Polycyclic aromatic hydrocarbons		20–60	2
Nitrosamines		0.04–0.4	2

[a] 1 = increased effort required; 2 = increased effort required in the longer term; 3 = reduced effort required in the longer term.

Source: adapted from Danish Veterinary and Food Administration *(16)*.

Havelaar et al. *(19)* attempted to estimate the number of DALYs lost annually in the Netherlands as a result of *Campylobacter*-related ill health. The Netherlands had a notified incidence of 18–24 cases per 100 000 population from 1994 to 1998. Making adjustments for unreported cases and allowing that such cases would be likely to be less serious, the authors estimated that *Campylobacter* causes the loss of about 1400 DALYs annually. Although this figure is small compared with the burden of major chronic diseases in the Netherlands, such as diabetes (87 500 DALYs) or stroke (169 600 DALYs) *(20)*, it nevertheless points to a significant burden of potentially avoidable disease related to foodborne infections, with social and economic consequences for communities and their health care systems.

Economic burden

Studies have attempted to put a monetary value on the burden of foodborne disease. The numerous contributory factors – such as the severity of the illness, lost productivity, the costs of health care and any laboratory investigation – introduce considerable variability into these estimates, but all point to a substantial overall total. In the United Kingdom, a single case of laboratory-confirmed salmonellosis was estimated to cost nearly £800 in 1990, including the need to hospitalize some patients, their loss of earnings, the disruption to the victim's family and lost economic output *(21)* (Table 2.4). The costs associated with vCJD are considerably higher. In the United Kingdom, care and treatment of people with vCJD is estimated to cost the health services about £45 000 per case *(22)*, and a further £220 000 may be paid to each family as part of the Government's no-fault compensation scheme *(23)*.

Table 2.4. Estimated average cost of a laboratory-investigated case of salmonellosis, 1990

Factor	Cost per case (£)
Local authority investigations	58
Laboratory investigations	48
General practice costs	29
Hospital costs	167
Prescribed medicines	6
Loss of production	413
Other costs	67
Total	788

Source: adapted from Sockett & Roberts *(21)*.

The infectious intestinal diseases study in England estimated that there were 9.4 million cases annually with a total estimated cost of £3–4 billion per year in 1994–1995 costs *(10)*. It estimated that less than half the cases were foodborne, but the cost of each foodborne case (including those not reported) was assessed at £79.

The costs of preventing a disease from entering the human population once it has been able to contaminate the food supply may also be high. The cost of eliminating BSE in cattle in Europe is estimated to be €13 billion.

Political consequences

Notable recent food safety issues have raised widespread concern and distrust of official scientific opinion in consumers. This, in turn, has led to increased political and government involvement in food regulation activities. These episodes have also highlighted the risk that food safety can be compromised if a single government department is responsible for both regulating the food and farming industries and promoting their interests.

Dioxin-contaminated animal feed from a single source in Belgium was distributed to more than 1500 farms in Europe over 2 weeks in 1999 *(24)*. The delay in informing EU officials led to criticism from the European Commission (EC), the institution of legal proceedings against the Government of Belgium and ministers' resignations *(25,26)*.

BSE, addressed in detail below, has probably led to more political and structural change in western Europe than any other food or agricultural issue.

In Germany, the emergence of BSE in early 2001 led to the resignation of both the agriculture and health ministers and the restructuring of the agriculture ministry to become more consumer-oriented *(27)*. In the United Kingdom, responsibilities for food control were transferred from the Ministry of Agriculture, Fisheries and Food and to a new, separate food authority: the Food Standards Agency. Elsewhere in Europe, similar national agencies have been created to ensure adequate regulation of food safety and restore public confidence *(12)*, and a European Food Safety Authority has been established.

BSE, along with other food concerns, also contributed to the reform of the EC structure, with the establishment of a single directorate responsible for consumer, food safety and health issues. The Scientific Steering Committee – the EC's main scientific advisory body, set up to advise on all aspects of consumer health – published some 106 opinions and related documents from January 1998 to October 2001, 96 of which are related to BSE (http://europa.eu.int/comm/food/fs/sc/ssc/outcome_en.html, accessed 6 October 2002).

Efforts to increase public confidence in the wake of BSE included moves to increase transparency in policy-making and to improve consumer access to the scientific risk assessment process at the national, EU and Codex Alimentarius Commission levels. A more precautionary approach to food safety issues is also apparent. Response to the possible link between *Mycobacterium avium* subsp. *paratuberculosis* in milk and Crohn's disease in human beings provides an example: an EU expert committee concluded that "There are sufficient grounds for concern to warrant increased and urgent research activity to resolve the issue" *(28)*. While uncertainty remains, it has nevertheless been proposed to improve hygiene and extend pasteurization times to reduce the incidence of *M. avium* subsp. *paratuberculosis* in milk *(10)*.

Microbial hazards in food

The rising incidence of microbial foodborne disease has focused attention on the sources of contamination. From 1993 to 1998, animal products (meat, poultry, eggs and milk) were directly responsible for just over half of the 22 368 investigated outbreaks in which food was identified as a cause (Fig. 2.2) *(7)*.

Primary contamination and its causes

Many foodborne pathogens such as *Salmonella*, *Campylobacter jejuni* and *E. coli* are zoonotic (of animal origin), whereas others such as *L. monocytogenes* are widespread in the environment. Thus, the illnesses they cause usually result from contamination at the point of production, often coupled with additional failures of hygiene practices further down the food chain.

Table 2.5 shows examples of surveillance data on the prevalence of selected pathogens among farm livestock in Europe. The methods for data collection

Fig. 2.2. Food involved in foodborne disease outbreaks
in the WHO European Region, 1993–1998

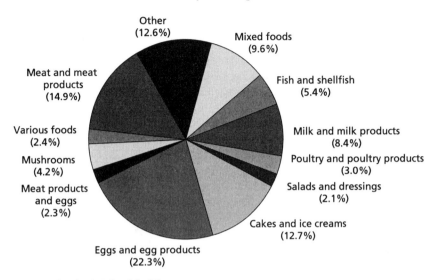

Source: Tirado & Schmidt (7).

were not consistent between samples, but the findings indicate how pools of infectivity can be found at the start of the food chain.

Farm animals commonly acquire microbial hazards as a result of horizontal transmission from their environment. The principal sources are other infected animals, feed, water and wildlife such as birds and rodents. Transfer between animals can be exacerbated by intensive husbandry, which increases contact between animals and hampers the maintenance of adequate hygiene. Studies of poultry farms in Europe and the United States show that *Campylobacter*-contaminated faeces can be spread in confined areas as dust and may be retained on walls, drinkers, feeders, water and feed *(30)*. Similarly, dust sampling can be an accurate indicator of the presence of *Salmonella* in poultry flocks and on equipment for handling and packing eggs *(31)*.

Manufactured feed has traditionally been an important source of *Salmonella*. Most feeds are now heat-treated, and contamination in products from modern, well managed feed mills is very low. Data from the United Kingdom's Veterinary Laboratory Agency in 1999 *(32)* showed that only 0.7% of extruded poultry feed samples and 1.5% of pig and poultry meal samples tested positive for *Salmonella*. Nevertheless, even low levels of contamination can be significant for newly hatched chicks, which are very susceptible to colonization.

In many European countries, poultry and egg products are the most common carriers of *Salmonella* in the food supply and have played a crucial role in the rapid increase in the incidence of *S. enteritidis* infection from the mid-

Table 2.5. Prevalence of microorganisms in livestock
in selected EU countries, 1998

Microorganism, country and livestock	Number in sample	Prevalence (%)
L. monocytogenes		
Germany, dairy cattle (herds)	1246	7
Germany, cattle (herds)	14	21
Germany, sheep and goats (herds)	648	11
Italy, sheep and goats (animals)	110	26
Portugal, sheep and goats (animals)	46	11
Finland, pigs (animals)	188	2
Campylobacter		
Denmark, poultry (flocks)	5943	47
Sweden, poultry (flocks)	3561	9
Netherlands, poultry (flocks)	189	31
Denmark, cattle (herds)	85	47
Denmark, pigs (herds)	318	69
Netherlands, cattle (herds)	192	48
Netherlands, pigs (herds)	38	97
Verocytotoxic *E. coli* or *E. coli* O157		
Italy, veal calves (herds)	282	11
Northern Ireland, cattle (animals)	166	21
Belgium, cattle (herds)	467	7
Germany, cattle (herds)	149	48
Sweden, cattle (herds)	125	6
Netherlands, cattle (herds)	419	5

Source: Federal Institute for Health Protection of Consumers and Veterinary Medicine *(29).*

1980s *(33).* In this instance, vertical transmission in the breeding flocks to their progeny has been a significant factor. The contamination in eggs was not of the same phage type as that found in feed, but it was found in the ovaries, in the faeces and in the environment where hens were kept, and could be traced back through parent and grandparent birds.

Provision of clean feed and water, along with closed poultry houses and the elimination of wild rodents and birds, has been a key part of enhanced biosecurity measures that have been shown to reduce *Salmonella* and *Campylobacter* infection in broiler chickens in Finland, Sweden and Norway.

In Sweden, egg-laying flocks, broiler flocks and breeder flocks (parent birds for broilers) have been subject to a series of voluntary and regulatory control measures for more than a decade (three decades for broilers). These include raised standards for poultry housing, staff training in hygiene measures to avoid the introduction of contamination, new controls on equipment and feed, and an extensive sampling and surveillance programme *(34).* Vaccines and antibiotics are usually not permitted, although coccidiostats are permitted for the treatment of necrotic enteritis. Any infected flocks are isolated and destroyed; the empty poultry houses are disinfected under supervision, and environmental samples must prove negative before new flocks can be introduced. Birds imported for breeding must repeatedly test negative before being released from quarantine.

As a result of the measures, notified *Salmonella* infections in broiler flocks fell from more than 30 per year in the early 1980s, when controls were first introduced, to less than 3 per year for most of the period 1995–1999 *(34)*. Similarly, infections in laying flocks dropped from over 30 flocks in 1991 to less than 6 flocks per year from 1997 to 1999 (Table 2.6).

Table 2.6. Number of farms with egg-laying poultry flocks in Sweden affected by *Salmonella* infection, 1991–1999

Year	Farms affected by:	
	S. enteritidis	*Salmonella* spp.
1991	2	34
1992	1	11
1993	0	6
1994	1	25
1995	1	11
1996	0	6
1997	0	5
1998	0	5
1999	1	5

Source: Wahlström *(34)*.

In other livestock, similar measures are also showing success. For example, *Salmonella* infection rates in cattle dropped from over 150 herds per year in the late 1970s to less than 10 in the late 1990s.

In the United Kingdom, human salmonellosis rates have fallen from a peak of nearly 33 000 reported cases in 1997 to less than 15 000 cases in 2000. A major factor has been an extensive vaccination programme for poultry breeder flocks *(35)*. Its aim is to prevent colonization of the reproductive tract by *S. enteritidis*, thus controlling vertical transmission and reducing intestinal colonization. Vaccination is part of the egg industry's voluntary Lion Code of Practice, which has received support from the major retail chains.

Crops in the field can be contaminated with pathogens carried by farm animals and human beings. The public health implications are especially serious when the products affected are those usually consumed without cooking such as salad fruits and vegetables.

Inadequately treated manure might be used as a fertilizer. It could also contaminate water used to irrigate, wash or cool a crop or adhere to poorly cleaned farm equipment used in harvesting or transport. In the Russian Federation, *Yersinia* was detected in 25.4% of water samples taken from wells situated in a zone irrigated with sewage water from a swine-breeding complex, whereas no *Yersinia* was isolated from wells remote from the zone. An epidemiological relationship was established between a case of *Yersinia* infection and the use of infected well water *(36)*. In eastern Slovakia, 8.2% of sampled rodents and 7.7% of cattle carried strains of *Leptospira* found in local reservoirs used for recreation *(36)*. When a marked peak in human cases of infection with the protozoan *Cryptosporidium* was noticed in the Sheffield area of the United Kingdom in 1986, epidemiological evidence pointed to a herd of cattle on a farm adjacent to a reservoir as the source *(36)*. Fruits, vegetables and milk that have been in contact with contaminated manure have all been identified as sources of infection by *Salmonella (36)* and *E. coli (37)*.

Similarly, human carriers who pick, sort and pack the product may contaminate crops, either directly or via sewage-contaminated water. In this way, products could become contaminated with pathogens that are specifically of human origin, such as the enteric viruses. Outbreaks of hepatitis A in Sweden and elsewhere caused by imported salad vegetables highlight the public health risks associated with importing vegetables from areas where hepatitis A is endemic to areas where it is not *(38)*.

Insects and wildlife may also transfer pathogens to crops. For example, *Campylobacter* was isolated from flies netted in the anterooms of barns containing positive broiler flocks in Sweden *(36)*.

Slaughter and primary processing

Slaughter and associated operations usually increase the levels of bacterial contamination of meat. The close proximity of animals during transport and lairage and the increased shedding of *Salmonella* induced by stress and by faecal material adhering to a bird's feathers or an animal's hide markedly increase the potential for cross-contamination.

Bacterial transfer can occur during dressing, cutting and washing of animal carcasses and scalding, plucking and evisceration of poultry. A study carried out in the Netherlands found *Salmonella* to be present in about one quarter of all broiler flocks, with 4% of the birds in these flocks actually carrying the organism – about 1% of the total. Nevertheless, tests of carcasses leaving abattoirs showed that about 50% were contaminated *(39)*. In some individual batches, contamination approached 100% of carcasses.

Antimicrobial agents and pathogens

Resistance to antibiotics currently used in the treatment of all types of bacterial infection in human beings is a major concern. Resistant strains of pathogenic bacteria emerge owing mainly to the large-scale use of human antibiotics for medical purposes but also to veterinary antibiotic usage. Intensive husbandry systems in both agriculture and aquaculture often use antimicrobial agents as veterinary medicines and, at subtherapeutic levels, as growth promoters and prophylactics. WHO has been one of several bodies that have voiced concern that this might contribute to the problem of increasing antibiotic resistance to human pathogens (40). If antibiotic-resistant bacteria are present in the intestinal tracts of a large proportion of food-producing animals, they would inevitably contaminate carcasses during slaughter, cutting and handling (41).

The EC Scientific Steering Committee has identified a number of issues resulting from the use of antimicrobial agents that may create food and environmental problems in the future (42). In reviewing recent evidence, the Committee noted the persistence in the environment of certain antimicrobial agents, the creation of environmental pools of resistance, the transfer of resistance between organisms and the increasing resistance of bacterial species that are not the primary targets of the antimicrobial agents (43,44). The Committee also noted that, for several veterinary antimicrobial agents, ending their widespread use appeared to remove the selection pressure for resistant organisms. For example, the prohibition of avoparcin, an antibiotic widely used in poultry-rearing, led to a fall in the presence of enterococci resistant to vancomycin, a related antibiotic used in human medicine (45).

Resistance to several different antibiotics is common. The frequency of reported multiresistant S. typhimurium DT104 increased during the 1990s in Europe, especially the strains resistant to ampicillin, chloramphenicol, streptomycin, sulfamethoxazol and tetracycline. For example, in the United Kingdom, S. typhimurium DT104 was the second most prevalent serotype isolated from salmonellosis cases in the late 1990s; in 1997, 58% of all isolates showed the typical pattern of resistance to these five antibiotics (46). Multiple resistance is emerging in other foodborne organisms: a sample of salami tested in Switzerland contained an isolate of Enterococcus faecalis that was resistant to at least 12 antibiotics (47). There is also evidence that resistance can be transferred between different pathogen species, such as E. coli and Salmonella (48).

WHO considers resistance to fluoroquinolones, a group of antibiotics originally developed to fill the void created by increasing resistance to other clinical antibiotics, to be of special concern (49). Since the late 1980s, the fluoroquinolone enrofloxacin has been increasingly used in Europe to treat poultry and pig infections, and fluoroquinolone-resistant Salmonella serotypes have been reported in France, Germany, Ireland, the Russian Federation, Spain and the United Kingdom (40).

Experience in Sweden has shown that Salmonella can be eliminated from poultry flocks without using antimicrobial agents, and good husbandry can enhance livestock growth rates without the need for antibiotics. The growth rate of fattening pigs achieved in Sweden on conventional farms with efficient production and without the use of antimicrobial agents was on average no less than that found in countries using antimicrobial agents *(50)*. The Scientific Steering Committee noted that farms with the poorest animal health and hygiene records were the farms where antibiotic growth promoters had their most growth-enhancing effect *(41)*. Similar observations have been made for aquaculture, where resistance problems have led to alternative solutions, including improved hygiene and the development of alternatives to antibiotics, such as vaccines *(41)*. In this context, closed, recirculating fish farm systems are a promising alternative for producing fish without using antimicrobial agents while minimizing the risk of environmental contamination.

The use of antibiotic resistance marker genes as indicators in trials of genetically modified plants has led to concern that resistance will spread through inadvertent release of the genes and their transfer to pathogenic bacteria. There is no evidence that those currently in use pose a health risk to human beings *(51)*, but the European Commission Scientific Steering Committee has proposed that, as a precautionary measure, such marker genes should be removed from plant cells before the plants are commercialized. The manufacturer should justify failure to do this *(41)*. A WHO expert report on modified microorganisms used for food production *(52)* made a similar recommendation.

Problems from harvest to consumption

Although raw materials may be contaminated with pathogens at the source, later points in the food chain are also important contributory factors in the spread of foodborne disease. The major contributing factor groups in the investigated outbreaks reported to the WHO Surveillance Programme for Control of Foodborne Infections and Intoxication in Europe are, in order of importance: inappropriate temperature, use of inadequate raw materials, environmental factors and inadequate handling.

Inappropriate temperature, such as inadequate refrigeration and inadequate cooking, reheating or hot holding, was involved in 44% of the outbreaks investigated. This distribution varies according to geographical location. For example, the main contributing factor is inadequate refrigeration in Mediterranean countries, but inadequate cooking, reheating or hot holding in northern Europe *(7)*. Use of inadequate raw materials was reported in 20% of the outbreaks. These raw materials were either chemically or microbiologically contaminated or contained contaminated ingredients (such as spices) or toxic mushrooms. Inadequate handling was reported in 14% of the investigated outbreaks, mostly cross-contamination, inadequate processing, insufficient hygiene and reusing leftovers. Environmental factors were involved in 13% of the outbreaks investigated. In this category, contamination by personnel was the most frequently reported contributing factor, followed by contaminated equipment and use of inadequate rooms *(7)*.

Contamination and cross-contamination leading to foodborne disease can occur in food-processing plants, butchers' shops and food retailers or in the kitchen immediately before consumption. Preparation of a meal using chicken in a domestic kitchen has been shown to lead to the wide dissemination of *Salmonella* and *Campylobacter* to surfaces with hand and food contact in the environment, and cleaning regimens based on detergent and water alone failed to reduce the frequency of contamination *(53)*.

Additional failures in good hygiene practice also frequently contribute to an outbreak. Common failures entail incorrect storage, allowing pathogens already present at low levels to multiply to dangerous levels, and inadequate cooking, allowing pathogens to survive. Identifying this type of contributing factor is essential in implementing adequate measures in the food industry and the catering sectors to prevent foodborne diseases (such as hazard analysis and critical control point – HACCP – plans) and to provide a basis for educating consumers.

Despite rising sales of food consumed outside the home, most food is still prepared and eaten domestically. Consequently, the private home is the location where most foodborne outbreaks occur in Europe: more than 40%. Outbreaks associated with mass catering kitchens in restaurants, cafeterias and catering services accounted for 22% of the total; schools, kindergartens and homes for children, 9%; hospitals, 3%; retail shops, 2%; institutions, 1%; homes for elderly people, 1%; and "other" or various places, the remaining 22% *(7)*.

The frequency distribution of the places where the outbreaks occurred varies throughout the European Region, depending mostly on differences in eating habits *(7)*. In Poland, for example, 57% of outbreaks occur at home, and these are frequently related to the preparation of dishes containing raw eggs contaminated with *Salmonella*. In Hungary, where up to 83.5% of outbreaks occur at home, many result from intoxication from wild mushrooms cooked in the home. In contrast, the largest percentage of outbreaks in the Netherlands is reported to occur outside the home, in restaurants, hotels or cafeterias, and many of these outbreaks result from the *Bacillus cereus* in rice dishes served in Chinese restaurants. In Switzerland, the incidence of outbreaks occurring at home is relatively low, which could be a consequence of the consumer education programmes launched in 1991 to reduce *Salmonella* infections.

Large, well run commercial food-processing operations are very conscious of the damage that any association with an outbreak of foodborne disease can do to them. As a result, they pay particular attention to establishing control systems that help ensure the production of safe food.

Chapter 4 (pp. 255–269) discusses control measures in more detail. The essence of good hygiene practices can be summarized in simple ways such as WHO's five keys to safer food – keep clean; separate raw and cooked; cook thoroughly; keep food at safe temperatures; and use safe water and raw materials *(54)* – or elaborated in detail in codes of good manufacturing or hygiene practice, produced by trade associations, regulatory bodies and international organizations such as the Codex Alimentarius Commission *(55)*. The most effective approach to ensuring food safety is based on the HACCP concept (see pp. 265–266), which systematically identifies the areas in a processing operation in which problems can arise and institutes measures to ensure that control is exercised at these points. Although applied initially in larger-scale commercial food-processing operations, HACCP principles are increasingly being applied throughout the food chain, from farm to table *(55)*.

Chemical hazards in the food chain

Chemical hazards may arise at various points during food production, harvest, storage, processing, distribution and preparation.

Primary contamination

Chemical contamination usually occurs at the very start of the food chain as a result of environmental contamination or agricultural practices. These can be controlled by enforcing environmental pollution regulation and effective codes of good agricultural practice.

Environmental contamination

Most food contamination arises from industrial contamination of air, soil and water. The chemical industry, the energy sector, the waste disposal industry and agriculture are common sources of contaminants in Europe. In addition, in some CCEE, mining and smelting are still an important source of pollution. Food and water are usually contaminated solely in polluted areas rather than throughout a country.

Heavy metals can enter the food chain through soil or water. Eating foods contaminated with toxic metals such as lead, cadmium or mercury may have serious health consequences. For example, dietary lead exposure among infants and children may adversely affect the nervous system and behaviour, and the EU and other European countries regulate the levels of lead and other heavy metals in commercial baby foods. People are mainly exposed to mercury, in the form of methylmercury, through fish; several European countries recommend that vulnerable groups, including pregnant women and nursing mothers, limit their intake of certain fish known to contain high levels of mercury.

Polyhalogenated hydrocarbons are a category of environmental contaminant that includes dioxins and PCBs. Dioxins are produced during various combustion and incineration processes or as unwanted by-products in the manufacture of certain industrial chemicals. PCBs were intentionally produced for electrical applications in many industrial countries from the 1930s until the 1970s, when production was drastically reduced. Despite the control of the sources, both dioxins and PCBs are very persistent in the environment and have made their way into the food chain. The main source of human exposure is fatty foods such as meat, milk and fish. The levels of dioxins and PCBs in foods are widely monitored and generally indicate reduced dietary exposure since the 1970s. For example, surveillance data from the United Kingdom indicated that the average dietary intake of PCBs declined from 1 µg per person per day in 1982 to 0.34 µg per person per day in 1992 *(56)*. Occasional incidents of serious contamination can occur such as the dioxin contamination of animal feed in Belgium noted previously, but overall the concentrations of both dioxins and PCBs in the diet are expected to continue to fall as further measures to reduce emissions into the environment take effect *(57)*.

Dioxins have a range of toxic effects and can be carcinogenic. Long-term exposure is linked to impairment of the immune system, the developing nervous system, the endocrine system and reproductive functioning. In June 2001, the Joint FAO/WHO Expert Committee on Food Additives *(58)* recommended a tolerable exposure to dioxins (70 pg per kg body weight) that is in the range of current exposure levels estimated in several European countries.

Agricultural applications

The use of pesticides, fertilizers and veterinary drugs is subject to strict controls aimed at protecting the consumer. For example, in the EU, Council regulation (EEC) no. 2337/90 *(59)* establishes a procedure for establishing maximum residue limits of veterinary medicinal products in foodstuffs of animal origin. A previous section discussed particular concerns about the abuse and misuse of antimicrobial agents in animal husbandry and the increase of antibiotic-resistant microorganisms. The use of hormones in meat production is strictly regulated in the EU.

Applications of organic and inorganic fertilizer may result in high concentrations of nitrates in groundwater and surface water in certain areas in Europe. Vegetables such as lettuce or spinach may have high concentrations of nitrate, especially if they are grown in greenhouses. Commission regulation (EC) no. 194/97 *(60)* sets maximum limits for nitrates in both lettuce and spinach.

Council directive 91/414/EEC *(61)* regulates the placing of plant protection products on the market. It requires pesticides to be evaluated for safety based on dossiers prepared by their manufacturers. If a pesticide is accepted, it is placed on a positive list of permitted pesticides and assigned a maximum residue limit before it is introduced in agriculture. Because of pesticides' inherent toxicity, good agricultural practices are extremely important when they are applied. In a number of situations, foods have been found to contain high levels of pesticide residues, for example, when the crops had been harvested too soon after applying pesticides or when excessive amounts are applied. A case study in this chapter focuses on residues of pesticides in food and water.

Secondary contamination – food processing and packaging

Food processing and food packaging may contribute to contamination of foods. Polycyclic aromatic hydrocarbons are genotoxic, immunotoxic and carcinogenic compounds produced during certain industrial processes. Although they are formed during the barbecuing or grilling of meats and thus can enter the food chain at a very late stage, human beings are mainly exposed through air pollution and cigarette smoke. Their presence has also been reported in some samples of olive-pomace oil (olive oil extracted using solvents). Other chemical contaminants can be introduced later in the food chain as a result of some aspect of food processing subject to regulatory limits and controls. For example, acid hydrolysis of proteins can produce carcinogenic chloropropanols. In 2000, a United Kingdom survey of imported soy sauce found levels of the chloropropanol 3-monochloropropane-1,2-diol in some samples that exceeded the EU limit value due to enter into force in April 2002. Their presence in soy sauce is avoidable and prompted a number of actions to remove the affected products, alert consumers and strengthen checks on suppliers (62).

Trans-fatty acids are described in Chapter 1 (p. 27). Some concerns have been expressed about effects on health, although the consensus of expert opinion is that the risk to health of *trans*-fatty acids intake at average consumption levels is small. Nevertheless, FAO has recommended that intake should not be increased (63), and the food industry has responded by modifying the hydrogenation process to reduce levels of *trans*-fatty acids in margarine (64). One further example is nitrosamines. These can be carcinogenic and are formed by the reaction of nitrite with secondary amines. They can be present in food or formed in the body as a result of ingestion of nitrates or nitrites in food and water. Factors affecting their production and dietary exposure have been investigated extensively.

Chemicals in food-contact materials can gain access to foods. The lead concentration in food from lead-soldered cans is about 5–10 times higher than that in food from other cans. The use of cadmium-plated and galvanized equipment in food processing, cadmium-containing enamel and pottery glazes and cadmium-based (or lead-based) pigments or stabilizers in plastics may also be significant sources of food contamination. As a result, the chemicals permitted for use in the manufacture of food-contact materials are restricted.

For example, food-contact plastics can only be manufactured using monomers and other starting substances on a list of approved chemicals. Many of the monomers and starting substances have either a prescribed specific migration limit or a prescribed limit on the residual quantity left in the material or article after manufacture. A similar list for plastic additives within the EU is being developed.

Chemicals added to food during processing are strictly regulated, although occasional problems can arise with unscrupulous or ill informed food processors.

Risk assessment

In food safety, risk assessment is a systematic, logical and transparent method of assembling information on foodborne disease to characterize the risk to human health associated with food (Fig. 2.3). It has long been used to assess

Fig. 2.3. Stages in microbiological risk assessment

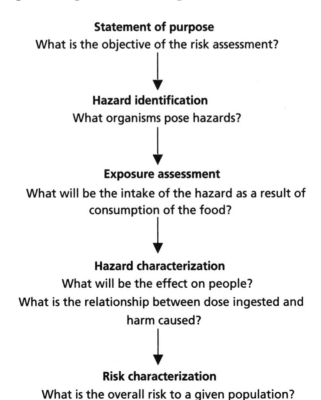

Statement of purpose
What is the objective of the risk assessment?

Hazard identification
What organisms pose hazards?

Exposure assessment
What will be the intake of the hazard as a result of consumption of the food?

Hazard characterization
What will be the effect on people?
What is the relationship between dose ingested and harm caused?

Risk characterization
What is the overall risk to a given population?

the risks associated with chemical exposure, but its formal application to food-borne pathogens is comparatively recent. Risk assessment can be qualitative – identifying, describing and ranking hazards associated with foods – but can also express risk quantitatively if sufficient data are available. Risk assessment provides the scientific basis for risk analysis; although it can be conducted independently, there is inevitable and desirable interaction with the other components of risk analysis: risk management and risk communication (see Chapter 4, pp. 258–265).

Risk assessment should be based on internationally agreed principles and consider other factors, such as health benefits, socioeconomic factors, ethical issues and environmental considerations. The basis for risk assessment should be communicated effectively, so that the public can be involved at the early stages of the process.

Food safety, diet and nutrition

Some foods and dietary patterns are associated with more specific risks than others, although common sources of microbial contamination show different distributions in different countries (Table 2.7).

Table 2.7. Sources of outbreaks of infectious intestinal diseases traceable to specific primary food types in six European countries

Food types	Percentage in:					
	Croatia	Norway	Portugal	Spain	United Kingdom	Yugo-slavia
Meat and meat products	40	20	35	6	38	13
Fish and shellfish		11	6	8	14	–
Eggs and egg products	14		6	37	10	38
Milk and dairy products	3	7	3	3	3	4
Ready meals and sauces	4	4	9	–	3	–
Rice dishes	–	–	–	–	4	–
Salads, fruits and vegetables	3	5	–	–	6	4
Cakes and pastries	–	–	26	6	–	–
Desserts and confectionery	34	–	–	–	14	29
Miscellaneous or uncertain	3	30	16	39	7	13
Water	–	23	–	–	1	–
Total	100	100	100	100	100	100

Source: Tirado & Schmidt *(7).*

In all countries shown, and most others in the WHO European Region, animal products (including dairy products) account for most infections from known food sources, with sweet foods (containing eggs) and processed foods making up most of the rest of the cases. The frequent involvement of animal products is hardly surprising, as most infectious pathogens are zoonoses, deriving from animals.

Fruits and vegetables comprise a small part of the total, although some zoonotic pathogens have been associated with plant-based foods. For example, *E. coli* O157 and *Salmonella* have been associated with products such as bean sprouts and lettuce. Fruits and vegetables can also be vehicles for environmental pathogens such as *L. monocytogenes* in coleslaw *(65)*.

Fruits and vegetables were the source of less than 5% of outbreaks of infectious intestinal disease in the United Kingdom *(66)*. The agents most often responsible were small, round, structured viruses and *S. enteritidis* (20% and 17% of outbreaks related to fruits and vegetables, respectively), and they were often present in the food because of obvious cross-contamination (34% of such outbreaks).

These figures relate to infectious foodborne disease. Data on the presence of non-infectious contaminants should also be considered. For example, a 1997 survey of pesticide residues in the EU found residues in 39.6% of more than 45 000 samples of fruits, vegetables and cereals. Most samples were below the maximum residue limit and therefore unlikely to be toxicologically significant *(67)*. Maximum residue limits were exceeded in 3.4% of the samples. Multiple residues were detected in over one third of the positive samples, and the toxicological effects of multiple residues need to be investigated further *(68)*.

Interactions between infection and nutrition

Infectious diseases – including foodborne diseases – spread most rapidly and show greater infection rates and severity of symptoms among poorly nourished populations. An infection, in turn, may worsen the nutritional status of the person infected.

Worldwide, each year infectious diseases kill more than 12 million children under 5 years old; 50% of these deaths are associated with malnutrition. Poorly nourished children have 3–4 episodes of diarrhoea and 4–5 severe respiratory infections each year *(69)*.

Not only are infection and poor nutritional status associated, but each may exacerbate the risk of the other. Infectious disease can worsen nutritional status by:

- reducing food intake, for example, through lack of appetite and painful mouth ulcers;
- reducing nutrient absorption, for example, through intestinal damage;
- changing nutrient levels and requirements, for example, as part of the effects of infection on metabolism;

- reducing the ability of the ill person to grow food or to earn an income to buy it; and
- directly removing nutrients, for example, through consumption of significant quantities of nutrients by some parasites, which makes them unavailable to the host.

Equally, a lack of adequate food can raise the risk of infection, including foodborne infection, by:

- leading to the consumption of unsafe foods; and
- reducing resistance to infection, because of a lack of the nutrients required for an optimally functioning immune system.

Further, malnourished people suffer more severe episodes of illness and more complications, and spend more time ill for each episode than well nourished people.

A cyclical model (Fig. 2.4) can help show how nutrition and infection can interact. The impact of infection on the nutritional status can vary according to the disease ecology, the age of the individual, patterns of eating and types of food consumed.

Fig. 2.4. Relationships between undernutrition and infection

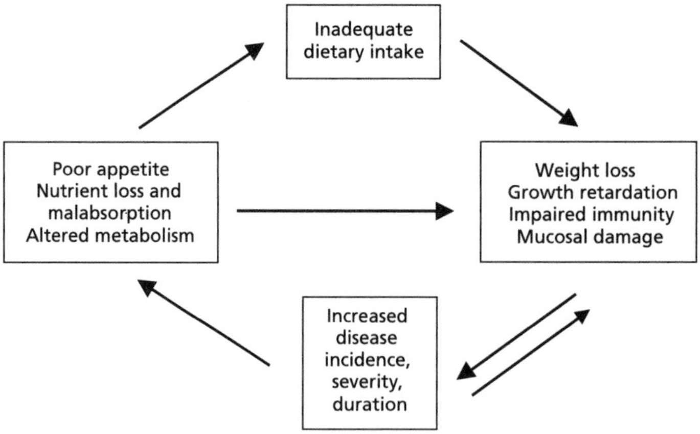

Source: adapted from Ulijaszek (70).

In practice, the infection and malnutrition complex can start in the womb, where pelvic and urinary infection and systemic illness all may contribute to low birth weight, either from prematurity or slow growth. Such infants are prone to infection, especially if they do not receive breast-milk. Underweight infants and children are especially susceptible to respiratory and intestinal infections. These infections, in turn, cause poor growth and micronutrient deficiency. Unless these problems are treated and nutritional recovery occurs, they continue into adolescence, leading to stunting, which is a risk factor for low-birth-weight babies, and the cycle may continue (see Chapter 1, pp. 48–49). Infections can be prevented through a range of public health measures, including immunization and those related to the environment. Nutritional status can be enhanced by improving diet, including increasing consumption of fortified foods or nutritional supplements. There are specific nutritional management regimens for infection. Combinations of approaches enable the infection–malnutrition cycle to be broken in individuals and communities.

Inequality in food safety

Little attention has been paid to the unequal distribution of food safety risks across socioeconomic groups. More research is needed in this area to substantiate claims, but there are several reasons to expect that different hazards may affect less affluent groups and more affluent groups.

People in low-income groups or countries are especially susceptible to the following hazards.

1. Food of poor quality or handled by untrained staff is more likely to be on sale at lower prices, attracting consumers with small budgets.
2. Food handled by untrained food vendors may more likely be of poor microbial quality (71).
3. People without easy access to transport may be unable to maintain a chilled food chain from the point of purchase to their homes.
4. Some low-income families may not be able to afford certain hygiene aids, such as refrigerators, freezers, insect- and rodent-proof storage containers, hot water or even freely available clean water. Data from Tajikistan, for example, show that 53% of all households and 78% of households in low-income areas do not have a refrigerator (72).
5. People on lower incomes may be more inclined to save leftover food for later consumption or to use food after its recommended consumption date, increasing the risk of foodborne disease.
6. Lower breastfeeding rates in low-income families (73) reduce infants' opportunities to gain immunity from breast-milk and increase the risk of infection from the use of substitute food and poorly cleaned feeding equipment.
7. The poorer nutritional status of low-income people may increase their risk of infection, including foodborne infection, as discussed above.

8. People with reduced access to general information on hygiene and food handling may inadvertently take risks, increasing their exposure to infection and increasing the opportunity for infection to spread to other members of the household or community (74).
9. People with reduced access to health facilities may not get quick and effective treatment for food poisoning, increasing the risk that the infection may spread to other members of the household or community.
10. Other factors may also play a part. Rapid urbanization, poor infrastructure, high levels of housing density and large family size may be linked to the spread of some infectious diseases, such as rotavirus (75). An inability to read and understand food label information, such as storage and cooking instructions and consume-before dates, may be linked to greater exposure to foodborne pathogens (76).

People in more affluent countries may enjoy greater public health investment, more rapid control of disease outbreaks and more funding to support laboratory and epidemiological surveillance. Nevertheless, affluence can have hazards.

1. Middle-income or higher socioeconomic groups may have increased exposure to foodborne hazards through foreign travel.
2. The prevalence of some important pathogens, such as *Salmonella* and *Campylobacter*, is likely to be higher in more affluent countries with more widespread industrialized animal production.
3. Certain agricultural practices related to the use of chemicals could be more widespread in more affluent countries, leading to a generally higher exposure to such chemicals. Here, accurate data might actually show otherwise, since the use of chemicals in poorer societies might be less effectively controlled.
4. The practice of eating food that is not fully heat-treated seems to be linked to more affluent societies and perhaps more affluent groups within a society. This has applied to certain types of meat, notably chicken and duck, and probably still applies to a number of vegetables, some of which represent important hazard exposure (such as sprouts).
5. The existence of efficient cold-chains in more affluent countries and among affluent groups could have increased the importance of certain frigophile microorganisms (such as *Listeria* and *Yersinia*).
6. The increased import of food from other regions with potentially new hazards could have influenced the disease burden in more affluent societies.

There appears to be little research into the links between food-handling practices and social class or educational level. Food handlers in Italy with higher levels of education knew substantially more about foodborne pathogens.

Although most food handlers expressed positive attitudes towards hygiene, those with better education or training in food handling more often put their knowledge into practice (77).

In the absence of detailed research into awareness of food hygiene among different social groups, evidence on general awareness of health and hygiene suggests that people in higher socioeconomic groups show more health promoting behaviour, starting in childhood. A study in Scotland found that children of higher social classes tend to undertake more personal hygiene tasks, to have healthier eating habits and to brush their teeth more frequently (78). Similarly, health-related behaviour corelated with final educational levels among young people in Finland (79). In western Norway, a study of 25-year-olds showed higher occupational status to be the strongest predictor of health-enhancing behaviour and lower occupational status to be the strongest predictor of health-damaging behaviour (80).

Case studies

This section briefly examines seven food safety topics that illustrate trends and issues and are widely discussed causes of concern: *Salmonella*, *Listeria*, BSE, enteroviruses, pesticide residues, breast-milk contaminants and food intolerance. The case studies indicate the broad range of food control issues that need to be considered in the wider context of food and nutrition policy.

These issues do not necessarily have the highest priority in any part of Europe: other concerns – including outbreaks of unusual diseases such as echinococcosis or human brucellosis or trichinosis or contamination with dioxin or radioactive substances – may be more important to some food control authorities.

Salmonella

As mentioned, *Salmonella* and *Campylobacter* are the two most common causes of food poisoning throughout most of Europe, with more than 160 000 and 120 000 reported cases, respectively, in EU countries in 1999 (81). Salmonellosis is typically acquired from foods of animal origin, although cross-contamination can lead to other foods acting as vehicles. It is characterized by an incubation period of 6–48 hours, followed by the onset of fever, headache, nausea, vomiting, abdominal pain and diarrhoea. Symptoms generally last for up to a week and occasionally give rise to sequelae such as reactive arthritis and meningitis. The incidence and control of salmonellosis are discussed above.

The numbers and trends in reported cases of *Salmonella* food poisoning show considerable disparities between countries (Table 2.8), although comparisons between countries may be unreliable owing to different recording and notification systems and different levels of access by individuals to the notification system. In addition, the proportion of cases reported varies between

Table 2.8. Reported salmonellosis cases, including imported cases,
per 100 000 population in European countries in 1988, 1993 and 1998

Country	Cases per 100 000		
	1988	1993	1998
Albania	NA[a]	25	22
Armenia	NA	24	11
Austria	30	150	89
Azerbaijan	NA	32	9
Belgium	NA	107	137
Bosnia and Herzegovina	NA	6	10
Bulgaria	NA	23	16
Croatia	87	158	95
Czech Republic	105	418	476
Denmark	62	74	73
Estonia	37	33	30
Finland	NA	50	54
France	NA	NA	30
Georgia	NA	< 1	2
Germany	80	176	139
Greece	NA	14	9
Hungary	140	163	179
Iceland	NA	32	36
Ireland	NA	8	36
Israel	NA	82	91
Italy	20	36	25
Kazakhstan	NA	41	19
Kyrgyzstan	NA	10	8
Latvia	NA	45	45
Lithuania	15	42	69
Luxembourg	NA	11	13
Malta	NA	15	24
Netherlands	NA	18	14
Norway	NA	27	35
Poland	92	50	69
Portugal	NA	6	6
Republic of Moldova	NA	44	33
Romania	NA	7	6
Russian Federation	47	68	41
Slovakia	106	221	400
Slovenia	NA	169	64
Spain	NA	NA	12
Sweden	NA	49	49
Switzerland	69	88	42
The former Yugoslav Republic of Macedonia	NA	35	18
United Kingdom	44	58	45
Yugoslavia	29	32	47

[a] NA: not available.

Sources: Tirado & Schmidt *(7)* and *Trends and sources of zoonotic agents in the EU in 1998 (29)*.

countries. The differences in figures do not necessarily reflect the level of competence of food control authorities. Indeed, some of the countries experiencing rapidly rising numbers have well developed surveillance facilities and substantial food hygiene control measures at the national and local level.

Control measures may have different effects on the pattern of food poisoning incidence, reducing one source of contamination but not others. Eggs and egg-containing foods were particularly associated with an epidemic of *S. enteritidis* infections from the mid-1980s to early 1990s in Europe *(7)*. Such measures as improved hygiene and vaccination against this particular serotype have resulted in substantially fewer cases in the United Kingdom. Figures from Denmark for 1988–1998 show changes in the importance of different sources of infection (Fig. 2.5). The overall incidence of human salmonellosis rose during this period.

Fig. 2.5. Changing sources of reported cases of salmonellosis in Denmark, 1988–1998

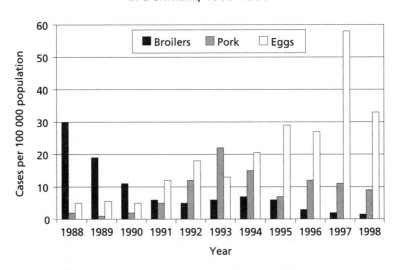

Source: Annual report on zoonoses in Denmark 1998 (82).

Food control strategies that focus on one source at a time may be responsible for the differentiation of incidence between *Salmonella* and other foodborne microorganisms such as *Campylobacter*. In some countries, such as Ireland, the incidence of both *Salmonella* and non-*Salmonella* enteritis is rising, while in others, such as Germany, the incidence of the former is falling and that of the latter is rising *(7)*.

Cases imported by visitors or residents returning to a country may undermine efforts to reduce the rates of infectious foodborne disease. In countries such as Finland and Sweden, imported cases account for the great majority of reported cases of salmonellosis *(7)*. During the 1990s, all people working in the food industry in Sweden had to be tested for *Salmonella* if they had stayed abroad for more than five days. This meant that more tests were carried out and more cases found and notified.

The EC has proposed a series of targets for reducing *Salmonella* contamination, with thresholds applied to breeding flocks of chickens from 2005, laying hens from 2006, broiler chickens from 2007 and turkeys and breeding pigs from 2008 *(81)*.

L. monocytogenes

Listeriosis is a severe disease. The main syndromes include miscarriage and stillbirth in pregnant women, infections of the central nervous system and/or bacteraemia in neonates and adults, and the case–fatality rate is high: 20–30%. Especially susceptible people include those with impaired T-cell-mediated immunity, such as neonates, elderly people, pregnant women, people treated with immunosuppressive therapy and people with AIDS.

L. monocytogenes differs from most known foodborne pathogens: it is ubiquitous and resistant to diverse environmental conditions, including low pH, high sodium chloride concentrations, low-oxygen atmospheres and cold conditions. Its various ways of entering a food-processing plant, its tenacity in the industrial environment and its ability to grow at temperatures as low as 4 °C and to survive in food for prolonged periods under adverse conditions make this bacterium a significant public health problem.

Listeriosis is reported mainly from industrialized countries, and the incidence in countries in Africa, Asia and South America is either unknown or low. Whether this reflects true differences in geographical areas, food habits and food storage, or diagnosis and/or reporting practices is not known. Since 1990, the annual incidence of listeriosis in Belgium, Denmark, Finland, France, Norway, Sweden, Switzerland and United Kingdom has ranged from 2 to 7 cases per million population, similar to the data for North America. Most recent trends indicate that the incidence of the disease has risen in 13 EU countries from 1.5 cases per million population in 1995 to 2.6 in 1998. It is not known whether this reflects a real increase or better reporting.

Although the incidence of listeriosis is much lower than that of salmonellosis, for instance, the total health care costs are comparable because listeriosis infections are relatively severe *(83)*. The indirect costs arising from unreported salmonellosis, however, probably far exceed those from listeriosis, as the severity of the disease makes underreporting of listeriosis less likely.

All European surveillance systems for listeriosis are passive, and the rate of underreporting is not known. All systems include mandatory notification, voluntary notification and laboratory analysis. Laboratory analysis is the only system that allows the precise identification of outbreaks. Because surveillance systems are diverse, data cannot be compared between countries. Little is known about the incidence of listeriosis in some countries, especially in the CCEE and NIS.

There is no vaccine against *Listeria*. The best approach for preventing listeriosis is reducing the exposure of susceptible populations to contaminated food. Thus, food contamination needs to be controlled and information provided to the people most at risk. In some countries, booklets and posters with information on foods known to be associated with listeriosis and reminders about elementary food hygiene have been distributed to populations at risk, mainly pregnant women and immunocompromised people.

BSE

BSE was first recognized as a transmissible spongiform encephalopathy of cattle in the United Kingdom in November 1986. The number of cases increased rapidly, but it was initially thought that BSE was unlikely to harm human beings, similar to scrapie, a well characterized transmissible spongiform encephalopathy of sheep. With the report of the first ten cases of vCJD in March 1996, however, BSE became the first known zoonotic transmissible spongiform encephalopathy.

The United Kingdom had a dramatic epidemic of BSE, totalling over 180 000 reported cases. Further, an estimated 800 000 infected cattle were slaughtered before showing overt clinical symptoms *(84)*. After peaking in 1992–1993, incidence has declined considerably, but more cases have been reported outside the United Kingdom, especially since the EU testing programme started in January 2001 (Table 2.9).

By December 1987, epidemiological studies concluded that animal feed made from ruminant-derived meat and bone meal was the most likely cause of BSE. Early control tactics in the United Kingdom included banning the use of ruminant-derived feed (which started by July 1988) and policies on partial herd slaughter. These measures reflected the initial assessment that BSE posed no hazard to human beings. Nevertheless, specified tissues with potentially high levels of BSE infectivity were prohibited from entering the food chain following measures announced during 1989. By then, more than 20 000 cases of BSE had occurred in the United Kingdom, which continued to export animal feed containing ruminant meat and bone meal.

In 1989, the EU initiated a partial ban on the export of cattle from the United Kingdom, expanding the ban during the next few years. In June 1994, the EC prohibited the feeding of mammalian protein to ruminants throughout the EU. By this date over 100 cases had been identified in other countries, including France, Ireland, Portugal and Switzerland.

Control measures introduced across the EU in 2001 include removing cattle older than 30 months from the food chain, unless the animals are negative

Table 2.9. BSE in selected European countries: total cases,
incidence in national herds and positive test results
in healthy adult cattle entering the food chain

Country	Cases, 1986 to 5 November 2002[a]	Incidence per million adult cattle, 2001[a,b]	Positive cases per 100 000 tests on healthy cattle, January–August 2002[c]
Austria	1	1.0	0
Belgium	90	28.2	3.4
Czech Republic	4	2.9	_[d]
Denmark	9	6.8	0.7
Finland	1	2.4	0
France	692	19.7	2.6
Germany	221	20.0	1.6
Greece	1	3.3	0
Ireland	1 091	61.8	7.3
Italy	54	14.1	3.0
Liechtenstein	2	–	–
Luxembourg	2	0	0
Netherlands	43	10.3	1.6
Poland	4	–	–
Portugal	688	137.9	66.8
Slovakia	10	18.3	–
Slovenia	3	4.3	–
Spain	190	24.2	8.0
Switzerland	420	49.1	–
United Kingdom	182 581	102.4	1.2

[a] Data from the International Office of Epizootics (http://www.oie.int/eng/info/en_esb-monde.htm and http://www.oie.int/eng/info/en_esbru.htm, accessed 5 November 2002).

[b] Data from the International Office of Epizootics (http://www.oie.int/eng/info/en_esbincidence.htm and http://www.oie.int/eng/info/en_esbruincidence.htm (United Kingdom as calculated), accessed 5 November 2002).

[c] Data from the EC (http://europa.eu.int/comm/food/fs/bse/testing/bse_test30_en.pdf (as calculated), accessed 5 November 2002).

[d] –: data not available

on a rapid test assessment. High-risk bovine material must be removed from the food chain and from cosmetic and pharmaceutical production. Measures to reduce the potential infectivity of human blood supplies have been introduced in some countries, and procedures for cleaning surgical instruments or for using disposable instruments are being introduced. WHO has issued guidance on the safe handling of potentially infected materials (85).

The inquiry into the handling of the BSE crisis in the United Kingdom *(86)* identified a number of concerns, including:

- the initial assumption that the disease would not transmit to human beings;
- the lack of information about the small doses required to transmit the disease orally to cattle;
- the lack of information about the use of bovine material in food, cosmetics and pharmaceuticals;
- poor review procedures to ensure that priority research was undertaken;
- poor monitoring and enforcement procedures to ensure that legislation was fully implemented;
- unacceptable bureaucratic delays in turning policy into practice; and
- poor risk communication to the public.

The CJD Surveillance Centre (http://www.cjd.ed.ac.uk/figures.htm, accessed 5 November 2002) gives the numbers of vCJD cases in the United Kingdom through October 2002:

1994	0
1995	3
1996	10
1997	10
1998	18
1999	15
2000	28
2001	20
2002	24

Five cases have been reported in France and one in Ireland.

The eventual toll in human lives from vCJD remains uncertain. Problems in estimation include the unknown incubation period, the absence of a laboratory marker of exposure and lack of information about the actual exposure among the populations affected and the dose of agent required for infection. Uncertainty remains about how human beings are exposed, although consumption of food contaminated by BSE is the most likely hypothesis.

Foodborne viruses

Many viruses can replicate in the human gut, and new viruses continue to be discovered. After successful replication in the cells lining the gut, viruses are shed via the stools and can then be transmitted by poor hygiene or the consumption of contaminated food or water. Enteric viruses differ in viral epidemiology, immune response, stability, infectivity and levels of shedding, however, and not all such viruses are commonly associated with foodborne transmission.

Illness caused by foodborne contamination is frequent for the Norwalk-like human caliciviruses, occasional for hepatitis A virus and rotaviruses and rare for astroviruses, adenoviruses and picornaviruses. Although the Norwalk-like human caliciviruses are a more common cause of foodborne illness, hepatitis A and E viruses give rise to more serious illness.

The Norwalk-like human caliciviruses are among the most common causes of sporadic cases and outbreaks of gastroenteritis, accounting for 11% of cases in all age groups, up to 80% of reported outbreaks in the Netherlands and 6% of sporadic cases in the United Kingdom (87,88). Foodborne transmission is common. Few data are available from most European countries, but Norwalk-like human caliciviruses are probably endemic all over the world. Unlike the other endemic enteric viruses, they are a common cause of illness in adults and children and commonly cause large outbreaks, with attack rates of 40–50% among people consuming contaminated food (87). Oysters are a common vehicle for foodborne transmission, as they are filter-feeding molluscs that concentrate viruses from polluted waters and are often eaten raw. A large international outbreak from contaminated oysters was detected in 1999 in eight European countries and has spread to Asia. Immunity to Norwalk-like human caliciviruses is poorly understood but appears to be short-lived at best.

The prevalence of hepatitis A infections differs by region, with low levels in northern Europe, intermediate levels in southern Europe and possibly high infection levels in the CCEE and NIS. In the United Kingdom, the number of notifications declined in the early 1960s, stabilized in the 1970s at 5–7 per 100 000 population but rose in the early 1990s to 14.6 per 100 000 population (89). In Italy, the incidence of hepatitis A virus declined from 10 per 100 000 in 1985 to 2 per 100 000 from 1987 to 1990 but increased after 1991. People aged 15–24 years had the highest attack rate. Large outbreaks of hepatitis A have been reported recently in Europe. Shellfish consumption is a reported risk for infection and was the most frequently reported source of infection in Italy from 1985 to 1994 (90).

In highly endemic regions, hepatitis A infections typically occur during childhood and 95% are asymptomatic. Following infection, immunity develops and outbreaks are uncommon. In other areas, most infections with hepatitis A virus are associated with travel among older people. An increasingly high proportion of the population is not immune and therefore at risk of infection, favouring the spread of hepatitis A virus once it is introduced.

There is no Europe-wide standardized surveillance for foodborne viruses. As a result, most information on their incidence and trends is extrapolated from a few detailed epidemiological studies and several anecdotal reports. Reliable methods with demonstrated efficacy for detecting viruses in food are not available. The viruses cannot be grown in cell culture, and there is no workable animal model. As a result, the effect of commonly used prevention measures and food-processing methods on viral infectivity is not known other than by extrapolation from data obtained for structurally similar viruses, such as poliovirus.

In the EU, directive 91/492/EEC *(91)* requires that shellfish for the market contain no more than 230 *E. coli* in 100 g of shellfish flesh. This is inadequate for the control of viral contamination, however, since the presence of viruses and the presence of coliform bacteria are not correlated. Hepatitis A virus has been detected in mussels that otherwise meet bacteriological standards.

An EU directive *(92)* requires the investigation and surveillance of zoonoses. In addition, a more recent EU decision *(93)* was issued to establish reference laboratories to monitor shellfish for viral contaminants.

Pesticide residues in foods

The use of pesticides to control pests for agricultural and other purposes frequently leads to the contamination of soil, surface water, groundwater and air. As a result, pesticide residues and/or their metabolites are found in food and drinking-water. Exposure to harmful levels of pesticides can cause cancer or damage the respiratory, nervous, reproductive, immune and endocrine systems *(33,94)*.

Pesticide use

Despite international efforts to promote the sustainable use of pesticides in agriculture and an actual reduction in use in several countries, overall pesticide use did not decline substantially in the WHO European Region during the 1990s. The pesticide groups most commonly used in the Region from 1992 to 1996 were fungicides, herbicides, insecticides and plant growth regulators. The main compound categories included dithiocarbamates, inorganics, phenoxy hormone products, urea derivates, triazine, organophosphates and carbamates (http://apps.fao.org/page/collections?subset=agriculture, accessed 5 November 2002).

Europe accounts for about two thirds of world pesticide application *(95)*. The use of pesticides varies widely, however, because different crops are grown in each country and different measurement methods are used. Fig. 2.6 shows pesticide use declining in some countries and increasing in others in the 1990s.

More marked has been the decline in use that accompanied the dissolution of the USSR, where pesticide use was once more intensive than in western

Fig. 2.6. Use of pesticides (kg active ingredient per hectare of agricultural land) in selected European countries, 1992–1994 and 1996–1998

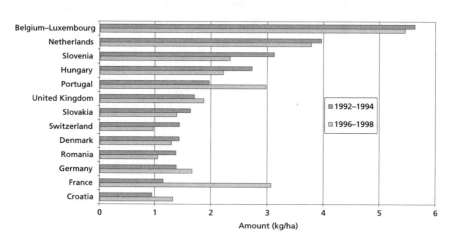

Source: FAO statistical database (http://apps.fao.org/page/collections?subset= agriculture, accessed 5 November 2002).

Europe *(96)*. Pesticide use was especially heavy on cotton crops grown with Aral Sea irrigation water, and in Kazakhstan and the Republic of Moldova *(97)*.

The intensive application of pesticides for cotton monoculture for nearly three decades has polluted the Aral Sea region, which includes the Autonomous Republic of Karakalpakstan in Uzbekistan and the provinces of Qyzylorda in Kazakhstan and Dashoguz in Turkmenistan. High levels of DDT and other organochlorine compounds (such as alpha- and beta-hexachlorocyclohexanes) and tetrachlorodibenzo-*p*-dioxins appeared in soil, water, air and every biological level of the food chain, notably in human beings. A broad panel of analytes (more than 60 organochlorine and congener-specific dioxins, furans and PCBs) was measured in breast-milk samples and in a variety of adult and infant foods collected in southern Kazakhstan. A recent pilot study in the Autonomous Republic of Karakalpakstan *(98)* has confirmed these findings, showing that perinatal exposure to such environmental pollutants in the Aral Sea region might be the principal reason that rates of anaemia, kidney and liver diseases, respiratory infections, allergies, cancer and tuberculosis are higher than in other NIS. Food produced in the Aral Sea region may be contaminated with environmental contaminants such as dioxins, furans and PCBs as well as organochlorine pesticides *(98)*.

Organochlorine pesticides, such as aldrin and DDT, do not readily decompose but persist and accumulate in the environment and in the food chain.

Their use is now largely prohibited in Europe. They were banned in the USSR in 1988 and in several other parts of Europe in the mid-1980s. A wide range of less persistent pesticides has been developed, including organophosphates (such as malathion, diazinon and dichlorvos), carbamates (such as aldicarb and carbaryl) and synthetic pyrethroids.

Residues in food and drinking-water

Qualitative and quantitative information about the presence of pesticide residues in foods in the WHO European Region is very limited. Monitoring programmes started only recently in some countries. The EU and Norway first collected common data on pesticide residue levels in fruits and vegetables in 1996 and in fruits, vegetables and cereals in 1997. In the 1997 monitoring programme, pesticide residues were present in 36% of the samples. Maximum residue limits were exceeded in 3.4% of cases, mainly in fruits and vegetables, and multiple residues were detected in about 16% of the positive samples. The residues found most often in the 1996–1997 programme were of fungicides followed by insecticides, including vinclozolin, iprodione, procymidone, dithiocarbamates, endosulfan, thiabendazole, chlorpyriphos, carbendazim, imazalil, captan, chlorothalonil and methamidophos, folpet and methidathion. Among these, some fungicides and organophosphate insecticides have acute toxicity and may cause irreversible health effects.

The extent of drinking-water contamination in the Region is largely unknown. In the EU, the established drinking-water standard of 0.5 µg/l total pesticides is exceeded in an estimated 65% of groundwater in all agricultural land (99).

Policies and prevention strategies

Current policies in the European Region for preventing health risks caused by exposure to pesticides vary considerably, for example, between EU countries and others. Many accession countries, however, are harmonizing their regulations with EU legislation. At the international level, countries that are members of the World Trade Organization (WTO) should comply with the Sanitary and Phytosanitary Measures Agreement, which recognizes the standards, guidelines and recommendations established by the Codex Alimentarius Commission as a basis for protecting human health and for international trade. The EU has established specific regulations on pesticide use and residues in food and water.

Policies may differ between countries in the Region, but national authorities use two general strategies to prevent or reduce exposure to harmful pesticides: regulation of the use of pesticides according to good agricultural practices and compliance with established maximum residue limits for foods and water. In this context, adequate methods for assessing the chronic and

acute hazards posed by pesticide residues need to be developed and harmo-
nized.

Regulation for proper pesticide use

Application in a way that prevents environmental pollution and residues in
food and drinking-water is the first step to protect human health from exposure to harmful pesticides. Initiatives to reduce the risks of pesticide use at the
international level include the development of the FAO International Code of
Conduct on the Distribution and Use of Pesticides, the Organisation for
Economic Co-operation and Development Pesticide Programme, the FAO
Inter-Country Programme on Integrated Pest Management and the WHO
Pesticide Evaluation Scheme. Although integrated pest management has been
recognized to be effective in controlling pests and reducing pesticide use, it is
not considered in the actual concept of good agriculture practices used to
establish current maximum residue limits.

In the EU, the Sixth Environmental Action Programme *(100)* aims to reduce the use of pesticides and promote a conversion to methods of integrated
pest management. Directive 91/414/EEC on the placing of plant protection
products on the market *(61)* refers to the application of good plant protection practices and integrated pest management methods in agriculture.
Although implementing the directive will eventually reduce the use of pesticides, there is concern about the time needed for its full implementation, and
new strategies for a future EU policy on plant protection have been considered, including promoting organic farming to reduce pesticide use. An EC
workshop *(99)* recommended additional policy instruments to reduce risk,
promote sustainable agriculture, protect human health and the environment
and promote the free circulation of goods, and that the reform of the Common Agricultural Policy (Agenda 2000) should contribute to meeting these
objectives.

Establishment of maximum residue limits

The Codex Committee on Pesticide Residues is responsible for developing
international standards (maximum residue limits), guidelines and other
recommendations on pesticide residues in and on foods. These become part
of Codex Alimentarius, once adopted by the Codex Alimentarius Commission. In developing maximum residue limits, the Codex Committee on Pesticide Residues relies on the FAO/WHO Joint Meeting on Pesticide Residues,
which evaluates residues and toxicological data and recommends proposed
maximum limits and acceptable daily intakes and, more recently, acute reference doses. National authorities are responsible for adopting and implementing these standards and guidelines, which are designed to protect consumers'
health and to facilitate trade.

In the EU, directives establish maximum residue limits in vegetables, fruits, cereals and animal products *(101–103)*. Inspections and monitoring are carried out in accordance with the provisions of two directives *(104,105)*. Another directive covers sampling *(106)*, and two *(107,108)* regulate the levels of pesticides in food products for infants and young children.

Risk assessment methods

The provisions of the Sanitary and Phytosanitary Measures Agreement on risk assessment requires governments to take account of the risk assessment methods developed by the relevant international organizations, such as FAO and WHO. In the EU, a directive *(61)* covers important provisions for assessing hazards posed by use of pesticide residues.

Dietary exposure assessment is an integral part of risk assessment to determine the adequacy of proposed maximum residue limits and the underlying good agriculture practices from a public health viewpoint. This includes ensuring that the estimated acceptable daily intake or acute reference dose of a pesticide is not exceeded. Exceeded maximum residue limits are strong indicators of violations of good agricultural practices; comparison of the exposure with acceptable daily intakes or acute reference doses will then indicate whether chronic or acute health risks, respectively, are possible.

GEMS/Food has provided international dietary exposure assessment calculations for pesticides considered by the FAO/WHO Joint Meeting on Pesticide Residues and the Codex Committee on Pesticide Residues. The revised guidelines for predicting dietary intake of pesticide residues, prepared by GEMS/Food and the Codex Committee, address methods for assessing the potential chronic hazards posed by pesticide residues to be implemented at the national and international levels *(109)*. Five GEMS/Food regional diets based on FAO food balance sheets are used internationally to predict the long-term daily dietary intake of residues. The GEMS/Food European diet is currently used in the risk assessment procedure in the WHO European Region. The revision and expansion of the 5 GEMS/Food diets to 13 cluster diets are being discussed. The last meeting of the Codex Committee on Pesticide Residues requested GEMS/Food to develop some examples of the effects on exposure assessment if the proposed cluster diets replaced the current European diet.

For pesticides that have acute toxic effects or may be able to induce long-term effects after a single dose, short-term dietary intake should be considered and compared with the toxic effects from short-term exposures that cause concern. This means using an acute reference dose instead of an acceptable daily intake. A 1997 FAO/WHO consultation developed a method for assessing acute dietary exposure *(110)*. This method is still being refined. Additional data on consumption have been requested and new procedures for acute risk assessment and management are being discussed by the FAO/WHO

Joint Meeting on Pesticide Residues, by the Codex Committee on Pesticide Residues and at the EU level. The EU Scientific Committee on Plants is considering the United Kingdom's policy on estimating the acute dietary intake of pesticide residues, which also takes account of the variability of residues between individual commodities *(111)*.

Special considerations in risk assessment and risk management

Risk managers should take account of aspects of assessing pesticide exposure that are especially relevant in protecting human health. For example, during the last meeting of the Codex Committee on Pesticide Residues, the EU and consumer representatives opposed increasing any maximum residue limits for pesticides for which there were concerns about acute and chronic exposure. The 1997 FAO/WHO consultation on Food Consumption and Exposure Assessment of Chemicals *(110)* recommended that dietary exposure assessment be based on the best use of available data and that risk assessors and risk managers consider:

- the importance of issues such as aggregated exposure (multiple routes of exposure) and cumulative effects of pesticides that are commonly toxic (such as cholinesterase inhibitors, including carbamates and organophosphates);
- in addition to estimating dietary intake, other possible sources of exposure such as drinking-water and occupational and environmental exposure; and
- differences in food consumption patterns and vulnerability to toxicity between and within populations, and the potential human health effects resulting from exposure to chemicals in food.

Methods to address these issues at the international level have not been resolved. For example, pending assessments of acute toxicity, there is no international consensus on how to address the risks of pesticide residues in food for infants and children. Compared with adults, infants and children can be more susceptible to some pesticides (such as organophosphates), have greater exposure to pesticides in their diet in relation to their body weight, have less diverse diets and have broader potential sources of exposure. Precautionary measures should be considered in developing future risk management policies to protect the health of the whole population in the European Region. One such approach is the EU limit value of 0.01 mg/kg for each individual pesticide in processed cereal-based foods and infant formula, pending toxicological evaluation of the substances to settle the doubts about the adequacy of the existing acceptable daily intake for infants and children *(112,113)*. Another example is the United Kingdom's approach to estimating dietary intake of pesticide residues *(111)*.

Data gaps and research needs

Major changes in the European Region since 1990 have influenced diets in the eastern part of the European Region. To allow all countries to participate fully in further developing the concept of a regional diet, newly established countries should be included in the regional diets as soon as data from food balance sheets are available. Data from countries experiencing dramatic economic changes should be updated as soon as possible. In addition, data on the actual levels of pesticide residues in foods and water are needed from many countries in the European Region to provide a sound basis for risk analysis.

Acute reference doses should be derived for all active substances where relevant, as soon as possible. To develop the GEMS/Food databases for the assessment of acute dietary exposure, the Codex Committee on Pesticide Residues has asked countries to provide data on large-portion consumption, the median weight of individual commodity units, the body weights and ages of the populations relevant to the data and the percentages of the commodities that are edible. New data on the unit-to-unit variability of residue levels for relevant combinations of commodities and pesticides are necessary to find more realistic default factors in variability.

Further research is required in new fields of pesticide toxicity, such as developmental neurotoxicity, immunotoxicity and endocrine and reproductive toxicity, to improve the criteria for the standard toxicological tests in use and the current toxicological databases and, ultimately, to protect human health.

Countries in the eastern part of the Region still have very limited capacity to assess dietary exposure. The 1997 FAO/WHO consultation *(110)* addressed these problems and made recommendations on the need for financial and technical assistance for training, for improving the integration of Codex Alimentarius work and for support from FAO and WHO and other organizations in improving data on food consumption.

Contaminants in breast-milk

The contamination of breast-milk merits particular attention. Universally acknowledged as the best food for infants and young children, breast-milk is recommended as the sole food for the first 6 months of life and is strongly encouraged for infant health during the first year or more of life. Further information is available in chapters 1 and 4 of this book and a WHO publication *(114)*.

Some of the most common contaminants found in breast-milk are chemicals used to promote food production: organochlorine pesticides. Although most are no longer used, these pesticides remain in the environment for many years owing to their great stability. Breast-milk may also contain persistent organic pollutants resulting from industrial processes. International efforts to reduce or eliminate the use and emission of such chemicals are being undertaken through the Stockholm Convention on Persistent Organic Pollutants signed in May 2001. Persistent organochlorines accumulate in fatty tissues, and because of its high fat content, breast-milk is a potential source of excessive organochlorine ingestion for infants. Recent studies of mother's milk have found high levels of organochlorines in Belarus *(115)*, the Czech Republic *(116)*, France *(117)*, Israel *(118)*, Kazakhstan *(119)*, Romania *(120)*, Spain *(121)*, Sweden *(122,123)* and Turkey *(124)*. The average levels of the insecticide malathion were also very high in Kazakhstan *(125)*. High levels of dioxins, lindane and metabolites of DDT have been reported in breast-milk from mothers around the Aral Sea region of Uzbekistan *(98)*.

A WHO survey *(126)* found that breast-milk is contaminated with a number of compounds, many at levels that approach or exceed the tolerable daily intake levels for adults. Because infants depend on breast-milk as the sole source of food, the level of contamination has more importance than if they consumed a variety of foods. Further, toxic effects in infants may be more serious than in similarly exposed adults. Physiological differences may lead infants to absorb a greater proportion of an ingested amount of a chemical contaminant, and they may have a less effective blood–brain barrier *(110)*.

The WHO survey *(126)* drew the following conclusions.

- Several contaminants were found at levels that caused concern, and countries should undertake basic monitoring of breast-milk for persistent organic pollutants.
- Primary prevention measures to control and reduce the introduction of organochlorines in the environment are the most effective way to eliminate and minimize exposure.
- Risk management should consider measures for limiting the intake of contaminated foods by girls and women of childbearing age (to lower the mothers' accumulated stores of such chemicals) rather than restricting breastfeeding.
- Risk assessment of contaminants in breast-milk should be considered for both routine and emergency assessment of food safety.
- Overall, breast-milk contains low levels of chemical contaminants that, under most circumstances, do not pose an appreciable risk to health, especially given the well established benefits of breastfeeding. Health authorities therefore can and should reassure mothers that breast-milk is by far the best food to give their babies.

Food intolerance and food allergy

Food has ingredients that trigger intolerance or allergic reactions in some people. The outcome of inadvertent exposure to an offending food ingredient can be extremely serious or even fatal, and regulatory authorities may need to give higher priority to the effects on public health of adverse reactions to food ingredients.

Although sometimes confused with food allergy, food intolerance refers to an abnormal physical response to a food or food additive that is not an allergic reaction. It differs from an allergy in that it does not involve the immune system. Food allergens are the part or parts of foods that cause allergic reactions, and are usually proteins. Most allergens can cause reactions even after cooking or digestion.

Food sensitivity reactions may be delayed or immediate. Over 170 foods have been identified as leading to immediate reactions, which may range from mild (such as stomach upset) to life threatening (such as asthma and anaphylactic shock) *(127)*. In delayed reactions, symptoms do not appear for at least 24 hours after ingestion. These include disorders such as coeliac disease, an inflammatory reaction to specific proteins found in certain cereal plants, especially gluten in wheat. Although it is not considered fatal, patients with coeliac disease are 50–100 times more likely to develop malignant lymphomas *(127)*.

Studies in the United Kingdom suggest that, although up to 20% of people believe they may have adverse reactions to some foods, objective tests have shown the prevalence to be less than 2%, rising to 8% among infants and young children. Adverse reactions are usually a response to natural ingredients in food, but reactions to synthetic additives may affect more than 0.3% of the population *(128)*.

Common allergens are cow's milk, eggs, fish, shellfish, peanuts, soya, tree nuts and wheat, and derivatives of these. Cow's-milk allergy is most common in infancy, with a prevalence of about 2% of infants *(127)*, and is usually outgrown. Intolerance to milk sugar (lactose) can develop after infancy, however, and is believed to affect about 70% of people worldwide, including an estimated 90% of the population of the central Asian republics, but little more than 10% of ethnically white groups in northwestern Europe. In Belgium, Ireland, the Netherlands, Sweden and the United Kingdom, only 5% of the population is thought to suffer any degree of lactose maldigestion from deficiency of lactase, a digestive enzyme. In other European countries, the prevalence of lactase deficiency ranges from 15% to 75%, although the exact figures are difficult to determine. Among black and Asiatic communities where milk is not traditionally consumed as part of the typical adult diet, lactase deficiency can develop in almost 100% of the population. Several researchers have suggested close clinical similarities between lactose intolerance and irritable bowel syndrome *(129)*.

Peanut allergy affects about 0.5% of the population in the United Kingdom and 1% in the United States, where peanut consumption is greater

(127). Rice allergy is relatively frequent in Japan and cod allergy in Sweden, leading to the conclusion that variation in early feeding practices and the age at which specific items are introduced into the diet may account for some of the observed geographical variation in patterns of allergy.

Fig. 2.7 shows the prevalence of self-reported adverse reactions to foods in several European countries. The data come from the European Community Respiratory Health Survey (ECRHS), a multicentre study comparing the prevalence of adult asthma between countries to identify risk factors associated with the international variation in Europe *(130)*.

Fig. 2.7. Prevalence of self-reported food allergy or intolerance in selected European countries

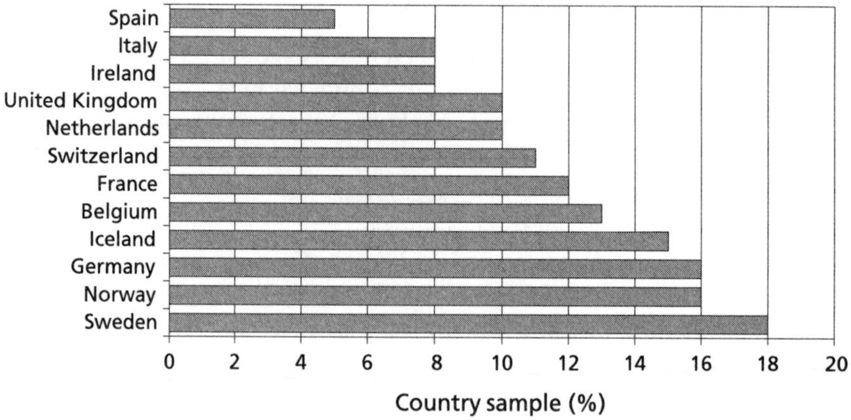

Source: adapted from Woods et al. *(130)*.

Food control authorities have recommended managing the problem by improving the labelling of foods likely to contain common allergens. Explicit warnings may help consumers to avoid the more common causes of intolerance, but all ingredients in foods must be listed to ensure that the people who suffer from reactions to less common ingredients can get the information they need to protect their health.

Precautionary labelling may also be recommended for products that may contain unintentional ingredients. Such labels currently include such phrases as "may contain traces of ..." or "manufactured on the same equipment as ...".

An emerging area of concern is the potential for genetically modified foods and food ingredients to contain compounds that provoke unexpected reactions in sensitive people. The evaluation of genetically modified foods increasingly includes tests for novel proteins and for allergenicity.

Evaluation of allergenicity in genetically modified foods

WHO and FAO held an expert consultation on procedures for evaluating the allergenicity of genetically modified foods. The report *(131)* acknowledges the need to "pay particular attention to allergenicity when assessing the safety of foods produced through genetic modification" when genes are derived not only from sources known to be allergenic but also from foods with no known allergenicity. The participants advocated continuing to identify allergens and their characteristics, developing databases on proteins and gene sequences, validating suitable animal models for allergy assessment and developing post-marketing surveillance procedures.

The report *(131)* also includes a revised decision tree (Fig. 2.8) that can be used to help assess allergens in novel foods, and provides further details on testing

Fig. 2.8. Decision tree for assessing the allergenic potential of foods derived from biotechnology

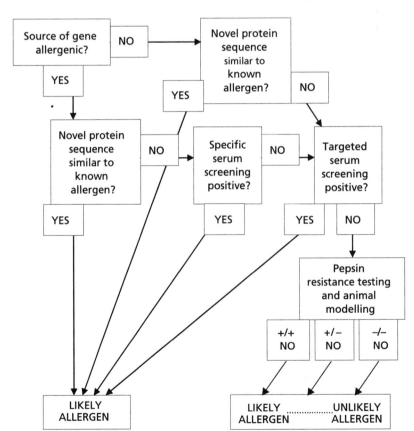

Source: Evaluation of allergenicity of genetically modified foods (131).

procedures. To ensure harmonization of testing for allergenicity, the participants called on United Nations agencies to provide technical support to Member States and to promote interaction between experts in different countries.

Emerging food control issues

This chapter has shown that food safety problems continue to be urgent and, in some cases, are increasing in urgency throughout the European Region. Public interest in the safety and quality of food is immense, and consumer concerns have increased pressure on governments to take greater responsibility for protection. One response is the considerable institutional changes (described here and in Chapter 4, pp. 255–269) made to develop more dynamic systems reflecting modern consumer concerns and trade issues.

Food control systems cannot deliver a completely risk-free food supply; zero risk is impossible. Improvements can be made, however, and scientific knowledge, technology and foresight improved. As described in Chapter 4, food control systems in countries have evolved over the past century in response to different local problems. There is now, however, considerable impetus towards harmonizing these systems. Two major drivers in this process have been the globalization of the world economy and the increasingly common nature of food safety problems faced by different countries.

Promoting free trade in a global economy requires any food-exporting country to have a reliable food control system. WHO and FAO support such efforts by providing expert advice on strengthening these systems (132). The objectives of a food control system may conflict. For instance, a high priority given to the free movement of food across national borders may conflict with strong consumer protection. Consumers in countries with a high level of protection against contaminated foods (such as protection from *Salmonella* in Sweden) may be exposed to extra risk if foods from countries with less stringent standards are imported under free trade agreements. All countries reserve the right to implement measures to protect public health, but under the Agreement Establishing the World Trade Organization these measures must be non-discriminatory and based on scientific risk assessment. WTO members are expected to accept measures that achieve the same level of health protection and are deemed equivalent, even if different from their own national procedures.

Over recent decades, the international philosophy of food control has changed in three important areas:

- an emphasis on the analysis of risk to human beings as a basis for food regulation;
- a shift of responsibility for food safety away from the official food control system towards quality control systems established by producers; and

- increasing awareness of the need to look upstream at the sources of the contamination, including the pressures put on food producers to meet changing trading conditions and increased competition.

In particular, HACCP-based systems have raised awareness of food safety issues and achieved significant advances, but the full potential cannot be realized without a trained food sector, detailed risk assessment and major changes in the way inspection and surveillance programmes are performed *(132)*.

From the perspectives of consumers and public health, international cooperation promises improved food safety in the long term. Concern has been expressed, however, that the decision-making process has been too far removed from consumers, to a forum in which industry dominates over consumer interests. Consumer organizations have increasingly demanded to be involved in the risk assessment process and in shaping its context and terms.

Food safety problems also tend to converge with economic development. In countries with less developed economies, the food producer and the consumer have a closer connection. There are fewer processed and packaged foods; most fresh food is traded in traditional markets, and street sellers and hawkers supply most food consumed outside the home. Food safety concerns in these countries typically include:

- the inappropriate use of agricultural chemicals;
- the use of untreated or partially treated wastewater, sewage or manure on crops;
- the absence of food inspection, including meat inspection;
- a lack of infrastructure, such as a functional cold-chain; and
- poor hygiene, including a lack of clean water supplies.

Much perishable food is prepared and consumed on demand, and there is only limited storage of prepared foods.

As a country's economy develops, its participation in the global food economy and its capital investment in the agricultural sector increase. Farmers in emerging economies can be expected to increase the use of intensive animal and fish production techniques and associated veterinary products, to make wider use of agricultural chemicals for crop production and to import animal breeds and plant strains offering better yields. Food production and processing tend to occur on a larger scale at greater distances from the consumer, and commercial pressures accumulate to reduce costs and increase markets. The effects of these changes on food safety in more affluent economies have already been noted and will continue in emerging economies.

At the same time, food production technology in more affluent economies will continue to develop, influenced by some of the trends shown in Table 2.10.

These trends – combined with the ability of biological hazards to mutate and the increasing proportion of the population comprised by vulnerable groups – will require a vigilant and agile system to protect public health and facilitate trade.

Table 2.10. Trends in the food industry in Europe

Drivers of innovation	Food industry response	Improvements in knowledge
Demand for cleaner foods, especially organic produce	Innovative packaging technology such as active films	Impact of genetic modification on public health
Need to eliminate the use of artificial ingredients and additives	Increased use of aseptic packaging and modified atmosphere packaging for minimally processed foods	Identification of new and emerging pathogens
Demand for minimally processed and fresher foods	New forms of food preservation, including pulsed light and high-pressure processing	Causation of foodborne viral infections
Demand for ready-to-eat food	Raw materials, production aids and cultures produced by genetic modification	Cost-effective and accurate biosensors to assess food safety
Functional foods and nutraceuticals	Probiotics and biocins (bacterial toxins)	Function and control of prions
Information and access to data	Fat substitutes	Use of phytochemicals
Need to reduce costs	Shelf life and food safety indicators	Extension of indicators to developing countries

Source: adapted from Background paper: developing a food safety strategy (14).

WHO and food safety

WHO has a mandate to protect public health. It recognizes that the right of every individual to adequate, nutritious and safe food is central to fulfilling this mandate and, to this end, WHO assists in a range of food-related activities. These include setting international standards for trade in food, assessing health risk and developing a framework for risk analysis, monitoring foodborne disease and providing technical assistance. In 2000, the Fifty-third World Health Assembly unanimously confirmed food safety as an essential public health priority and committed WHO to expanding its responsibilities in food safety (http://www.who.int/gb/EB_WHA/PDF/WHA53/ResWHA53/15.pdf, accessed 11 October 2002). The outcome of this has been a global food safety strategy with the objective of reducing the health and social burden of foodborne disease (14). It is intended that the objective will be achieved by:

• advocating and assisting in the development of risk-based, sustainable, integrated food safety systems;

- developing science-based measures along the entire food chain that will prevent exposure to unacceptable levels of chemical and microbial hazards; and
- assessing, communicating and managing foodborne risks in cooperation with other sectors and partners.

The strategy *(14)* identifies the major food safety concerns outlined elsewhere in this chapter and includes the following approaches.

1. Surveillance systems for foodborne diseases need strengthening. Detailed and accurate knowledge is essential for effective action to reduce the problem.
2. Working with FAO, WHO will develop and disseminate tools for improved risk assessment. These will serve as an agreed basis for setting national and international standards, national food priorities and management strategies.
3. WHO will promote a holistic approach to the production and safe use of foods derived using new technology, including genetic engineering.
4. WHO will support a thorough review and optimization of the work of the Codex Alimentarius Commission and greater participation of the health sector in Codex work, and urge that the Commission's decisions be based on protecting the health of consumers.
5. The results of risk analyses should be communicated in a readily understandable form that will promote useful dialogue between stakeholders and enable them to participate in the risk analysis process.
6. WHO will work to establish an international coordination group on food safety to ensure a consistent, effective approach.
7. To build capacity, WHO will formulate regional food safety strategies based on not only the global strategy but also specific regional needs, such as technical support, training and education.

Strengthening food safety in Europe

FAO and WHO jointly convened a Pan-European Conference on Food Safety and Quality in 2002 *(133)*, to enable European countries to survey and discuss important issues in food safety and quality in the Region and to consider how the transparency and reliability of European food chains could be improved to strengthen consumer confidence. Particular attention was given to identifying opportunities for: harmonizing food safety policies across the Region, cooperating in developing policy and science, and improving information and communication systems on food safety and quality.

Working groups at the Conference made recommendations on how these objectives might be achieved, focusing on three main areas: policy, cooperation and strategy *(134)*. The participants recognized the need for integrated, multidisciplinary, prevention-oriented food safety policies, supported with the necessary human and financial resources, and applied with the cooperation and participation of stakeholders throughout the food chain, from farm to table.

In addition, international collaboration and harmonization should be improved in a number of aspects of food safety policy to promote capacity building, to avoid duplication of effort, to improve public health protection and to facilitate trade.

Finally, food safety strategies should be risk-based, giving priority to the problems that pose the greatest health threat and the preventive measures that are expected to result in the greatest reduction in foodborne illness. In addition to risk assessment, strategies should consider consumers' religious or ethical concerns and the desire to promote more sustainable food production practices. In cases of scientific uncertainty or inconclusive risk assessment, provisional risk management procedures may be adopted based on the precautionary principle.

The Conference participants also recommended that independent, transparent and effective national food safety authorities be established for scientific advice, risk assessment and risk communication.

References

1. *International trade statistics.* Geneva, World Trade Organization, 2000.
2. JONES, J.M. *Food safety.* St Paul, MO, Eagen Press, 1992.
3. *Foodborne disease: a focus for health education.* Geneva, World Health Organization, 1999.
4. MOSSEL, D.A.A. ET AL. *Essentials of the microbiology of foods.* Chichester, John Wiley & Sons, 1995, pp. 119–121.
5. NACHAMKIN, I. ET AL. *Campylobacter jejuni* infection and the association with Guillain-Barré syndrome. *In*: Nachamkin, I. & Blaser, M.J., ed. *Campylobacter*, 2nd ed. Washington, DC, ASM Press, 2000, pp. 155–175.
6. ARCHER, D. & YOUNG, F.E. Contemporary issues: diseases with a food vector. *Clinical microbiology reviews*, 1: 377–398 (1988).
7. TIRADO, C. & SCHMIDT, K., ED. *WHO Surveillance Programme for Control of Foodborne Infections and Intoxication in Europe, 7th report 1993–1998.* Berlin, Federal Institute for Health Protection of Consumers and Veterinary Medicine–FAO/WHO Collaborating Centre for Research and Training in Food Hygiene and Zoonoses, 2000.
8. Food safety. *In*: *Overview of the environment and health in Europe in the 1990s* (http://www.euro.who.int/document/e66792.pdf). Copenhagen,

WHO Regional Office for Europe, 1999, pp. 51–52 (accessed 6 October 2002).

9. *Dioxins and their effects on human health* (http://www.who.int/inf-fs/en/ fact225.html). Geneva, World Health Organization, 1999 (Fact Sheet 225, accessed 6 October 2002).

10. FOOD STANDARDS AGENCY. *A report of the study of infectious intestinal disease in England.* London, The Stationery Office, 2000.

11. ADAMS, M.R. & MOSS, M.O. *Food microbiology,* 2nd ed. Cambridge, Royal Society of Chemistry, 2000.

12. *Improved coordination and harmonization of national food safety control services: report on a joint WHO/EURO–FSAI meeting, Dublin, Ireland 19–20 June 2001* (http://www.euro.who.int/document/E74473.pdf). Copenhagen, WHO Regional Office for Europe, 2001 (accessed 6 October 2002).

13. *Food safety strategic planning meeting: report of a WHO strategic planning meeting, WHO headquarters, Geneva, Switzerland, 20–22 February 2001* (http://whqlibdoc.who.int/hq/2001/WHO_SDE_PHE_FOS_01.2.pdf). Geneva, World Health Organization, 1997 (accessed 6 October 2002).

14. *Background paper: developing a food safety strategy* (http://www.who.int/ fsf/BACKGROUND%20PAPER.pdf). Geneva, World Health Organization, 2001 (accessed 6 October 2002).

15. SARI KOVATS, R. ET AL., ED. *Climate change and stratospheric ozone depletion: early effects on our health in Europe.* Copenhagen, WHO Regional Office for Europe, 2000 (WHO Regional Publications, European Series, No. 88).

16. *Denmark: top priority on food safety.* Copenhagen, Danish Veterinary and Food Administration, 2000.

17. *Determinants of the burden of disease in the European Union.* Stockholm, National Institute of Public Health, 1997.

18. MURRAY, C.L.J., & LOPEZ, A.D., ED. *The global burden of disease. A comprehensive assessment of mortality and disability from diseases, injuries, and risk factors in 1990 and projected to 2020.* Cambridge, MA, Harvard School of Public Health, 1996.

19. HAVELAAR, A.H. ET AL. Health burden in the Netherlands due to infection with thermophilic *Campylobacter* spp. *Epidemiology and infection,* **125**: 505–522 (2000).

20. MELSE, J.M. ET AL. A national burden of disease calculation: Dutch disability-adjusted life-years. *American journal of public health,* **90**: 1241–1247 (2000).

21. SOCKETT, P.N. & ROBERTS, J.A. The social and economic impact of salmonellosis. A report of a national survey in England and Wales of

laboratory-confirmed *Salmonella* infections. *Epidemiology and infection*, **107**: 335–347 (1991).

22. *Food Standards Agency review of BSE controls* (http://www.bsereview.org.uk/data/report.htm). London, Food Standards Agency, 2000 (accessed 6 October 2002).

23. *Compensation scheme for variant CJD victims announced* (http://www.doh.gov.uk/cjd/press/pr011001.htm). London, Department of Health, 2001 (Press Release 2001/0457, accessed 6 October 2002).

24. *PCB and dioxin contamination in the feed and food chain in Belgium* (http://dioxin.fgov.be/pe/ene00.htm). Brussels, Federal Government of Belgium, 1999 (accessed 6 October 2002).

25. *Initiation of infringement proceedings against Belgium for failure to meet its Community obligations in the dioxin crisis* (http://www.fst.rdg.ac.uk/foodlaw/news/eu-99-45.htm). Brussels, European Commission, 1999 (Press Release IP/99/406, accessed 6 October 2002).

26. Dioxin crisis topples Belgian government (http://ens-news.com/ens/jun1999/1999-06-15-03.asp). *Environmental news service*, 15 June 1999 (accessed 15 January 2003).

27. *Renate Künast and Ulla Schmidt new federal ministers?* (http://www.bundesregierung.de/dokumente/Pressemitteilung/ix_28378.htm?script=0). Bonn, Federal Government of Germany, 10 January 2001 (Press Release 6/01, accessed 6 October 2002).

28. SCIENTIFIC COMMITTEE FOR ANIMAL HEALTH AND ANIMAL WELFARE. *Possible links between Crohn's disease and paratuberculosis*. European Commission, Directorate-General for Health and Consumer Protection, 2000 (SANCO/B3/R16/2000).

29. FEDERAL INSTITUTE FOR HEALTH PROTECTION OF CONSUMERS AND VETERINARY MEDICINE. *Trends and sources of zoonotic agents in the EU in 1998*. Brussels, European Commission, 2000 (SANCO/409/2000).

30. BERNDTSON, E. ET AL. *Campylobacter* incidence on a chicken farm and the spread of *Campylobacter* during the slaughter process. *International journal of food microbiology*, **32**: 35–47 (1996).

31. DAVIES, R. & BRESLIN, M. Environmental contamination and detection of *Salmonella enterica* serovar *enteritidis* in laying flocks. *Veterinary record*, **149**: 699–704 (2001).

32. *Salmonella in livestock production*. New Haw, Athelstone, Veterinary Laboratories Agency, 1999.

33. WHO EUROPEAN CENTRE FOR ENVIRONMENT AND HEALTH. *Concern for Europe's tomorrow: health and the environment in the WHO European Region*. Stuttgart, Vissenschaftliche Verlagsgesellschaft, 1995.

34. WAHLSTRÖM, H., ed. *Zoonoses in Sweden up to and including 1999* (http://www.sva.se/pdf/zoonosinsweden.pdf). Uppsala, Swedish Zoonoses

Centre, National Veterinary Institute of Sweden, 2001 (accessed 6 October 2002).

35. WARD, L. Salmonella *infections at lowest level since 1985*. London, Public Health Laboratory Service, 2001.

36. ADDIS, P.B. ET AL. *Generic environmental impact statement on animal agriculture: a summary of the literature related to the effects of animal agriculture on human health* (http://www.mnplan.state.mn.us/pdf/1999/eqb/scoping/humsum.pdf). Minneapolis, Environmental Quality Board of the Minnesota Legislature, 1999 (accessed 6 October 2002).

37. O'BRIEN, T. *Factory farming and human health*. Petersfield, Compassion in World Farming Trust, 1997.

38. Imported rocket salad partially responsible for increased incidence of hepatitis A cases in Sweden 2000–2001. *Eurosurveillance*, 6(10): 151–153 (2001).

39. RICHMOND, M. *The microbiological safety of food. Part 1. Report of the Committee on the Microbiological Safety of Food*. London, H.M. Stationery Office, 1990.

40. *The medical impact of antimicrobial use in food animals: report of a WHO meeting, Berlin, Germany, 13–17 October 1997* (http://www.who.int/emcdocuments/antimicrobial_resistance/whoemczoo974c.html). Copenhagen, WHO Regional Office for Europe, 1997 (accessed 6 October 2002).

41. SCIENTIFIC STEERING COMMITTEE. *Opinion of the Scientific Steering Committee on antimicrobial resistance* (http://europa.eu.int/comm/food/fs/sc/ssc/out50_en.html). Brussels, European Commission, 1999 (accessed 6 October 2002).

42. SCIENTIFIC STEERING COMMITTEE. *2nd opinion on anti-microbial resistance*. Brussels, European Commission, 2001.

43. WINCKLER, C. & GRAFE, A. Characterisation and use of waste from intensive livestock farming with reference to different soil types. Research report 297 33 911 – UAB-FB 000074; Use of veterinary drugs in intensive animal production – evidence for persistence of tetracycline in pig slurry. *Journal of soils and sediments*, 1(1): 58–62 (2001).

44. JØRGENSEN, S.E. & HALLING-SØRENSEN, B, ED. Special issue on drugs in the environment. *Chemosphere*, 40(7): 691–793 (2000).

45. VAN DEN BOGAARD, A.E. ET AL. The effect of banning avoparcin on VRE carriage in the Netherlands. *Journal of antimicrobial chemotherapy*, 45: 146–148 (2001).

46. *Information statement on* Salmonella typhimurium *DT 104*. London, Professional Food Microbiology Group, Institute of Food Science and Technology, 1997.

47. *Gefährliche Rohwurst?* (http://www.ethlife.ethz.ch/tages/show/0,1046,0-8-913,00.html). Zurich, Federal Institute of Technology, 2001 (accessed 6 October 2002).

48. WINOKUR, P.L. ET AL. Evidence for transfer of CMY-2 AmpC beta-lactamase plasmids between *Escherichia coli* and *Salmonella* isolates from food animals and humans. *Antimicrobial agents and chemotherapy,* **45**: 2716–2722 (2001).

49. *Use of quinolones in food animals and potential impact on human health: report of a WHO meeting, Geneva, Switzerland, 2–5 June 1998* (http://whqlibdoc.who.int/hq/1998/WHO_EMC_ZDI_98.10.pdf). Geneva, World Health Organization, 1998 (accessed 6 October 2002).

50. WIERUP, M. Preventive methods replace antibiotic growth promoters: ten years experience in Sweden. *UPUA newsletter,* **16**: 1–5 (1998).

51. *Safety aspects of genetically modified foods of plant origin: report of a Joint FAO/WHO Expert Consultation on Foods Derived from Biotechnology, WHO headquarters, Geneva, Switzerland, 29 May to 2 June 2000* (http://whqlibdoc.who.int/hq/2000/WHO_SDE_PHE_FOS_00.6.pdf). Geneva, World Health Organization, 2001 (accessed 6 October 2002).

52. *Safety assessment of foods derived from genetically modified microorganisms: report of a Joint FAO/WHO Expert Consultation on Foods Derived from Biotechnology, World Health Organization, Geneva, Switzerland, 24–28 September 2001* (http://www.who.int/fsf/GMfood/GMMConsult_Final_.pdf). Geneva, World Health Organization, 2001 (accessed 6 October 2002).

53. COGAN, T.A. ET AL. The effectiveness of hygiene procedures for prevention of cross-contamination from chicken carcases in the domestic kitchen. *Letters in applied microbiology,* **29**: 354–358 (1999).

54. *The five keys to safer food* (http://www.who.int/fsf/Documents/5keys-ID-eng.pdf). Geneva, World Health Organization, 2001 (accessed 14 January 2003).

55. JOUVE, J.-L. Good manufacturing practice, HACCP and quality systems. *In*: Lund, B.M. et al., ed. *The microbiological safety and quality of foods.* Gaithersburg, MD, Aspen Publishers, 2000, pp. 1627–1655.

56. *Polychlorinated biphenyls in food – UK dietary intakes* (http://archive.food.gov.uk/maff/archive/food/infsheet/1996/no89/89pcb.htm). London, Ministry of Agriculture, Fisheries and Food, 1996 (Food Surveillance Information Sheet No. 89, accessed 8 October 2002).

57. INSTITUTE OF FOOD SCIENCE & TECHNOLOGY. Dioxins and PCBs in food (http://ifst.org/hottop22.htm). *Food science & technology today,* **12**: 177–179 (1998) (accessed 8 October 2002).

58. *Joint FAO/WHO Expert Committee on Food Additives, Fifty-seventh Meeting, Rome, 5–14 June 2001. Summary and conclusions* (http://www.who.int/

pcs/jecfa/Summary57-corr.pdf). Geneva, World Health Organization, 2001 (accessed 8 October 2002).

59. Council regulation (EEC) no. 2377/90 laying down a Community procedure for the establishment of maximum residue limits of veterinary medicinal products in foodstuffs of animal origin. *Official journal of the European Communities*, L **224**(18 August): 1–18 (1990).

60. Commission regulation (EC) No. 194/97 of 31 January 1997 setting maximum levels for certain contaminants in foodstuffs (text with EEA relevance). *Official journal of the European Communities*, L **31**(1 February): 1–18 (1997).

61. Council directive 91/414/EEC of 15 July 1991 concerning the placing of plant protection products on the market. *Official journal of the European Communities*, L **230**(19 August): 1–18 (1991).

62. *Some soy sauce products to be removed* (http://www.foodstandards.gov.uk/news/pressreleases/soysaucerecall). London, Food Standards Agency, 20 June 2001 (accessed 8 October 2002).

63. *Fats and oils in human nutrition: report of a joint expert consultation* (http://www.fao.org/docrep/V4700E/V4700E00.htm). Rome, Food and Agriculture Organization of the United Nations, 1994 (accessed 8 October 2002).

64. Trans *fatty acids (TFA)* (http://ifst.org/hottop9.htm). London, Institute of Food Science & Technology, 1999 (accessed 8 October 2002).

65. NGUYEN-THE, C. & CARLIN, F. Fresh and processed vegetables. *In*: Lund, B.M. et al., ed. *The microbiological safety and quality of foods*. Gaithersburg, MD, Aspen Publishers, 2000, pp. 620–684.

66. O'BRIEN, S. ET AL. *The microbiological status of ready to eat fruit and vegetables*. London, Public Health Laboratory Service, 2000 (ACM/476).

67. *Monitoring for pesticide residues in products of plant origin, in the European Union and Norway – report 1997* (http://europa.eu.int/comm/food/fs/inspections/fnaoi/reports/annual_eu/fnaoi_rep_norw_1997_en.html). Brussels, European Commission, 1999 (accessed 6 October 2002).

68. COMMITTEE ON TOXICITY OF CHEMICALS IN FOOD, CONSUMER PRODUCTS AND THE ENVIRONMENT. *Draft report of the Working Group on Risk Assessment of Mixtures of Pesticides* (http://www.foodstandards.gov.uk/science/ouradvisors/toxicity/COTwg/wigramp/draftreport). London, Food Standards Agency, 2002 (accessed 15 January 2003).

69. BRUNDTLAND, G.H. Nutrition and infection: malnutrition and mortality in public health. *Nutrition reviews*, **58**: S1–S4 (2000).

70. ULIJASZEK, S. Transdisciplinarity in the study of undernutrition–infection interactions. *Collegium antropologicum*, **21**: 3–15 (1997).

71. GARIN, B. ET AL. Multicenter study of street foods in 13 towns on four continents by the Food and Environmental Hygiene Study Group of the

International Network of Pasteur and Associated Institutes. *Journal of food protein*, **65**: 146–152 (2002).

72. FALKINGHAM, J. *A profile of poverty in Tajikistan*. London, Centre for Analysis of Social Exclusion, London School of Economics, 2000 (CASE Paper 39).

73. BARTON, S.J. Infant feeding practices of low-income rural mothers. *MCN American journal of maternal/child nursing*, **26**: 93–97 (2001).

74. ARANGO, J. ET AL. [Sanitary conditions of community dining halls in greater Buenos Aires, Argentina]. *Revista Panamericana de salud pública*, **2**: 225–231 (1997).

75. SETHI, D. ET AL. A study of infectious intestinal disease in England: risk factors associated with group A rotavirus in children. *Epidemiology and infection*, **126**: 63–70 (2001).

76. JOHNSON, A.E. ET AL. Food safety knowledge and practice among elderly people living at home. *Journal of epidemiology and community health*, **52**: 745–748 (1998).

77. ANGELILLO, I.F. ET AL. Food handlers and foodborne diseases: knowledge, attitudes, and reported behavior in Italy. *Journal of food protection*, **63**(3): 381–385 (2000).

78. SCHOU, L. ET AL. Using a "lifestyle" perspective to understanding toothbrushing behaviour in Scottish schoolchildren. *Community dentistry and oral epidemiology*, **18**: 230–234 (1990).

79. KOIVUSILTA, L. ET AL. Health related lifestyle in adolescence predicts adult educational level: a longitudinal study from Finland. *Journal of epidemiology and community health*, **52**: 794–801 (1998).

80. ÅSTRØM, A.N. & RISE, J. Socio-economic differences in patterns of health and oral health behaviour in 25 year old Norwegians. *Clinical oral investigations*, **5**: 122–128 (2001).

81. *Report to the European Parliament and to the Council on the measures to be put into force for the control and prevention of zoonoses*. Brussels, European Commission, 2001 (COM(2001) 452).

82. *Annual report on zoonoses in Denmark 1998*. Copenhagen, Ministry of Food, Agriculture and Fisheries, 1998.

83. ROBERTS, T. & PINNER, R. Economic impact of disease caused by *Listeria monocytogenes*. *In*: Miller, A.J. et al., ed. *Food-borne listeriosis*. Amsterdam, Elsevier, 1990, pp. 137–149.

84. DONNELLY, C.A. ET AL. The BSE epidemic in British cattle. *Ecosystem health*, **5**: 164–173 (1999).

85. *WHO infection control guidelines for transmissible spongiform encephalopathies: report of a WHO consultation, Geneva, Switzerland, 23–26 March 1999* (http://www.who.int/emcdocuments/tse/whocdscsraph2003c.html). Geneva, World Health Organization, 1999 (accessed 6 October 2002).

86. LORD PHILLIPS OF WORTH MATRAVERS ET AL. *The BSE inquiry.* London, The Stationery Office, 2000.

87. KOOPMANS, M. ET AL. Molecular epidemiology of human enteric caliciviruses in the Netherlands. *Journal of infectious diseases*, 181: S262–S269 (2000).

88. DE WIT, M.A.S. ET AL. Sensor, a population-based cohort study on gastroenteritis in the Netherlands: incidence and etiology. *American journal of epidemiology*, 154: 666–674 (2001).

89. MAGUIRE, H.C. ET AL. A collaborative case control study of sporadic hepatitis A in England. *CDR review*, 5: R33–R40 (1995).

90. MELE, A. ET AL. Incidence and risk factors for hepatitis A in Italy: public health indications from a 10-year surveillance. *Journal of hepatology*, 26: 743–747 (1997).

91. Council directive 91/492/EEC of 15 July 1991 laying down the health conditions for the production and the placing on the market of live bivalve molluscs. *Official journal of the European Communities*, L 268(24 September): 1–14 (1991).

92. Council directive 92/117/EEC of 17 December 1992 concerning measures for protection against specified zoonoses and specified zoonitic agents in animals and products of animal origin in order to prevent outbreaks of food-borne infections and intoxications. *Official journal of the European Communities*, L 62(15 March): 38–49 (1993).

93. Council decision 1999/313/EC of 29 April 1999 on reference laboratories for monitoring bacteriological and viral contamination of bivalve molluscs. *Official journal of the European Communities*, L 120(8 May): 40–41 (1999).

94. HEALTH CANADA. *Contaminant profiles* (http://www.hcsc.gc.ca/ehp/ehd/catalogue/bch_pubs/98ehd211/con_profiles.pdf). Ottawa, Government of Canada, 2000 (accessed 6 October 2002).

95. FORASTIERI, V. The ILO programme on safety and health in agriculture: the challenge for the new century – providing occupational safety and health services to workers in agriculture *In*: *Top of the agenda: health and safety in agriculture*. Geneva, International Labour Organization, 2000.

96. LIBERT, B. *The environmental heritage of Soviet agriculture*. Wallingford, Centre for Agriculture and Biodiversity International, 1995, p. 104.

97. FESHBACH, M. & FRIENDLY, A. Harvest of neglect. *In*: *Ecocide in the USSR*. New York, Basic Books, 1992, pp. 49–68.

98. ATANIYAZOVA, O.A. ET AL. Levels of certain metals, organochlorine pesticides and dioxins in cord blood, maternal blood, human milk and some commonly used nutrients in the surroundings of the Aral Sea (Karakalpakstan, Republic of Uzbekistan). *Acta paediatrica*, 90: 801–808 (2001).

99. *Second Workshop on a Framework for the Sustainable Use of Plant Protection Products in the EU* (http://europa.eu.int/comm/environment/ppps/work-shp.pdf). Brussels, European Commission, Directorate-General for the Environment, Nuclear Safety and Civil Protection, 1998 (accessed 10 October 2002).

100. *Environment 2010: our future, our choice. The Sixth Environment Action Programme of the European Community, 2001–2010* (http://europa.eu.int/comm/environment/newprg/index.htm). Brussels, European Commission, 2001 (COM(2001)31, accessed 10 October 2002).

101. Council directive 90/642/EEC of 27 November 1990 fixing the maximum levels for pesticide residues in and on certain products of plant origin, including fruit and vegetables. *Official journal of the European Communities*, L **350**(14 December): 71–79 (1990).

102. Council directive 86/362/EEC of 24 July 1986 fixing the maximum levels for pesticide residues in and on cereals. *Official journal of the European Communities*, L **221**(7 August): 37–42 (1986).

103. Council directive 86/363/EEC of 24 July 1986 fixing the maximum levels for pesticide residues in and on animal products. *Official journal of the European Communities*, L **221**(7 August): 43–47 (1986).

104. Council directive 89/397/EEC of 14 June 1989 on the official control of foodstuffs. *Official journal of the European Communities*, L **186**(30 June): 23–27 (1989).

105. Council directive 93/99/EEC of 14 June 1989 on additional measures concerning the official control of foodstuffs. *Official journal of the European Communities*, L **290**(24 November): 14–17 (1989).

106. Council directive 79/700/EEC of 24 July 1979 establishing Community methods of sampling for the official control of pesticide residues in and on fruit and vegetables. *Official journal of the European Communities*, L **207**(15 August): 26–28 (1979).

107. Commission directive 91/321/EEC of 14 May 1991 on infant formulas and follow-on formulas. *Official journal of the European Communities*, L **175**(4 July): 35–49 (1991).

108. Commission directive 96/5/EEC of 16 February 1996 on processed cereal-based foods and baby foods for infants and young children. *Official journal of the European Communities*, L **49**(28 February): 17–28 (1996).

109. *Guidelines for predicting dietary intake of pesticide residues* (http://whqlibdoc.who.int/hq/1997/WHO_FSF_FOS_97.7.pdf). Geneva, World Health Organization, 1997 (accessed 6 October 2002).

110. *Food consumption and exposure assessment of chemicals: report of a FAO/WHO consultation, Geneva, Switzerland, 10–14 February 1997.* Geneva, World Health Organization, 1997 (document WHO/FSF/FOS/97.5).

111. *Data requirements handbook* (http://www.pesticides.gov.uk/applicant/registration%5Fguides/data_reqs_handbook/residues.pdf). London, Pesticides Safety Directorate, 2001 (accessed 6 October 2002).

112. *Opinion on a maximum residue limit (MRL) of 0.01 mg/kg for pesticides in foods intended for infants and young children.* Brussels, Scientific Committee for Food, 1997.

113. *Further advice on the opinion of the Scientific Committee for Food on a maximum residue limit (MRL) of 0.01 mg/kg for pesticides in foods intended for infants and young children.* Brussels, Scientific Committee for Food, 1998.

114. MICHAELSEN, K. ET AL. *Feeding and nutrition of infants and young children. Guidelines for the WHO European Region, with emphasis on the former Soviet countries* (http://www.euro.who.int/InformationSources/Publications/Catalogue/20010914_21). Copenhagen, WHO Regional Office for Europe, 2003 (WHO Regional Publications, European Series, No. 87, accessed 25 September 2003).

115. BARKATINA, E.N. ET AL. Organochlorine pesticide residues in breast milk in the Republic of Belarus. *Bulletin of environmental toxicology,* **60**: 231–237 (1998).

116. KALOYANOVA-SIMENEONOVA, F.P. *Review of the recent data on effects of persistent organochlorine pesticides. In: Proceedings of the Subregional Awareness Raising Workshop on Persistent Organic Pollutants (POPs), Kranjska Gora, Slovenia, 11–14 May 1998* (http://www.chem.unep.ch/pops/POPs_Inc/proceedings/slovenia/simeonova.html). Geneva, United Nations Environment Programme, 1998 (accessed 6 October 2002).

117. BORDET, F. ET AL. Organochlorine pesticide and PCB congener content of French human milk. *Bulletin of environmental toxicology,* **50**: 425–432 (1993).

118. RICHTER, E.D., & SAFI, J. Pesticide use, exposure and risk: a joint Israeli–Palestinian perspective. *Environmental research,* **73**: 211–218 (1997).

119. HOOPER, K. ET AL. Analysis of breast milk to assess exposure to chlorinated contaminants in Kazakhstan: PCBs and organochlorine pesticides in southern Kazakhstan. *Environmental health perspectives,* **105**: 1250–1254 (1997).

120. HERTZMAN, C. *Environment and health in central and eastern Europe. A report for the Environmental Action Programme for Central and Eastern Europe.* Washington, DC, World Bank, 1995.

121. HERNANDEZ, L.M. ET AL. Organochlorine insecticide and polychlorinated biphenyl residues in human breast milk in Madrid (Spain). *Bulletin of environmental toxicology,* **50**: 308–315 (1993).

122. MEIRONYTE, D. ET AL. Analysis of polybrominated diphenyl ethers in Swedish human milk. A time-related trend study, 1972–1997. *Journal of toxicology and environmental health part A*, **58**: 329–341 (1999).

123. NOREN, K. & MEIRONYTE, D. Certain organochlorine and organobromine contaminants in Swedish human milk in perspective of past 20–30 years. *Chemosphere*, **40**: 1111–1123 (2000).

124. KARAKAYA, A.E. ET AL. Organochlorine pesticide contaminants in human milk from different regions of Turkey. *Bulletin of environmental toxicology*, **39**: 506–510 (1987).

125. ELPINER, L.I. Public health in the Aral Sea coastal region and the dynamics of change in the ecological situation. *In*: Glantz, M.H., ed. *Creeping environmental problems and sustainable development in the Aral Sea Basin*. Cambridge, Cambridge University Press, 1999, pp. 128–156.

126. SCHUTZ, D. ET AL. *GEMS/Food international dietary survey: infant exposure to certain organochlorine contaminants from breast milk – a risk assessment* (http://whqlibdoc.who.int/hq/1998/WHO_FSF_FOS_98.4.pdf). Geneva, World Health Organization, 1998 (accessed 6 October 2002).

127. TAYLOR, S.L. Emerging problems with food allergens. *Food, nutrition and agriculture*, **26**: 14–21 (2000).

128. COMMITTEE ON TOXICITY OF CHEMICALS IN FOOD, CONSUMER PRODUCTS AND THE ENVIRONMENT WORKING GROUP ON FOOD INTOLERANCE. *Adverse reactions to food and food ingredients*. London, Food Standards Agency, 2000.

129. VERNIA, P. ET AL. Lactose malabsorption, irritable bowel syndrome and self-reported milk intolerance. *Digestive and liver disease: official journal of the Italian Society of Gastroenterology and the Italian Association for the Study of the Liver*, **33**: 234–239 (2001).

130. WOODS, R.K. ET AL. International prevalence of reported food allergies and intolerances. Comparisons arising from the European Community Respiratory Health Survey (ECRHS) 1991–1994. *European journal of clinical nutrition*, **55**: 298–304 (2001).

131. *Evaluation of allergenicity of genetically modified foods: report of a Joint FAO/WHO Expert Consultation on Allergenicity of Foods Derived from Biotechnology, Food and Agriculture Organization, Rome, Italy, 22 to 25 January 2001* (http://www.who.int/fsf/GMfood/Consultation_Jan2001/report20.pdf). Geneva, World Health Organization, 2001 (accessed 6 October 2002).

132. *Guidelines for strengthening food control systems*. Geneva, World Health Organization, 2002.

133. *FAO/WHO Pan-European Conference on Food Safety and Quality, 25–28 February 2002, Budapest, Hungary. Final report*. Rome, Food and Agriculture Organization of the United Nations, 2002 (PEC/REP1).

3. Food security and sustainable development

The Introduction identified three interacting parts of food policy: nutrition policy, food safety policy and policies ensuring that food supplies are plentiful and widely distributed. This chapter examines the adequacy, availability and sustainability of the supply of safe and nourishing food.

More attention is being paid to how food production policies affect food safety and nutrition. Agricultural policies that emphasize high production may increase the quantity of food produced but not necessarily the quality of the diet – in terms of its biochemical diversity, nutritional adequacy or safety.

Policy-makers are looking at the upstream sources of problems in the food supply. This chapter looks in more detail at these issues, the trends in production and the evidence for a concordance between ecologically sustainable supplies and healthy diets.

Food security

Sometimes confused with food safety, the term food security means ensuring that all members of a population have access to a supply of food sufficient in quality and quantity, regardless of their social or economic status. A secure food supply satisfies the consumer's needs without jeopardizing the production process in the short or long term. It ensures the sustainability of supplies while considering the safety of the methods of production and the nutritional suitability of the food produced. In addition, food security means that everyone always has both physical and economic access to enough food for an active, healthy life. The concept encompasses the following principles (see The First Action Plan for Food and Nutrition Policy, Annex 1):

- The ways in and means by which food is produced and distributed respect the natural processes of the earth and are thus sustainable.
- Both the production and consumption of food are grounded in and governed by social values that are just and equitable as well as moral and ethical.
- The ability to acquire food is assured.

- The food itself is nutritionally adequate and personally and culturally acceptable.
- The food is obtained in a manner that upholds human dignity.

Food production and health policies

In the early to mid-20th century, food policy focused on two sets of factors: those affecting the capacity to increase food output and those ensuring adequate food distribution. To the extent that public health policies were concerned with food production, the objectives were to increase the abundance of food and to improve access to it throughout the population, primarily in response to the prevailing deficiency diseases and outright hunger among lower-income households. Both WHO and FAO, which were established in the reconstruction period following the Second World War, adopted these approaches. Food was supposed to be plentiful and cheap.

In the latter half of the 20th century, diseases linked to nutrient deficiency were being replaced by those linked to nutrient or dietary imbalances, especially in western Europe (see Chapter 1). Public policy emphasized health education and the distribution of messages to encourage individuals to alter their eating and other lifestyle patterns: encouraging healthier choices. Few attempts were made to review strategies for producing and distributing food.

More recently, food production policies have begun to be reconsidered. As reflected in the international resolutions in Agenda 21 *(1)*, endorsed by the 1992 United Nations Conference on Environment and Development, and in subsequent statements, the relationship between agricultural production and its impact on the surrounding environment is receiving new and more urgent attention. With growing populations and limited land surface, the need to take an ecologically integrated view of food production is gaining ground with policy-makers.

Health and the environment

In an international workshop on ecology and health, WHO recognized the need for closer analysis of the links between the maintenance of ecological integrity and the maintenance of human health *(2)*. The participants recognized that:

- human populations depend on healthy ecosystems;
- where local populations have lost their ecological integrity, as in urban areas, they depend on healthy ecosystems elsewhere to support them; and
- present demands on the ecosphere exceed its capacity and therefore cannot be sustained in the long run.

The participants noted a broad range of concerns: loss of biodiversity, desertification and ecological degradation, water and air pollution, the social and psychological effects of depleted environments, and issues of social justice and human rights and food production. Others have raised similar concerns about the growth of trade in food and the risks of reduced biodiversity and increased ecological damage and subsequent threats to food security and nutritional health *(3–5)*.

The understanding of the relationship between food and health is considerably more complex than just a few decades ago. Evidence is accumulating that the nature of food production is inherently able to influence health, as discussed in this chapter.

The policies adopted in the 20th century were designed to improve food supplies and prevent ill health and succeeded in increasing the quantities of food produced. These same policies are now seen as potential causes of ill health. Agricultural policies that increased the yield of food are now criticized for failing to ensure environmental sustainability, for jeopardizing food safety and for neglecting food quality, especially nutritional quality (Table 3.1).

Table 3.1. Changing understanding of food and nutrition security

Term	20th-century model	21st-century model
Food security	Abundance of food through: • increased yields • increased global trading • processing and storage techniques	Sustainable production methods: • reduced input • ecologically sensitive production Reduced risk of foodborne hazards
Nutrition security	Public health dietary targets Health education messages	Production to meet dietary needs More equal access to food Control of misleading messages

In 1998, Hartwig de Haen, Assistant Director-General of FAO said *(6)*:

> Globally there is enough food to feed the world, but it is not equally distributed and many people do not have the means to buy it. … Even where food supplies are adequate at the national level, access to food is often a serious problem. Within countries and even within households, food is not always equally distributed. To ensure nutritional well being, every individual must have access at all times to sufficient supplies of a variety of safe, good-quality foods.

Poverty reduces access to adequate food supplies. Under Agenda 21 *(1)*, countries are committed to reducing poverty and social inequality. Food and health policies need to be formulated to ensure that food supplies are both adequate and equitably distributed, so that everyone can enjoy food and nutrition security.

In 2001, the WHO Regional Committee for Europe adopted resolution EUR/RC51/R6   (http://www.euro.who.int/AboutWHO/Governance/

20011123_1, accessed 20 January 2003), which recognized the links between poverty and ill health and emphasized the responsibility of the health sector "to contribute to the reduction of poverty, as part of comprehensive multisectoral efforts". A paper on poverty and health submitted to the Committee (http://www.euro.who.int/AboutWHO/Governance/RC/RC51/20010830_5, accessed 20 January 2003) pointed out the close links between lower social status and a higher risk of both malnutrition and of nutrition-related chronic diseases, including ischaemic heart disease, stroke, high blood pressure and obesity.

This chapter focuses on the need to improve:

- food security, especially among lower-income households in both urban and rural settings;
- nutrition security through production policies that meet dietary needs; and
- the sustainability of food production for the rising urban population of the European Region.

Food and nutrition insecurity

Some people in the European Region enjoy access to shops overflowing with food from all over the globe and have money in their pockets to buy it. Others lack both advantages and endure days when they eat one meal or no meal at all. Their food supplies are insecure and are likely to be unsafe and lacking in essential nutrients. Such inequalities can be found in every country in Europe.

Defining and measuring poverty is complex, as it can be experienced in many ways, and at different levels of social organization, such as the community, the household and the individual (7). Poor people experience insecure income, lack of or poor quality of food and poor quality of shelter and clothing. They have few household assets (such as furnishings and implements) and few productive assets (such as tools and land). These conditions create difficulty maintaining health and wellbeing, and increase dependence, feelings of helplessness and vulnerability to crime and antisocial behaviour. Poor households lack collective means to provide for children and support networks, and depend on outsiders, especially the public sector. Poor communities lack infrastructure, have few services, and show instability and disunity.

Poverty in Europe

The CCEE and NIS have experienced a startling economic decline: between the late 1980s and the mid-1990s, the numbers of people in poverty rose from an estimated 14 million to 168 million: 40% of the population (8). Among these were 50 million children. These figures are based on measures of absolute poverty in terms of the purchasing power of household income.

Measures of absolute poverty

The United Nations Development Programme has estimated the proportion of the population living in poverty in most countries in the European Region. Fig. 3.1 and 3.2 show the proportion of the population living below absolute levels of income defined in US dollars, and Fig. 3.3 shows estimates of the proportion living below locally defined poverty lines.

The World Bank *(11)* has estimated that more than 50 million children in the European Region live in low-income households, with nearly 20 million in extreme poverty, defined as less than US $2.15 per child per day.

Measures of absolute poverty are useful for comparing countries but indicate little about inequality within a country. For this task, measures of relative poverty and distribution of income are more accurate. A common measure is the Gini coefficient, which indicates the unequal distribution of national income among the population. A country with absolute equality of income would have a Gini coefficient of 0, and a country with gross inequality would have a Gini coefficient approaching 1. In the eastern half of the Region, the Gini coefficient rose strongly from 1989 to 1999: by 20–40% in Bulgaria, Poland, Romania and the Russian Federation *(13)*.

Fig. 3.1. Proportion of the population in selected CCEE and NIS with personal income below US $4.30 per day, latest available years

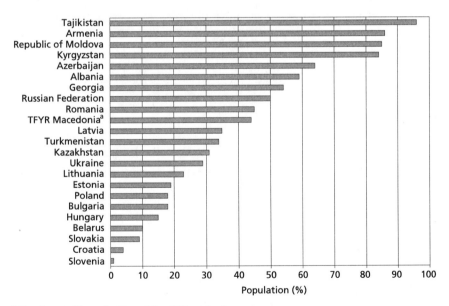

[a] The former Yugoslav Republic of Macedonia.

Note: The Czech Republic and Slovenia have values below 1%.

Sources: Human development report 2000 (9), Human development report 2001 (10), World development report 2000–2001 (11) and Falkingham *(12)*.

Fig. 3.2. Proportion of the population in selected western European
countries with personal income below US $14.40 per day,
latest available years

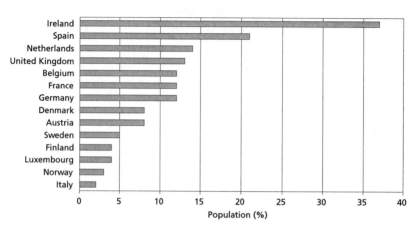

*Sources: Human development report 2000 (9), Human development report 2001
(10), World development report 2000–2001 (11)* and Falkingham *(12).*

Fig. 3.3. Proportion of the population in selected European countries
below the national poverty line, latest available years

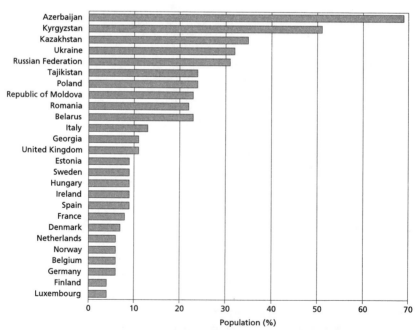

*Sources: Human development report 2000 (9), Human development report 2001
(10), World development report 2000–2001 (11)* and Falkingham *(12).*

A high level of relative poverty or income inequality may imply a high level of social exclusion. For example, low-income families may not be able to afford to participate in activities enjoyed by other families in the same culture or even the same neighbourhood. These may include food- and health-related activities such as inviting friends or neighbours to share meals, using a car to go shopping, eating in restaurants or taking exercise.

When poverty leads to suboptimal nutrition or outright hunger, the effects can harm both the individual and the community. Children may not be able to concentrate on school lessons and may disrupt their classes. Women may give birth to sickly children requiring medical attention and long-term care. Poorly fed men and women may lack the energy to improve family income by seeking work, perpetuating the problems of poverty. These problems affect large numbers of families: 26 million people in the CCEE and NIS are estimated to be undernourished *(14)*.

Agricultural workers tend to have higher poverty rates than industrial workers, approaching those found among unemployed households in some EU countries (Fig. 3.4). Agricultural workers also face declining employment

Fig. 3.4. Proportion of households in relative poverty among unemployed people and agricultural workers in selected EU countries and the EU as a whole, latest figures available in 1996

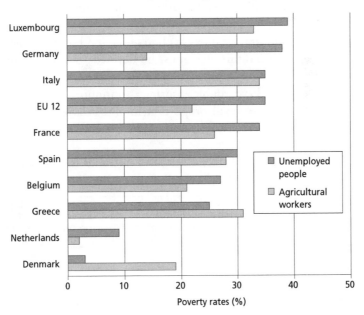

Poverty rates (%)

Note: EU 12 is the average for the 12 EU countries before Austria, Finland and Sweden became members in 1995.
Source: adapted from *Social portrait of Europe (15)*.

prospects as farms are merged and production intensified through capital investment (see p. 204–205). Poverty is also prevalent in rural areas in the CCEE and NIS. The relative rates of poverty in rural areas range from 2% higher than the compared national average in Tajikistan to 60% higher in Poland *(13)*.

Data for the EU *(16)* also show relatively high poverty rates among about 36% of households with single parents and young children and about 30% of households with single people living alone who are younger than 30 years or older than 65.

Food insecurity

Classic measures of national food security examine the supply of staple foods grown in the country as a percentage of the population's need for these staples. This reflects the country's ability to feed itself. National food security is often approximated by measures of cereal production as a proportion of cereal consumption.

Food insecurity can thus be measured at the national level as the proportion of cereal imports as a percentage of consumption, although this raises some questions. Apart from whether cereals are a good approximation of staple food supplies, there is the question of whether a national figure for food security can adequately reflect the number of people who may find it hard to obtain enough food. National production and consumption measures for staple foods do not necessarily reflect the distribution of food or access to food at the household level.

An alternative indicator is a proxy for household food security: the proportion of household expenditure that must be devoted to food to ensure adequate consumption. A high proportion of income on food indicates that households are likely to have trouble ensuring a continuing supply of adequate food and nourishment. A small proportion implies relatively easy access to food. Table 3.2 contrasts the two measures of insecurity.

Table 3.2. Indicators of household and national food insecurity
for countries in the European Region

Country	Household food insecurity: average expenditure on food as a percentage of total household expenditure *(17)*	National food insecurity: cereal imports as a percentage of national consumption[a] *(18)*
Tajikistan[b]	75	50
Uzbekistan	71	31
Azerbaijan	61	29
Romania	51	–6
Republic of Moldova	49	–1
Kyrgyzstan	48	9
Armenia	47	55
Yugoslavia	47	–3

Table 3.2 cont

Russian Federation	47	4
Lithuania	45	5
Latvia	44	11
Ukraine	43	−4
Bulgaria	43	−1
Bosnia and Herzegovina	41	30
Estonia	41	22
The former Yugoslav Republic of Macedonia	41	23
Hungary	40	−28
Poland	40	8
Turkey	39	5
Georgia	38	42
Greece	36	12
Ireland	35	10
Croatia	34	0
Kazakhstan	30	−52
Malta	28	_c
Slovakia	26	−11
Czech Republic	26	−5
Spain	24	24
Iceland	24	100
Portugal	24	61
Slovenia	23	48
Finland	23	−10
Israel	22	94
Italy	22	20
Germany	21	−16
Sweden	21	−17
Switzerland	19	29
Belgium	18	60
Netherlands	18	76
Denmark	18	−25
United Kingdom	18	−13
Austria	17	−7
France	17	−86
Norway	14	31
Luxembourg	13	−

[a] Negative values indicate net cereal exports.
[b] Data for Tajikistan came from Falkingham *(12)*.
[c] –: data not available.
Note: Household income and expenditure data are collected differently in different countries. The figures here are an estimate based on several years of data of the proportion of the average household budget spent on food and drink (alcoholic and non-alcoholic beverages) and on eating outside the home, when these data are available. The figures are for available years in the period 1990–1996, based on statistical information for countries in *Encyclopaedia britannica*. Data on cereals are for the period 1995–1997.

Table 3.2 shows national averages: half the population spends an even greater proportion of its income on food than the figure given. For example, the share of income spent on food in Tajikistan is 75% on average, but 60% for the richest fifth of households and 79% for the poorest fifth *(12)*. Even in western Europe the range can be broad.

Households with low incomes may have few appliances for food preparation and storage, such as a refrigerator or cooker. This may lead to the purchase of processed foods with a long shelf life, rather than fresh, perishable foods for home cooking.

Further, household food purchases may be insufficient for all family members to eat an optimum diet *(19,20)*. As a result, some – often the women in the household – may get inadequate nourishment *(21)*.

Although low-income householders are usually very efficient in obtaining staple foods for the small amount of money they have, such families may spend less on protective foods such as fruits and vegetables and more on energy-dense food *(22)*. In contrast, higher-income families eat more fruit and vegetables and spend a smaller share of their total income on food (see Fig. 1.33, p. 68) *(23)*. In countries with large supplies of mass-produced foods, the cost per unit of food energy is lowest for fat, oil, white bread and sugary foods.

Cheap food energy

Inexpensive food energy is less likely to meet dietary guidelines.

In developed economies, the cheapest sources of energy are usually processed foods with high levels of fat and refined carbohydrate and low levels of protective nutrients. Fresh fruits and vegetables are expensive in relation to the food energy they provide (Table 3.3).

People in more extreme poverty, such as that found in central Asia, may not be able to afford processed foods, and rely more on home-grown produce. Figures from Tajikistan show that, of the poorest fifth of households, 78% do not own refrigerators and 65% do not own electric or gas stoves, but 83% have access to garden plots for vegetable growing *(12)*. A lack of storage facilities prevents the keeping of perishable foods: in Tajikistan the poorest fifth of households keep in store barely 800 g of vegetables per person, compared with over 2300 g per person among all other households.

Food insecurity can thus selectively reduce the consumption of protective foods, such as fruits and vegetables. This problem may be alleviated, however, if householders have access to garden plots and smallholdings for domestic and local market production. In several NIS, more than half of households possess land. In Kazakhstan, one third of food is produced at home *(25)*. In the early 1990s, home production rose steeply in Romania (see p. 171).

Table 3.3. Retail price of food energy in the United Kingdom, March 2000

Food	Price (£ per 420 kJ(100 kcal))
Fresh oranges	0.28
Processed orange juice	0.19
Soft drink	0.12
Strawberries	0.98
Strawberry jam	0.11
Strawberry-flavoured ice cream	0.08
Frozen white fish	0.98
Frozen fish finger sticks	0.22
Fresh pork	0.27
Pork sausages	0.09
Whole-grain bread	0.05
White bread	0.03
Ready-washed watercress	8.25
Fresh tomatoes	1.00
Salad lettuce	0.45
Margarine	0.02
Sweet biscuits	0.02
Table sugar	0.01
Cooking oil	0.01

Source: adapted from Food Commission *(24).*

Reducing inequality in food and nutrition

Household food security and the nutritional security of family members depend on many factors: macroeconomic policies, local accessibility and affordability, and the influences on food choice, which are determined by both social influences and individual preferences. Fig. 3.5 identifies these influences, and shows how nutrition security is affected by international, national and local policies, rather than being a simple matter of individual lifestyle choices.

Improving nutrition security: local initiatives

For centuries, religious, voluntary and neighbourhood organizations have helped low-income families to gain access to healthier food, shelter and work and thus to promote social cohesion and preserve social capital. Such local initiatives work for:

- empowerment, by increasing people's control over local decision-making;
- increasing choice, by providing additional services, such as transport, retailing and catering, at the community level;
- improving income, by improving the uptake of welfare services and providing debt counselling, low-interest loans, job-application support and child care;

- improving skills and knowledge, by organizing demonstrations, discussion groups and recipe exchanges; and
- encouraging partnerships, by involving retailers and planning authorities in local decisions on food provision and assisting small retailers in isolated areas.

The WHO Regional Office for Europe produced the Urban and Peri-urban Food and Nutrition Action Plan *(26)*, which contains elements for community action to promote social cohesion and to reduce inequality through local food production for local consumption.

Fig. 3.5. Influences on food choices

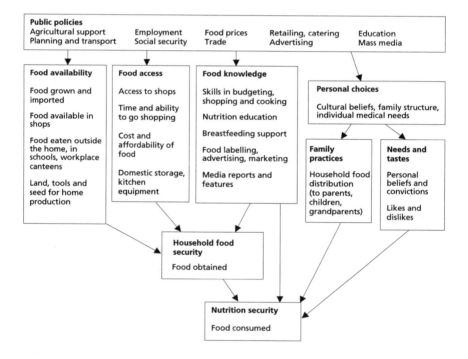

Evaluating the effectiveness of such initiatives requires tools that are sensitive to political and social processes and consider nutritional indices and the incidence of foodborne diseases. A review of factors affecting the success of such projects *(27)* acknowledged that participants may have difficulty determining measurable outcomes and noted that the chance of success was greater if the projects were securely funded and the people involved were well trained.

In some European countries, the private sector provides food aid in the form of food banks: schemes to collect, store and distribute to people in need the surplus food provided by food manufacturers, retailers and caterers. Surplus food resulting from the EU Common Agriculture Policy, such as beef and butter, has been distributed through charitable agencies, schools and hospitals. Although such schemes may appear an attractive means of providing food to many people who are least able to afford it, they have been criticized for reasons similar to those used to criticize food aid to underdeveloped countries. Such food aid may institutionalize a culture of dependence, fail to address the wasteful creation of surpluses and the inequitable distribution of food, and marginalize the recipients within an affluent society *(28,29)*. Although acceptable as a short-term palliative measure in times of crisis, food aid cannot be relied on to ensure nutrition security.

Improving nutrition security: national strategies

Local initiatives cannot by themselves provide the comprehensive coverage or fully integrated policies of the sort indicated in Fig. 3.5. Such solutions are better sought at the national level.

A review of national strategies on household food and nutrition security in the United Kingdom *(30)* emphasized the need for a coordinated approach involving several ministerial departments, including agriculture, environment and rural affairs, health, social welfare, education, employment and economic affairs. The problems that needed to be addressed across departments included minimum wage legislation, unemployment support and measures to create jobs, child care and support for working women, housing and fuel policies and insufficient education on food topics in schools. In addition, a national approach to food and nutrition insecurity requires integrating centralized, national policies with regional authorities' policies, especially measures related to transport, planning, food control and food distribution, such as retailing and catering.

National efforts are also appropriate for collecting and evaluating data. As indicated in previous chapters, there are considerable gaps in the data on incidence of foodborne diseases and on the influence of agricultural policies on household food security and individual nutrition security. The surveillance of food availability and nutrition status should be improved to monitor the conditions and outcomes in households vulnerable to poverty and inequality. Further, few studies have attempted to analyse trends over time for specific groups such as single parents, migrant families or older people on low incomes. More attention should be paid to how people manage when their social and economic circumstances deteriorate *(31)*. Prices and price differentials between foods need to be researched and monitored. Where appropriate, this information can be fed into the formulas needed for minimum income legislation, family budget standards and welfare benefit levels *(32,33)*.

In addition, national policies affect the provision of food eaten outside the home, especially in institutions under government control, such as schools, hospitals, prisons and military bases. National and local policies can affect catering in the high street, the workplace and in private institutions. In these situations, decision-makers should consider public health guidance on safe and healthy diets and the use of pricing policies and other incentives to encourage them. In Finland, for example, all meals provided by local authorities include vegetables. Mass catering is an excellent means of influencing food intake in Finland, since the average Finn eats about 125 meals per year outside the home. The intake of both fruits and vegetables has more than doubled in Finland in the last decade (see Chapter 1).

Finally, local and national strategies need to be developed to improve levels of physical activity. Barriers include the lack of facilities, such as safe walking and cycling routes, unpleasant or hazardous environments, lack of shelter from poor weather and the cost of using leisure facilities *(34)*. In addition, people with disabilities, who may be living on low incomes, are less likely to take part in physical activities *(31)*.

Low-income households may have more difficulty than the better off in gaining access to rural environments for leisure. The cost of having and fuelling a car, or of public transport for several family members may prohibit those on a tight budget from leaving their immediate neighbourhood for leisure purposes. Hiring a video would be less expensive.

Current trends in food supply

Modern food production has been based on increasing intensification and capitalization of the process, the concentration of ownership in fewer hands and a resulting reduction in retail price. While this has increased abundance and reduced cost, recent concern about the food safety risks of production methods and evidence of environmental damage resulting from modern agricultural practices have renewed interest in less intensive, less environmentally harmful forms of agriculture.

This section looks more closely at these contradictory tendencies and their implications for food and nutrition security.

Modern food production and distribution

Contemporary methods of food production resulted from scientific developments in agricultural research: the genetic selection of crop strains and animal breeds; the application of nutrients to crops and animal feed; the increase of yield through the use of biochemicals, such as pesticides and growth enhancers; and the use of veterinary medicine to prevent disease outbreaks in groups of confined animals and to promote their growth and productivity.

These technical developments have been matched by increased financial investment in farming and food production to gain from economies of scale. This has led to reduced labour costs; increased mechanization; the development of monoculture cropping patterns; increased field, herd and flock sizes; reduced crop biodiversity; longer transport distances; increased food processing and use of additives; greater concentration of retailing outlets; and increased marketing and advertising activity.

These are the trends throughout the industrialized world, not only in Europe. National governments have made policies to support farming and food production as a means of securing food supplies and preventing economic depression in rural areas. These policies have proved highly successful in increasing the quantity of food produced. The yields of cereals, milk and beef have almost doubled in the last four decades (http://apps.fao.org/page/collections?subset=agriculture, accessed 20 January 2003).

In the EU, farming support has taken the form of the Common Agricultural Policy (CAP), which costs the 15 EU countries about €40 billion annually. CAP has consisted of price support to strengthen markets and encourage production. For some products, such as milk and sugar, market support is given up to a certain total quantity of output (national quotas). For others, such as fruits, vegetables and fish, CAP has subsidized the withdrawal of products from the market to maintain high prices. These policies have been subject to several reviews and a series of reforms, and changes are being made to redirect support towards other objectives, such as reducing the intensification of animal production, improving environmental protection and developing rural economies. (For more on CAP and public health, see pp. 183, 223–224.)

Further, national governments provide subsidies and tax exemptions for transporting food and animal feed by road and air freight. Food and feed travel greater distances than in the past, as animal feed companies, food-processing companies, food retail chains and other purchasers in the food chain seek the most economical mass producers. The most economical producers tend to operate on a large scale, often overseas in regions with relatively low costs for land, labour or environmental protection.

In terms of food security, increased capitalization of the food chain reduces the number of local and small food businesses; it increases the concentration of business in the hands of fewer operators, who look across the globe for low-cost, large-scale suppliers. This process has already reduced the number of small farms and food producers in western Europe and can be expected to affect the CCEE and NIS. Small producers, such as family farms, and small processors, such as local abattoirs or vineyards or specialist meat processors or cheese makers, find their markets undercut by larger producers with reduced costs. Concentration in one part of the food chain can affect the viability of small businesses in another. For example, in retail and to some extent catering (such as fast food), concentration into fewer, more powerful companies can reduce the marketing opportunities for small businesses and the prices they can ask.

Within food manufacturing, the more traditional methods of canning, dehydrating, curing and pickling have been joined in the last few decades by new technologies for processing food and making it attractive to customers. These include the mechanical recovery of meat fragments, the high-pressure extrusion of starch pastes, and the use of food additives to enhance the taste, texture or appearance of processed foods, of modified-atmosphere packaging, and of cook-chill, cook-freeze and *sous-vide* preservation. Much of the drive towards increased sales of processed foods has relied on the nutrition transition: the shifting patterns of consumption that occur when disposable income increases in a population (see later in this chapter and Chapter 1, p. 17–19).

The increased concentration of food retailing in the hands of fewer companies leads to a loss of small independent traders and a reduction in street markets. The negative effects fall primarily on people whose access to retail outlets is thereby reduced: those living in rural or small towns that lose local shops and those without independent transport, who cannot easily travel to the nearest or cheapest retailer.

Economies in transition

Farm restructuring in the CCEE was expected to improve productivity and efficiency, mainly as a result of improved incentives from competitive markets *(35)*, but has not done so.

Following the dissolution of collective farms in the CCEE and NIS in the 1990s, much of the land reverted to ownership by families or cooperatives, as exemplified by Romania (Table 3.4).

Table 3.4. Agricultural land holdings in Romania, 1997

Owners	Number	Average size (ha)	Share of total agricultural land (%)
Commercial companies	490	3 657	12
Agricultural societies (cooperatives of members and non-member workers)	3 875	451	12
Farmer associations (informal cooperatives)	12 089	103	8
Families	3 500 000	2	59

Source: Rizov et al. *(36)*.

Limited access to capital and problems in gaining a market for their goods have hindered small-scale entrepreneur farmers from fully using their capabilities. Providing appropriate support would help these labour-intensive operations to increase their productivity, and would contribute to the development of surrounding rural areas *(36)*.

Small, family farms can play an important role in ensuring food security. An analysis of the technical efficiency of different farming systems in Bulgaria and Hungary *(35)* noted that family farms were distinctly more efficient than corporate farms in crop production using conventional measures, although efficiency in dairy farming differed little.

After 1991, former state farms in the Russian Federation were turned into commercial or cooperative farms but lacked investment. Food production declined by over 20% from 1991 to 1994, while industrial production fell by 44%. The rapid growth in small-scale family farming was the main reason why food production did not decline as rapidly. By 1994, family farms produced 89% of potatoes, 68% of vegetables, 44% of cattle and poultry and 40% of milk in the Russian Federation *(37)*.

Household production can be valuable during times of food insecurity. In Romania, the proportion of food produced at home by households with at least one person in employment increased from 21% to 31% from 1990 to 1992 *(25)*. In peasant households, the proportion of home-produced food rose from 68% to 80% in the same period.

The food industry in the CCEE and NIS has followed the patterns experienced by other parts of these countries' economies *(38)*. At the start of the transition, production was predominantly in the hands of large state-owned monopolies. Efficiency was low and methods relatively primitive. With a lack of competition and a focus on volume of output, product quality was low. These products found a market either domestically or in other CCEE and NIS, which comprised a net food importer as a whole. According to projections by the International Food Policy Research Institute, the CCEE and NIS will become major net exporters of cereal by the year 2020 *(39)*.

The privatization of the food industry in the CCEE is now nearly complete. In Poland, which was relatively slow to privatize, 85% of food industry production had transferred to private ownership by 1997, and 88% of food employment was in private enterprises a year later *(40)*. Nevertheless, privatization is only the first stage in establishing a modern food-processing industry. Restructuring is needed because the fall in agricultural output during transition left considerable excess capacity in first-stage processing such as grain milling, slaughterhouses and dairies. Significant investment is needed to replace obsolete machinery and to raise quality standards. The spread of western supermarkets in the CCEE and NIS may mean that consistent, high standards will be required of suppliers, although it may also undermine the marketing systems used by smaller producers.

Foreign investment has been concentrated in the sectors of the food industry with high value added, such as beverages and confectionery. This is where margins and demand growth are higher and the multinationals' expertise in production technology, product innovation and marketing can best be used. For example, in Poland in 1998, foreign investment was heavily concentrated in confectionery, beer, mineral waters and soft drinks, with large investment by food companies headquartered in the United States and western Europe *(40)*.

The areas with the greatest problems are unlikely to attract such investment. Thus, primary food processing is dominated by older production technologies, with low margins and poor growth prospects, which in turn limits the expansion of local production. The investment there is will probably come from western European food companies with modern techniques that demand uniform production quality and economies of scale *(39)*.

Ten eastern countries of the Region will join the EU, but CAP cannot simply be extended to them. The opportunity arises for new and more appropriate policies to be applied. In meetings between the EC and agricultural interests from accession countries, Franz Fischler, European Commissioner for Agriculture, Rural Development and Fisheries, has suggested initiatives to encourage sustainable agricultural practices and to supply the rising demand for organically produced food.

The development of a new set of agricultural policies for an enlarged EU, which can assist in these changes and encourage sustainable practices, would help countries meet their commitments under Agenda 21. Again, family farms may prove more responsive to such subsidies: in larger enterprises, especially those with absentee landlords, agricultural subsidies may be diverted to non-agricultural uses, limiting the social and environmental benefit they are designed to help provide.

Food distribution

Global trade in agricultural products has increased rapidly in the last few decades. In the last five decades, the volume of agricultural exports has risen by 550% and total agricultural production, 320% *(41)*. The difference shows that an increasing proportion of food is grown for export rather than local consumption. The volume of exports has increased significantly, but their value has increased even more dramatically, rising an estimated 1730% in the period, indicating a significant increase in the per-unit value of the foodstuffs being shipped, as a result of refrigeration techniques and faster delivery using air transport.

At an estimated US $544 billion in 1999, the international trade in agricultural goods comprises virtually half (48.4%) of total world trade in primary products. The European Region accounts for nearly half of all the world's agricultural exports and more than half of the agricultural imports. World trade in food products, excluding animal feed and other agricultural products, was worth US $437 billion in 1999, and the European Region was similarly dominant in both exports and imports (Table 3.5).

The transport of goods on roads in Europe has been increasing rapidly, especially in the EU, where transport increased from 420 billion tonne-km in

Table 3.5. European trade as a proportion of world trade
in agricultural (and especially food) products

Area	Proportion of world trade (%)			
	Agricultural exports	Agricultural imports	Food exports	Food imports
Western Europe	41	46	46	47
CCEE and NIS	4	5	4	6
Rest of world	55	49	50	45
Total	100	100	100	100

Source: International trade statistics (41).

1970 to 1318 billion tonne-km in 1999 *(42)*. Of this, food, animal feed and live animals accounted for about one fifth of national road transport and nearly one third of international road transport; in both cases, these products have comprised an increasing proportion of road-hauled goods over the last decade *(43)*. The EC estimates that 32% of road-hauled goods in the EU are agricultural products, such as food, feed and animals.

In terms of food security, it can be argued that increasing trade increases access to food by the world's population by widening the distribution of food crops and the variety of foods available from different regions. Further, trade is assumed to create wealth for traders, including primary producers, and a rise in wealth improves access to food supplies and the diet.

Several problems associated with increased food trading, however, may threaten the sustainability and security of the food supply. These include the selection of the commodities traded; the concentration of trade among a few dominant multinationals; the effects of transport, storage and packaging on the environment; and the need for traceability in the food chain. For the primary growers and producers, global trading provides markets in distant lands, but just as easily removes them when purchasers change their requirements, the relative values of currencies change or international political circumstances impinge on trade.

Retailing

The European Region shows two trends in general retailing. In one, largely in western Europe, large stores, serving more people and combined into single-company chains, are gradually replacing small, often specialist retail outlets. A few Mediterranean countries still show the more traditional patterns, with less than 100 people per general store, such as Spain (59 people per store) and Greece (66 people) *(44)*. The second pattern is largely derived from the formerly state-controlled economies in CCEE and NIS, in which a small number of retailers served large numbers of people, sometimes over 200 per store: 233 people per store in Estonia and 465 in the Russian Federation *(44)*.

North-western Europe in particular has seen an increasing concentration of retailers, especially food retailers. A few chains of large stores have replaced a larger number of small, independent shops and market stalls. In the 1990s, this concentration caused a dramatic reduction in the number of food outlets in the EU *(45)*.

These changes are reflected in the degree of concentration of retailing. Fig 3.6 shows the estimated proportion of retail sales controlled by the largest five firms – a standard means of estimating concentration of ownership – for several European countries *(46)*.

Fig. 3.6. Shares of food sales controlled by the five largest companies in selected European countries

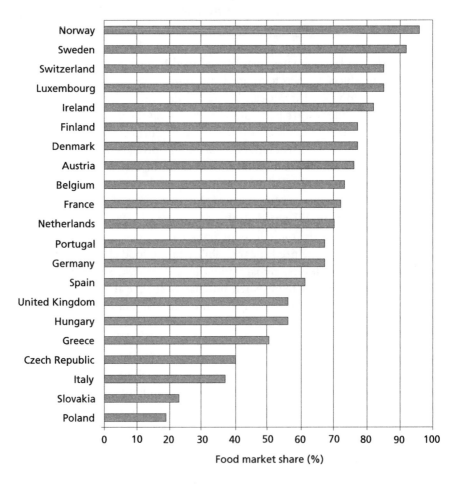

Source: Combined food market share of the top five grocery retailers in selected European countries (46).

The high concentration of ownership has implications for a secure supply of nourishing food: it may affect the prices and range of foods available and the accessibility of stores to consumers. Several studies have noted the policy of some large chains to adjust their prices according to store location. This includes reducing the range of foods available and increasing the price of socalled healthy (low-fat or low-sugar) versions of foods in areas where low-income families predominate (47).

A decline in the numbers of stores can lead to reduced access, especially for people with limited means of transport. Food deserts (areas with very few food retailers) can be found in some urban and many rural areas. The EU reviewed the problems faced by small retailers in rural areas in 1999, with recommendations to encourage greater investment in modernization in rural retailing and to focus public resources on activities with a high potential to create jobs (48).

Sustaining the European Region's food supplies

The massive increases in yield, the global trading of food commodities and the concentration of ownership of food distribution raise questions about the nature and sustainability of food production in the Region. European research, some of which is summarized here, is beginning to explore the potential costs, including damage to health and the environment.

Hidden costs of modern food supplies

An analysis of the impact of modern agriculture suggests that food production entails costs not borne by the producer and hence not reflected in the price of the goods. These costs (called externalities) include damage to health and the environment. Other sectors of the economy bear these costs. Health costs fall on individuals, their families and health and social services, as well as on the community through lost productivity. The costs of environmental pollution may be borne by, for example, water suppliers, who must remove some of the pollutants from water. Many environmental costs, such as lost amenities, soil erosion and lost biodiversity, are losses of natural capital that can only be recovered at some expense in the future.

Pretty et al. (49,50) have examined some of the externalities in modern farming (49):

> In practice, there is [sic] little or no agreed data on the economic cost of agricultural externalities. This is partly because the costs are highly dispersed and affect many sectors of economies. It is also necessary to know about the value of nature's goods and services, and what happens when these largely unmarketed goods are lost. The current system of economic calculations grossly underestimates the current and future value of natural capital.

The more obvious costs – such as the impact of pesticide use and the effect on environmental air quality and ozone depletion – have been estimated. Table 3.6 presents figures for the United Kingdom and Germany.

Table 3.6. Annual external costs of modern agriculture in the United Kingdom and Germany, 1996 prices

Cost category	Costs (£ million)	
	United Kingdom	Germany
Damage to natural capital		
Water:		
• pesticides in sources of drinking-water	120	58
• nitrate, phosphate and soil in sources of drinking-water	71	NA[a]
• zoonoses (especially *Cryptosporidium*) in sources of drinking-water	23	NA
• eutrophication, pollution incidents, effects on fish and costs of monitoring	17	33
Air: emissions of methane, ammonia, nitrous oxide (N_2O) and carbon dioxide (CO_2)[b]	1112	1125
Soil:		
• off-site damage caused by erosion, flooding, blocked ditches and lost water storage, damage to industry, navigation and fisheries	14	NA
• organic matter and CO_2 losses from soils	82	NA
Biodiversity and landscape:		
• biodiversity and wildlife losses	25	4
• hedgerows and drystone wall losses	99	NA
• bee colony losses and damage to domestic pets	2	1
Damage to human health		
Pesticides	1	9
Microorganisms and disease agents:		
• bacterial and viral outbreaks in food	169	NA
• BSE and vCJD	607	NA
• overuse of antibiotics	NA	NA
Total	2342	1230

Cost category	United Kingdom (£)	Germany (£)
Total cost per ha arable and grassland	208	71
Cost per ha arable land only	228	166
Cost per kg pesticide active ingredient	8.6	3.9

[a] NA: not available.
[b] Costs in Germany do not include data for ammonia, which accounts for 4% of the cost in the United Kingdom.

Sources: Pretty et al. *(49,50)* and Fleischer & Waibel *(51)*.

The data in Table 3.6 include only the costs to the rest of society that result from the actions of farmers, not additional private costs borne by farmers. These include costs arising from increased pest or weed resistance from the overuse of pesticides. Further, unmeasured distributional problems remain: for example, insect outbreaks arising from pesticide overuse can affect all farmers, even those not using pesticides.

In addition, Table 3.6 does not consider the environmental goods that may arise from farming practices but do not give rise to a monetary input to offset the costs. These might include measures for environmental protection, the training of farm workers, the preservation of farming skills and other forms of non-financial capital (for more on these forms of capital, see pp. 203–204).

Environmental degradation

The EU now gives considerable attention to the environmental consequences of agricultural practices and the need for reform. Policy changes in the EC level indicate a willingness to accept responsibility for the loss of landscape, biodiversity and damage to soil, water and air that have occurred (52):

> Technological developments, and commercial considerations to maximise returns and to minimise costs, have given rise to a marked intensification of agriculture in the last 40 years. The role of the common agricultural policy (CAP) in contributing to intensification has also to be mentioned.
>
> A high level of price support favoured intensive agriculture and an increasing use of fertilisers and pesticides. This resulted in pollution of water and soils and damage done to certain eco-systems; resulting high treatment costs had to be borne by consumers or taxpayers.
>
> Among the environmental developments, which the CAP helped to speed up ... [were] the destruction of hedgerows, stonewalls, and the ditches and the draining of wet lands [which] have contributed to the loss of valuable habitats for many birds, plants and other species. Intensification in certain areas led to an excessive use of water resources and to increased soil erosion.

These problems are not confined to the affluent economies of western Europe. The intensification of agriculture to increase output in the CCEE and NIS has also caused unwanted side effects. An FAO review (53) indicated that the environmental problems in these countries that result from intensive agricultural methods threaten the sustainability of the production process (Table 3.7).

An analysis by the Swedish Farming Federation of the environmental costs of milk and meat production traced the contributions to soil acidification and to eutrophication (oxygen depletion in lakes and reservoirs following fertilizer and slurry pollution) at various stages in the food chain (54). In milk production, the study found that 90% of acidification and 80% of eutrophication were linked to ammonia produced in manure on dairy farms. The same applied to beef production, but in much greater quantities (54).

Table 3.7. Environmental problems from intensive agriculture in the
CCEE and NIS, expressed by participants at an FAO conference, 1999

Country	Main environmental problems	Exacerbating hazards	Elements promoting sustainability
Bulgaria	Soil acidification Decreasing soil fertility	Restoration of individual property rights	Good natural and human resources
Croatia	Soil degradation	Pressure to increase production Lack of awareness	Low level of contamination Favourable legislative basis
Czech Republic	Water pollution Soil degradation	Property rights do not favour conservation	Nongovernmental organizations EU integration policy
Estonia	Groundwater pollution	Privatization of land	Supportive economic regulations Increase in quality of management
Hungary	Liquid-manure ponds Old machines and technology	Lack of awareness Lack of capital	Pressure from the EU High level of education
Latvia	Heritage of former period	Lack of economic basis for sustainable agriculture	Good, diverse natural resources
Lithuania	Degradation of drainage systems Afforestation	Lack of financial resources	Culture, ethics
Poland	Soil erosion Water pollution	Consumer habits Lack of institutional interest in sustainability	Transition process
Romania	Soil degradation Water pollution	Weak legislation Lack of policy coherence	Nongovernmental organizations International agreements
Slovakia	Industrial emission Soil erosion Soil acidification	Financial limitations Conflicts between industrial and environmental objectives	Increase in gross domestic product Good agricultural policy
Ukraine	Loss of natural fertility	Lack of national policy	Privatization of land Ecological and economic regulations

Source: Proceedings of the First Workshop of the Central and Eastern Europe Sustainable Agriculture Network, FAO, Godollo, Hungary, 2–7 March 1999 (53).

Energy

Energy is critical for food production. Agenda 21 *(1)* is a comprehensive international framework and action programme for sustainable development, and many sections address energy. It describes a programme whose objectives are:

a. Not later than the year 2000, to initiate and encourage a process of environmentally sound energy transition in rural communities, from unsustainable energy sources, to structured and diversified energy sources by making available alternative new and renewable sources of energy;

b. To increase the energy inputs available for rural household and agro-industrial needs through planning and appropriate technology transfer and development;

c. To implement self-reliant rural programmes favouring sustainable development of renewable energy sources and improved energy efficiency.

As rural communities intensify their agricultural production, they tend to increase their dependence on external energy sources. Modern agriculture relies substantially on fossil fuels. Nitrogen fertilizers, feed concentrates, pumped irrigation and power machinery such as tractors account for much of the energy used on farms. Additional energy is needed to transport farm produce and inputs such as animal feed, and to process, package and distribute food.

Kooijman *(55)* compared the energy used for packaged vegetables with that used for fresh, minimally packaged vegetables. Fresh food from local sources used the least energy (less than 10 MJ per kg), and vegetables in aluminium cans the most (40 MJ per kg).

The form of farming system can significantly affect the energy used to produce food. An analysis of apple orchards tended by conventional, organic or an intermediate, integrated pest management system, showed the organic system to have the highest output-to-input ratio (1.18), 7% better than the conventional system and 5% better than the integrated system *(56)*. Other comparisons of energy input in conventional and organic arable, vegetable and animal production have shown a consistent advantage for organic production systems (Fig 3.7) *(57)*.

Fig. 3.7. Energy used in conventional and organic agricultural systems

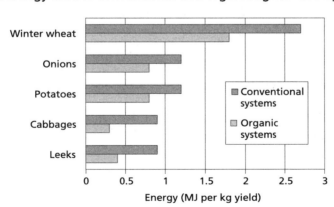

Source: adapted from Agricultural Development and Advisory Service *(57)*.

Water

Virtually all food production is based on the growth of plants, which depend on water. A corn crop that produces 7.5 tonnes of grain per ha needs about 5 million litres of water per ha during the growing season. Different crops need different amounts of water, from 500 litres per kg potatoes to 100 000 litres per kg beef *(58)*. High-yield crops require more water than low-yield varieties, and this is one reason why the worldwide agricultural consumption of water has nearly tripled since the 1950s *(59)*.

As with the energy required to produce food, more water is required to produce meat products. Moving towards more sustainable food production implies moving away from meat production, replacing meat with products that require less water.

Climate change

A WHO review of the health effects of climate change in the European Region *(60)* noted the potential impact on food security through (see Chapter 2, p. 101):

• geographical shifts in optimum crop-growing conditions
• yield changes in crops
• reduced water resources for irrigation
• flood and storm damage
• loss of land through a rise in sea level
• salinization of coastal land.

The review also noted potential problems in marine food supplies through changes in: water temperatures and currents, flows of fresh water and nutrient circulation. Indirect effects on agriculture include changes in soil quality, in the incidence of plant diseases and in the populations of weeds and insects.

Modelling exercises assume that farmers will adapt to changes in climate by, for example, changing crop varieties or the dates of planting. Human populations would respond to significant changes in food supplies by migration. The review *(60)* expresses concern at:

> the rapid commercial and political changes that have encouraged the production of standardized crops for unseen, remote markets using large-scale, heavily mechanized agricultural production methods. This has occurred to the extent that food has gradually become an international commodity rather than a source of nutrition for local populations.

The review also notes that there may be political implications. For example, as the land suitable for the cultivation of key staple crops or productive fishing grounds change location, political conflict may arise. Similarly, the control of sources of irrigation water may cause or exacerbate political conflict, especially in semi-arid countries such as Israel or Turkey.

Climate change results in part from increasing gaseous emissions from vehicles, primarily road and air traffic. Ironically, the food trade has been a large and increasing contributor to such pollution in the last few decades (see the next section).

An analysis of the impact on climate change caused by beef and dairy production by the Swedish Dairy Association *(61)* showed that producing 1 litre milk led to the release of the equivalent of nearly 1 kg CO_2 into the atmosphere, and the production of 1 kg beef led to the emission of 14 kg CO_2 equivalent.[3] Similarly, bulk transport, the production of packaging for beef products and the packaging process also produce far more CO_2 per unit of final product than the equivalent for milk production *(61)*.

Transport of food

In a case history studying the movement of potatoes in France *(62)*, the average distance travelled by the average potato increased 43% between 1985 and 1995. Such increasing transport adds to air pollution and road hazards. It also adds to road congestion, which further increases pollution levels. Air pollution is another cost externalized from food production: borne by the community as a health cost *(63)*, not reflected in the price of the food.

External transport-related costs – costs not paid for by those creating them – are estimated to be about 10% of gross domestic product: €658 billion in western European countries *(64)*. These figures include accidents, pollution and congestion but exclude the effects on physical activity and psychosocial factors.

Transport is the dominant source of air pollution in European cities and causes substantial damage to health *(65)*. It also contributes significantly to global climate change through the release of greenhouse gases such as CO_2. Estimates suggest that transport is responsible for over 25% of CO_2 emissions in the United Kingdom *(66)*. Air transport causes the release of more CO_2 than other forms of transport per tonne of food carried. Boat and rail cause the least pollution. Estimates of the amount of CO_2 released in long-distance air freight (for example, from New Zealand to the United Kingdom) show that as much as 1 kg may be released for each 1 kg food transported *(67)*.

A detailed study of the greenhouse-gas emissions generated in the life cycle of tomatoes and carrots consumed in Sweden gave contrasting results. For carrots, emissions were lowest if the crop was produced in or near Sweden; total

---

[3] These figures assume that 1 kg methane is equivalent to 21 kg CO_2 and that 1 kg N_2O is equivalent to 310 kg CO_2.

emissions for tomatoes – which may require heated greenhouses for production in Sweden – were lower if they were grown in Spain *(68)*.

These figures imply that food production and transport policies need to be analysed carefully to minimize environmental damage. Farm products may need to bear a greater burden of their environmental costs in their market price. An increase in food transport by air and road may be unsustainable in the longer term.

Agricultural policies and diet

As the previous section indicates, agricultural policies have focused largely on increasing yields and quantities, expanding international trade and developing and concentrating the means of food distribution.

Their costs to health are more difficult to assess than those to the environment. The former include directly attributable costs, such as the effects of agricultural chemicals as residues in food or food poisoning arising from contamination (see Chapter 2).

This section looks more closely at the nutritional implications of agricultural policies that may have encouraged the production of foods in quantities that may not be best suited to optimum dietary health. For example, considerable financial encouragement has been given to the production of meat and milk, which are not only relatively expensive in environmental and financial terms but also rich in saturated fat. In so far as this policy could be justified nutritionally, it was based on the experience of dietary deficiencies and the poor health and growth of children in the 1920s and 1930s *(69)*.

Policies providing direct support

In western Europe, the largest share of CAP funds has supported cereal, meat and milk farming. About half of the cereal produced is used for animal feed (Fig. 3.8).

Payments under the various budgetary headings need to be put in the context of the overall farming budget, for example, in terms of the value of farm output in the various food sectors. Some sectors receive far greater support than others as a proportion of the total European production value of those foods. For example, although the European Agricultural Guidance and Guarantee Fund appears to spend comparable amounts on sugar and on fruits and vegetables, this support amounts to 47% of the output value for the former but only 4% for the latter *(71)*.

These differences in support may lead to substantial distortions in the market. In a series of papers on the workings of CAP, the European Court of Auditors has criticized the butter *(72)*, sugar *(73)* and milk *(74)* regimes for protecting and promoting surplus production.

Fig. 3.8. CAP spending by the European Agricultural Guidance and Guarantee Fund according to product sector, 2001

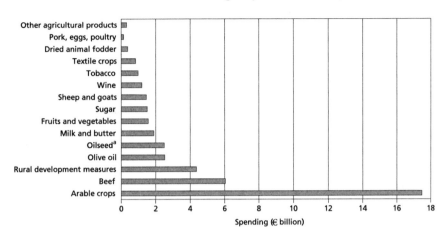

a Oilseed cake is used for animal feed.
Source: adapted from 31st financial report on the European Agricultural Guidance and Guarantee Fund EAGGF, Guarantee Section – 2001 financial year (70).

By subsidizing the production of certain foods, CAP has separated the producer from the consumer in the marketplace. It has created an artificial market for producers that may not reflect consumers' preferences and may encourage the consumption of food that undermines health (see also Chapter 4, p. 223–224) *(75)*:

> The CAP has become more health-oriented since 1996 in terms of food safety. However, risk factors of cardiovascular disease, cancer, diabetes and alcohol-related diseases, together accounting for 41 per cent of the disease burden in the European Region or 3 million premature deaths annually, are still not taken into consideration as required under the Amsterdam Treaty. Examples of the latter are: ... half a million tonnes of surplus butter, corresponding to one third of EU consumption, are sold with subsidies to the food industry; one million tonnes of quality fruits and vegetables destroyed yearly with the aim of keeping prices up ... . From a public health perspective, the tax money transferred to agriculture could be of greater benefit to citizens if spent in other ways.

A comparison of trends in the production of foods supported by CAP with trends in household purchases shows how this separation of producers and consumers can take place. In the United Kingdom, where records of household food purchases have been kept since the 1940s, trends can be shown for the purchase of, for example, sugar and fruit, and these can be compared with local quantities of farm production, as recorded by FAO since 1961 (Fig. 3.9 and 3.10).

Fig. 3.9. Trends in the production and household consumption of sugar in the United Kingdom, 1961–2001

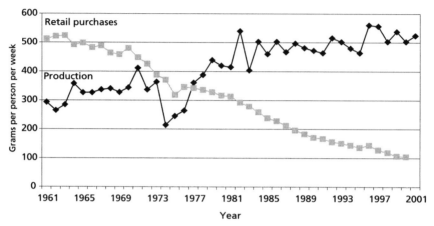

Sources: FAOSTAT agriculture data (http://apps.fao.org/page/collections?subset=agriculture, accessed 20 January 2003) and Department for Food, Environment and Rural Affairs *(23)*.

Fig. 3.10. Trends in the production and household consumption of fruit in the United Kingdom, 1961–2001

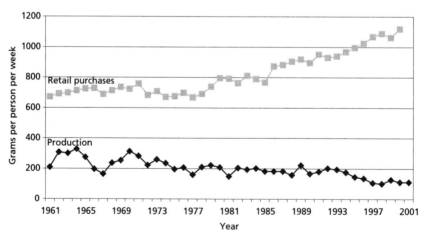

Sources: FAO food balance sheets (http://apps.fao.org/lim500/wrap.pl?FoodBalanceSheet&Domain=FoodBalanceSheet&Language=english, accessed 20 January 2003) and Department for Food, Environment and Rural Affairs *(23)*.

While factors such as external trade may influence production and the consumption of more processed food and more meals outside the home affects household purchasing figures, trends in production appear to have become divorced from those in home consumption in the United Kingdom. Joining CAP in the early 1970s appears to have done little to align the two.

A distortion of agricultural production in favour of certain foodstuffs can lead to chronic surpluses and to need to dispose of them through various channels. Highly perishable foods (such as fish, fruits and vegetables) have usually been removed from the market and destroyed, although recent moves have encouraged producer organizations to find alternatives, such as converting fruit into processed foods or industrial alcohol.

The EU has a small budget for food promotional activities and, until 1999, devoted it almost entirely to promoting meat (especially beef) and dairy products (especially butter and full-fat milk) *(75,76)*. The EU has also supported distribution schemes, offering low-price foods to hospitals, schools and other institutions. These, too, have focused on meat and dairy products, although some fruit and vegetable distribution has taken place.

The financial support for animal-derived products has led to a shift in agricultural land use towards livestock rearing rather than crops for human consumption. Three quarters of agricultural land in the EU is now used for animal feed and grazing *(77)*. Among five EU countries in southern Europe, the land area devoted to fruit and vegetable production has declined by over 20% in the last four decades, while that for grain production for animal feed has increased by 20% (Table 3.8).

Table 3.8. Land area devoted to crop production in France, Greece, Italy, Portugal and Spain as a whole, 1961–2000

Crops	Land area (ha thousands)								
	1961	1965	1970	1975	1980	1985	1990	1995	2000
Fruits and vegetables	8 720	8 636	8 132	8 075	7 916	7 573	7 317	6 695	6 680
Barley and maize	7 554	7 324	9 428	10 639	10 619	11 169	10 059	8 834	9 063

Source: FAOSTAT (http://apps.fao.org/page/form?collection=LandUse&Domain=Land&servlet=1&language=EN&hostname=apps.fao.org&version=default, accessed 20 January 2003).

A shift in consumption patterns has matched this change in land use. The typical diet includes greater quantities of animal products, resulting in the consumption of more animal fat (Table 3.9).

These figures should not be taken to imply that agricultural policy solely determines the consumption of foods and hence the population's dietary patterns and nutritional status. The relationship is complex. Rising income is the main driver of the nutrition transition: a move from plant- to animal-based foods (see Chapter 1, p. 17). As populations improve their standard of living, sales of animal-based foods increase.

Table 3.9. Meat and dairy supplies in France, Greece, Italy, Portugal and Spain, 1961 and 1999

Country	Beef and veal (kg/person)		Milk (kg/person)		Animal fat (kg/person)	
	1961	1999	1961	1999	1961	1999
France	28.6	26.2	220	265	28.8	39.6
Greece	5.1	22.3	101	257	9.5	20.8
Italy	14.6	25.6	145	261	12.0	25.4
Portugal	6.4	16.8	62	207	8.6	28.0
Spain	6.0	14.0	83	165	14.5	23.0

Source: FAOSTAT (http://apps.fao.org/page/form?collection=FS.NonPrimaryLive-stockAndProducts&Domain=FS&servlet=1&language=EN&hostname=apps.fao.org&version=default, accessed 20 January 2003).

This is not a simple relationship between rising wealth and rising demand: the available supplies and the suppliers' marketing activities shape demand. As more people move from plant to animal products, for example, animal production increases, leading to falling prices. Animal products become more widely available at lower prices, which encourages their consumption. The same applies to the creation of mass-produced processed foods, such as snack foods, soft drinks and confectionery. These are sold in increasing amounts thanks to aggressive marketing, especially aimed at children.

Food technology aids this process: for example, the use of chemical preservatives and other techniques can increase the shelf life and extend the distribution of foods. Similarly, a wide array of techniques is available to help create and market mass-produced processed foods.

In addition to these technical and economic changes, food companies actively promote their products through a wide range of advertising and marketing techniques (see Chapter 4, p. 252–254). Thus, the nutrition transition is not inevitable, but shaped by policies on food supply, pricing and technology; activities to promote products; and public health messages (see Fig. 3.5).

In trying to establish the optimum supply of foods that would meet nutritional needs, national governments may consider comparing their national dietary targets to their agriculture and food supply statistics. The task is complex, with assumptions needing to be made about the conversion of supply figures into consumption figures, about wastage and about the effects on agricultural and food-processing businesses. Nevertheless, a national food and nutrition policy requires such an evaluation.

Table 3.10 spells out some of the food supplies required to satisfy most of these recommendations, compares them with the actual food supplies in Ireland and Italy and shows the supply patterns of both countries in 1965 and 1999. The population of Ireland was supplied with high levels of fat and sugar and insufficient fruits and vegetables. Italy increased its fat supplies well beyond the maximum that might be recommended for health, but the amounts of fruit and vegetables were comfortably above the minimum.

Table 3.10. Comparison of dietary recommendations with food supplies to the populations of Ireland and Italy, 1965 and 1999

| Component | Population goals (78) | Theoretical food supplies required (per person per day) (78) | Actual food supplies (per person per day) (79) | | | |
| | | | Ireland | | Italy | |
			1965	1999	1965	1999
Total fat	< 30% of total energy	< 80 g fat	119 g	136 g	90 g	152 g
Saturated fat	< 10% of total energy	< 60 g fat from animal products	100 g	89 g	38 g	70 g
Sugar	< 10% of total energy	< 65 g raw sugar equivalent	146 g	116 g	73 g	81 g
Fruits and vegetables	> 400 g/day	> 600 g fruit and vegetables (> 400 g edible)	245 g	390 g	720 g	858 g

The food supply figures do not take account of distribution factors. In particular, they do not consider how income inequality and other influences – such as cultural preferences, pricing policies or catering practices – may affect consumption patterns among different sections of the population. Nevertheless, the data illustrate the value of comparing food supply policies with dietary need. Besides the overall quantities of food supplied, however, additional questions need to be asked about their nutritional quality and the potential for nutritional values to be ignored when quality changes. The next section considers this in more detail.

Specific effects of food production practices on nutrition quality

The nutrient density (nutrients per unit of food energy) and the biochemical diversity of food supplies can indicate how well foods can meet the needs of populations. There are four *a priori* reasons why the biochemical diversity and nutrient richness of human diets may have deteriorated in recent years.

1. The biodiversity of the diet has declined. There is good evidence that pre-Neolithic hunter–gatherers used hundreds of different fungal, plant and animal species in their diet. The post-Neolithic diet is largely restricted to agricultural products based on a narrow range of species. Staple crops are based on grains, which are biochemically less varied than the seeds of, for example, legumes and umbellifers *(80)*. Despite an apparent variety of foods in modern supermarkets, nutritionally the diet may be unvaried: "variety of brand name does not imply variety of underlying chemistry" *(80)*.

2. Species selection has favoured volume or weight yields over nutrient content or biochemical diversity. Modern crops have been selected and bred over many centuries largely for yield. Yield is to some extent incompatible with biochemical diversity, since selection for high yield favours plants that produce starch and cellulose and can hold water, which reduces the nutrients per unit weight and per unit of food energy. Livestock breeding has emphasized maximum muscle growth, while the biochemical diversity and nutrient richness of animals are found less in muscles than in, for example, the liver *(80)*.

3. Methods of storing and processing food tend to reduce rather than enhance the nutritional content. Nutrients that are volatile and easily oxidize or otherwise lose their potency are likely to diminish during storage, processing (such as physical grinding or crushing) or heating (during cooking or extrusion). Some processes, such as freezing and inert-gas packing, can help to preserve volatile nutrients during storage. Other processes, such as bulking or sweetening foods, dilute nutrient density.

4. Stocks of non-farmed, high-nutrient sources of food are threatened. Access to wild foods that tend to have higher nutrient density declined sharply in the last century. Wild berries, nuts and fungi thrive in relatively unmanaged woodland and open heathland, but their extent has declined markedly in the last few generations, and the proportion of the population living in urban areas, without easy access to woodlands, has increased. Stocks of wild fish are also under threat, especially in the last few decades, and fish farming is unlikely to be able to provide the same number or variety of species.

Farming policies that encourage the production of high volumes of food have substantially affected the nature of the crops and livestock produced. Crops are selected for specific characteristics – such as heavy cropping, fast growth, early fruiting, resistance to disease, frost and pesticides, responsiveness to fertilizer, bruise-resistant skin for transport, long storage and shelf life – not for their nutritional qualities. Species and strains of crops for processed foods – such as types of sugars, starches and oils – are selected for how well they fulfil the technical needs of the process, rather than the dietary needs of the consumer.

Similarly, animals are likely to be selected for fast muscle growth, high milk yield, frequent egg production, low aggression or best response to growth-promoting chemicals and antibiotics. Rarely are they selected for the nutritional qualities of the food produced from them.

Biodiversity

Studies of dietary balance and health indicate that greater dietary diversity is associated with reduced mortality from all causes *(81)* and from cancer and CVD *(82)*. Wahlqvist *(83)* suggests that the available evidence "indicates that, taking a week as a time frame, at least 20, and probably as many as 30 biologically distinct types of food, with the emphasis on plant food, are required" to ensure optimum dietary health.

Biodiversity not only contributes directly to dietary diversity but may also increase food security by safeguarding against climatic and pestilential disasters that may affect one or more food source. Intact, diverse ecosystems also act as a buffer against the spread of invasive plants, animals, pathogens and toxins *(83)*.

About 75% of the genetic diversity of agricultural crops worldwide was lost during the 20th century *(84)*. Newly introduced varieties and breeds have almost always displaced traditional ones. Although about 10 000 plant species have been used for human food and agriculture, not more than 120 cultivated species now provide over 90% of human plant food *(85)*. Over the last 15 years, 300 of 6000 farm animal breeds have become extinct, and a further 2000 are at risk of disappearing *(85)*.

Agricultural biodiversity is declining in European countries, leading to a potential loss of biochemical diversity in the diet, as shown by the following examples (Table 3.11) *(84)*. In Europe, half of all breeds of domestic animal (horses, cattle, sheep, goats, pigs and chickens) became extinct during the 20th century, and one third of the remaining 770 breeds are in danger of extinction by 2010. In Provence, France, the number of plant species in the diet

Table 3.11. Examples of reduced biodiversity in food production in Europe

Country	Crop/Crop-growing land	Varieties used
France	71% of apple production	1 (Golden Delicious)
	30% of bread wheat	2
	70% of bread wheat	10
Netherlands	80% of potato-growing land	1
	90% of wheat production	3
	75% of barley production	1
United Kingdom	68% of early potatoes	3
	71% of wheat area	4

Source: adapted from Pretty *(84)*.

fell from 250 to 30–60 in the 20th century. Similarly, 90% of local wheat varieties in Greece have been lost since the 1920s.

Plant production

Few data compare the nutritional values of wild plants with varieties grown as commercial crops, but a study of edible vegetables eaten in Crete *(86)* found that wild, green-leafed plants used in traditional cuisine are rich in phytonutrients, such as antioxidant flavonols and flavones. The study noted that over 150 varieties of edible wild greens are believed to be consumed in Greece, often in the form of traditional green pies made with virgin olive oil. Analyses of these pies showed that the concentrations of antioxidants were considerably higher than in well recognized rich sources, such as red wine. These findings may reveal the secret of the well known health benefits of the so-called Mediterranean diet.

In most food supplies, the size and quality of a plant crop are determined largely by the species, variety and cultivar of the plant, the conditions in which it is grown, such as the nutrient levels in the soil, and post-harvest treatment. Soil fertility has long been recognized as an important influence on crop production. Seeking to maximize the use of land for crop production, many farmers have abandoned the practice of leaving fields fallow for a season to allow some natural regeneration in their fertility. (CAP payments to farmers to set aside land – that is, remove it from production – have usually led to the reduced use of poor-quality land and even greater exploitation of the land remaining in production.)

Arable land may be routinely used for two crops per year. The rotation of crops to encourage maximum fertility – for example, alternating nitrogen-fixing crops with nitrogen-depleting crops – has given way to the replacement of soil nitrogen by applying nitrogen-rich fertilizer. In addition, the drive to increase animal and dairy production has led to the increasing use of fertilizers to promote the growth of selected fast-growing grasses on pasture land, in place of traditional multispecies meadows.

There appear to be no systematic studies of the effects on the nutritional content of plant crops when trace elements in the soil are not replenished. It may be argued that, at least in some areas, sufficient quantities of trace elements remain in the soil to ensure high levels in plants and hence in human nutrition. Nevertheless, deficiency may be found and appropriate action taken in some areas. For example, providing iodine in irrigation water during one season led to a fivefold increase in the iodine levels in locally grown crops, vegetables and meat for the following three years, and resulted in fewer infant deaths and stillbirths *(87)*.

There is evidence that the quantity of essential minerals in commonly grown crops in the United Kingdom has declined significantly in the last 50 years. In a comparison of the mineral composition of 20 types of fruits and vegetables analysed in the 1930s and in the 1980s, the levels of calcium, magnesium, sodium and copper in vegetables, and potassium, iron, magnesium and copper in fruit were found to have declined significantly *(88)*. Phosphorus showed no change. Other minerals were not measured in both surveys. Water content increased. Care must be taken in interpreting the figures, as these could be influenced by changes in analytical techniques and in the sources of fruit and vegetables and their varieties.

Different apple varieties have significantly different vitamin C levels. Some types have three or even five times more of this vitamin than others, although the heaviest cropping varieties (especially Golden Delicious) have some of the lowest levels *(89)*.

There is increasing evidence that various plant chemicals such as phenols and flavonoids may play a role in nutrition, acting as protective agents against degenerative diseases. Few studies of the effects of agricultural systems on these plant chemicals have been undertaken. Researchers at the University of Copenhagen have suggested that plants produce some of these compounds as a defence mechanism against attack from pests and that high levels of fertilizer use weaken these defence mechanisms, necessitating in turn greater use of pesticides to protect the crops *(90)*.

Sunlight and ultraviolet light can affect flavonoid levels in plants. Reducing sunlight can dramatically reduce the amounts of quercetin, naringenin and caffeic acid in tomatoes. For example, phenol levels in cherry tomatoes declined by 50% when sunlight was reduced by 60% and a similar decrease when ultraviolet B light was reduced *(91)*.

These findings have implications for the growing of crops under glass or plastic sheeting, which may reduce flavonoid levels. Covered production of fruit and vegetables has increased dramatically in recent years. The findings also have implications for moves in agriculture to grow crops that mature early. Flavonoids and anthocyanins are reported to be several hundred per cent higher in red onions harvested in July than in those harvested in April *(91)*.

Nutrients in organically produced crops

Some controversy has attached to claims that organically produced crops are nutritionally superior. The evidence from the limited research undertaken to date is equivocal, with some data showing that conventionally grown crops tend to be higher in water content and hence lower in nutrients per unit of weight. A recent study of apples grown under three regimes found several environmental advantages in the organic system, but the nutritional data showed "inconsistent differences" *(56)*. A taste panel considered the organic produce to be the tastiest, which might encourage greater consumption of nutrients if a greater quantity is eaten.

Research into comparative nutritional values is hampered by difficulties in comparing like with like. For example, different crop varieties may be best suited to high-yield intensive agriculture and to organic production. The United Kingdom Soil Association reviewed the literature in 2002 *(92)*.

One possible line of research is the suggestion that a plant's response to attack by pests may increase the concentration of useful phytochemicals in the plant, such as antioxidants. Plants grown in conventional systems using high levels of anti-pest measures may thus have lower levels of these biochemicals than plants grown in less protective systems. Further, it might follow that fruit with blemishes, such as scar tissue on apples, might show higher levels of such biochemicals than unblemished fruit. Research is needed on these hypotheses.

Animal production

The links between yield-enhancing farming methods and the nutrient value of the product have been explored for livestock as well as arable farming. For instance, the growth of cattle largely depends on a combination of high-energy and high-protein feed, lack of exercise and genetic selection.

These factors combine to produce flesh of particular nutritional quality. In comparisons of the meat of free-living buffalo compared with farmed beef cattle, buffalo carcass meat is typically found to be less than 3% fat, whereas farmed beef is typically 20–25% fat *(93)*. Even so-called lean commercial beef is about 8% fat. In chicken, the evidence suggests that over the last century, the carcass fat content has risen by nearly 1000% *(94)*.

Not only do farmed animals tend to have far more fat than free-living animals, but the fat contains higher levels of saturated fatty acids. For example, the fat of wild hogs is typically one third polyunsaturated fatty acids, versus less than one tenth in farmed pigs *(93)*. The fat of wild game birds is 60% polyunsaturated fatty acids, whereas farmed chickens have less than 20% *(93)*. In cattle, the polyunsaturated fraction comprises nearly 50% of the fat content of free-living buffalo, but barely 2% of the fat of domesticated cattle reared for beef. Milk and butter from farmed cattle show a similarly low proportion of polyunsaturated fat: typically less than 3% of the fat *(93)*.

Further, the nature of the polyunsaturates appears to differ between free-living and farmed animals. Free-living animals typically show 10 times the amounts of very long-chain derivatives of both linoleic and linolenic fatty acids, such as C20:4, C20:5, C22:5 and C22:6, and correspondingly smaller amounts of shorter-chain fatty acids *(95)*.

Nature of fat in different species

Wild animals in their usual habitats have a greater proportion of their fat as polyunsaturated fatty acids compared with domesticated varieties (Fig. 3.11).

Human body fat and human milk tend to reflect the fat consumed in the diet.

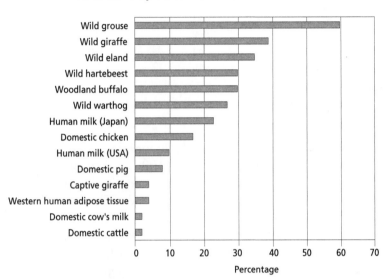

Fig. 3.11. Polyunsaturated fatty acids as a proportion
of total fatty acids from various sources

Source: adapted from Crawford *(92).*

Attempts to alter the fatty acid profile of animal products have had mixed results *(96).* Fish oil fed to cattle flavoured the milk unacceptably. It also tainted pig meat, but an increased content of long-chain fatty acids in egg yolks has proved commercially feasible.

Fish and aquaculture

Fish are a valuable source of the omega-3 family of long-chain polyunsaturated fatty acids, which make a unique contribution to health. An alternative rich source of these nutrients in human diets is animal brain tissue, but this source has become unpopular and, following the rise in BSE, is now little used in western Europe.

Stocks of wild fish have declined, which has increased demand for farmed fish. Marine oil supplies are becoming more limited and their prices are rising. As a result, fish farmers have turned to other oils for feeding their stock. Soya, palm and rapeseed (canola) oils dominate world commodity markets, together accounting for more than 50% of edible oil production, while marine oils account for less than 2%. The pattern of fatty acids in fish closely parallels the pattern of fatty acids in the food that the fish eat, so the choice of oil for fish feed affects the nutritional value of the fish produced (Table 3.12).

Table 3.12. Fatty acids in the flesh of farmed trout
according to their feed

Type	Fatty acids (g per 100 g fatty acids) in trout fed:	
	marine oils	marine and vegetable oils
Polyunsaturated		
Omega-3	31	16
Omega-6	9	19
Monounsaturated	42	38
Saturated	19	28

Source: Sargent & Tacon *(97).*

Food storage and transport

The increasing transport of food has implications for nutrient levels. Long storage leads to a reduction of the more volatile nutrients in food. Preservation methods are designed to prevent deterioration in the appearance of the product, spoilage from microorganisms and rancidity from oxidation, but not specifically to preserve nutrients.

In times of scarcity, storage techniques are a welcome means of providing food when none would otherwise be available. They have proved essential for travel and exploration and in the growth of urban populations. Dehydration, salting, pickling, curing, canning and chilling have extended the range of foods available and the locations where they can be consumed, improving the nutritional diversity of the diet.

When food is plentiful, there may be reason to question the widespread use of food preservation techniques. If fresh equivalents are available, they are usually nutritionally superior to preserved foods. Yet preserved food can be stored and transported in quantity, allowing the food to be supplied more economically. Food preservation techniques thus give less nutritious foods an economic advantage in the marketplace. Only in the case of rapid freezing methods might a preserved food be likely to be as nutritious as its fresh counterpart.

Food manufacturing processes

Studies of the nutritional impact of various processing techniques, which turn raw commodities into processed foodstuffs, have a long history. Table 3.13 gives some characteristic examples of the impact of processing on nutrition.

Potato products give an example of the effects of food processing (Fig. 3.12). Nutrient density declines as processing increases. Similar trends can be shown for fruit (from fresh through to fruit juices, desserts and fruit flavoured soft drinks) and chicken (from fresh through to chicken nuggets and chicken-flavour snacks).

Table 3.13. Examples of the effects of processing
on the nutrient value of foods

Processes (examples)	Effects
Modified atmosphere packaging (salad leaves)	Reduces loss of antioxidants and extends availability of nutrient-dense foods
Freezing (vegetables, meat, offal and fish)	Prevents loss of volatile nutrients and extends availability of nutrient-dense foods
Irradiation (beef patties, shellfish and fruit)	Extends availability and leads to some loss of volatile nutrients
Refining (flour extraction and juice extraction)	Leads to loss of fibre, vitamins, minerals and antioxidants
Concentration (fruit juice refining and vegetable dehydration)	Leads to loss of volatile vitamins and antioxidants
Hydrogenation (hardening marine and vegetable oils for margarine)	Creates *trans*-saturated fatty acids
Bulking (using starches in baby foods and water in meat products)	Reduces nutrient density
Adding salt and flavourings (savoury snacks)	Increases the sodium load and raises consumption of fatty foods
Substitution (colouring and flavouring used in place of fruit in juice drinks)	Leads to loss of nutritious ingredients and reduces nutrient density

Fig. 3.12. Loss of vitamins and increase in fat as potatoes are processed

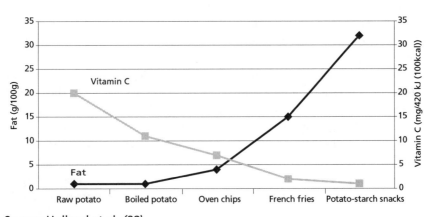

Source: Holland et al. *(98).*

Recent moves to offer nutritionally improved processed foods (with lower fat or sugar levels) and functional foods (with specific health-enhancing properties) demonstrate the potential for food manufacturers to consider nutritional criteria as part of product formulation. Further, good practices in nutrition labelling are being developed, in conjunction with consumer groups, and are being considered as part of the Codex standards for internationally traded foods *(99)*.

Retailing practices

Retailers may suggest that they sell only what their customers want to buy, but the relationship between supermarkets and shoppers' choices is complex. Supermarkets help to shape purchasing patterns; their decisions about shelf space allocation, pricing differentials, end-of-aisle promotion, special offers and other marketing methods can significantly, if transiently, affect customers' purchasing decisions (see p. 175).

In addition to their promotional activities, supermarkets have increasingly become food manufacturers. Supermarkets have launched brands of packaged foods with their own labels, and have incorporated their own butchery departments, bakeries, fishmongers and greengrocers. Some supermarkets now sell more of their own brands than of all other brands of food *(45)*. Increasingly, the supermarket can control all the steps from primary producer to final customer. In such a position, retailers can strongly influence consumer choices, and act to improve nutrition security. From the perspective of a food and nutrition policy, supermarkets' growing power and influence clearly comprise one of the priorities that public health policy-makers need to address *(100,101)*.

Similar trends can be seen in food served ready to eat in restaurants and cafés. The rise of fast-food chains has come to symbolize modern food trends. In a fast-food outlet, the customer selects food from a limited range of easily cooked foods, allowing the store staff to assemble the dishes rapidly from standard ingredients.

The owner determines the menu choices available, according to criteria including cost, preparation time, ease of cooking, storage needs and shelf life. In recent years, fast-food companies have started to declare the nutritional composition of their products, and this has helped companies review the nutritional value of their foods. Recent moves by leading fast-food chains have included nutrition-motivated changes in some cooking practices, such as a decline in the use of saturated and hydrogenated fat for deep frying of French fries and lower fat levels in their specifications for burger meat *(102)*.

Policies for food and nutrition security

An emerging policy challenge is to find ways to maintain and enhance food production while improving the positive functions of agricultural and environmental management and eliminating the negative ones. This has entered EU policy with the November 1999 communiqué of the EU Agricultural Council *(103)*:

(1) sustainable agriculture ensures that agriculture's natural base remains productive and agricultural production can be competitive in the future and that farming works to promotes positive environmental impact.

(2) the role of agriculture is broader than that of simply producing food and non-food products. Agriculture is multifunctional and clearly has effects on the environment and rural landscape. Furthermore, it has a fundamental role to play in the viability of rural areas.

...

(4) agriculture plays an important role in contributing to the maintenance of employment in rural areas and in the whole food and non-food production chain.

...

(10) economical, environmental, social and cultural services provided by farmers must be recognised; for these services farmers should be adequately remunerated. ...

To this can be added: the food being provided should be safe and nutritious.

The challenge is to link schemes that encourage more sustainable agriculture with those that improve nutritional quality, so that farmers and food manufacturers provide the food that is needed for nutritional reasons and do so in a sustainable way.

The evidence in this chapter shows the importance of seeing food production as an integral part of protecting and promoting health and protecting the environment. This section suggests approaches to food policy that combine the various elements into a more coherent whole.

Diet and sustainable production

Three quarters of all agricultural land in the EU is devoted to producing animal feed *(78)*. In addition, several million ha land outside the EU are used to provide animal feed imports, amounting to 14 million tonnes of cassava, 17 million tonnes of soybeans and 22 million tonnes of soya cake in 1999 (http://apps.fao.org/page/form?collection=Production.Crops.Primary&Domain=Production&servlet=1&language=EN&hostname=apps.fao.org&version=default, accessed 20 January 2003). As farmers replace meat and bone meal with vegetable protein sources, in response to BSE control measures, the demand for land for producing animal feed may grow.

A study by the Swedish Environmental Protection Agency *(104)* examined the implications of reducing land requirements, energy demands and fertilizer input and compared Sweden's current dietary pattern with a more ecologically sustainable one. The latter was then compared with dietary targets for the health of populations recommended by WHO. This showed that reducing the ecological impact of food production would help to meet health goals (Table 3.14).

Table 3.14. Actual daily consumption of various food groups in Sweden and that recommended to reduce ecological impact

Food	Level of consumption (g/day)	
	Actual	Recommended for reduced ecological impact
Margarine, butter, oil	50	50
Milk products	400	300
Cheese	45	20
Meat, poultry, sausage	145	35
Fish	30	30
Egg	25	10
Bread	100	200
Cereal	15	45
Potatoes	140	270
Vegetables	150	190
Root vegetables	25	100
Fruit	150	175
Dried legumes	5	50
Snacks/Sweets	200	140
Soft drinks	150	80

Source: A sustainable food supply chain (104).

The study also noted that animal products tended to be more energy dense than grains and vegetables and that a reduced intake of animal foods could result in a greater volume of food being eaten (104). This in turn might require more transport resources, but the study concluded that these potential increases were small compared with the benefits.

The current world population uses about one third of the world's land to grow food and feed. About one third remains forested and the remaining third is unsuitable for crops, pasture or forest because it is too cold, dry, steep, stony or wet or because the soil is too infertile or shallow to support sufficient plant growth (58). Animal production also requires more land. Research from Sweden on beef and dairy production shows that every litre of milk produced requires 1.5 m^2 of arable land (for pasture and for cereal and other cattle feed input) for a year (104). Beef production requires even more land: each 1 kg Swedish beef requires 33 m^2 of land (for grazing and for cereal and other feed input) for a year. Of these, 2.3 m^2 lie outside Sweden, where feed material is cheaper.

In view of population trends over recent decades, increases in food supply using conventional farming methods are not expected to be able to feed the world's population beyond 2050 *(105)*. Such methods are likely to cause escalating environmental problems. Extensification (bringing marginal or forested land into production) risks loss of biodiversity and rapid soil depletion, as the land is usually unsuitable for agriculture, and conventional intensification (increasing yields per unit area) currently relies on high levels of fertilizer, pesticide and other agrochemical and veterinary input. Biotechnology might offer a faster means of developing higher-yield varieties of plants and animals through genetic engineering, but its environmental and health effects remain to be fully assessed, and some consumers and some farmers resist using it for ethical, environmental, safety and other reasons.

An alternative means of increasing food supply is to change the pattern of foods produced, reducing the high level of animal products and increasing the use of land for food crops. As shown earlier in this chapter, the water resources needed to produce livestock-based foods are at least one order of magnitude greater than those needed to produce plant-based foods.

Pimentel et al. *(58)* have graphically shown the links between environmental and dietary factors. Fig. 3.13 indicates that foods from organisms high on the food chain, such as animals and dairy foods, have more harmful effects on the environment than foods from lower down the food chain, such as plants.

Fig. 3.13. Environmental sustainability and the food chain

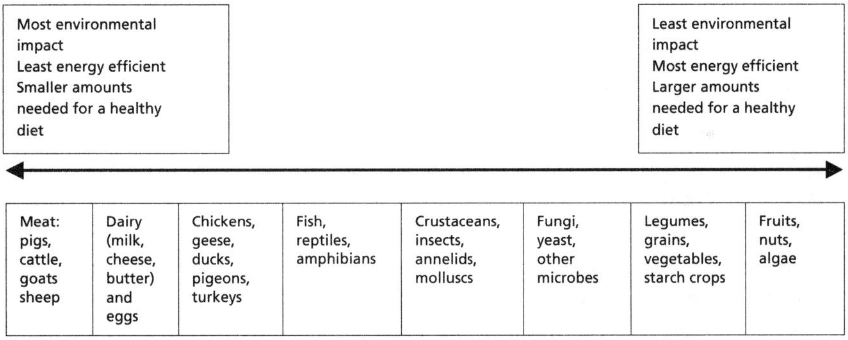

| Most environmental impact
Least energy efficient
Smaller amounts needed for a healthy diet | | | | Least environmental impact
Most energy efficient
Larger amounts needed for a healthy diet | | | |

←———————————————————————————————————————→

Meat: pigs, cattle, goats sheep	Dairy (milk, cheese, butter) and eggs	Chickens, geese, ducks, pigeons, turkeys	Fish, reptiles, amphibians	Crustaceans, insects, annelids, molluscs	Fungi, yeast, other microbes	Legumes, grains, vegetables, starch crops	Fruits, nuts, algae

Source: adapted from Pimentel et al. *(58)*.

A study of the environmental impact of dairy farming in the EU examined the ecological damage caused by different forms of dairy farming *(106)*. It noted that low-input methods could provide yields as high as 5500 litres of milk per cow per year, with organic systems achieving 7000 litres per cow per year, on a par with intensive non-grazing systems in southern Europe and with intensive grazing systems (2 animals per ha plus silage and maize) in France. Highly intensive non-grazing systems in northern Europe gave substantially better yields (about 9000 litres per cow per year), but at high environmental cost in feed requirements and pollution. The study also noted the loss of traditional breeds of cattle: 35 breeds were endangered and 36 critical.

Influencing consumption patterns

A policy that reduces income inequality is likely to increase the purchasing power of low-income households. Increasing affluence has tended to lead to greater demand for animal products in most of the European Region in the last five decades, although consumption of red meat has declined in western Europe in the last decade or so. The consumption of red meat, poultry and dairy food is predicted to increase in much of the rest of the Region (107).

Global policies that encourage animal production have been criticized for benefiting wealthier consumers at the expense of poorer ones by increasing the demand for land and grain. Some analysts, however, suggest that competition for cereal foods need not necessarily drive up world grain prices, and that livestock rearing by low-income families offers a source of income to alleviate their poverty (108). Presumably this would not apply in most urban settings in the Region.

Allowing unfettered increases in meat production to meet demand is still a risky long-term option. Alternative policy developments that encourage a largely plant-based diet might be preferable. These require changes in agricultural support mechanisms, taxation and cost internalization.

World Bank discussion papers argue against giving public financial subsidies to large-scale livestock and dairy enterprises, at least in countries receiving its financial assistance (109). The EU CAP has supported meat and dairy production but is facing reform towards more environmentally oriented support mechanisms (52,107).

Accounting for health and environmental costs in retail prices (internalization) is a means of dealing with the problem. As mentioned earlier, the direct cost to the purchaser seldom includes all the costs of production, including the health and environmental effects. Some have argued that, for the market to operate effectively, the true costs of dietary preferences need to be internalized so that food sources that most damage the environment carry a concomitant financial cost to the purchaser (58).

Costs may be internalized in part through stricter charging by bodies that clean up the pollution caused by agriculture (such as water authorities, food control authorities and sanitary and epidemiological departments) and an increase in the price of nonrenewable fuels, but other costs are hard to pass back to the producer. Already, the producer is squeezed from all sides, especially in terms of the margin between the ex-farm price and what the consumer pays at the checkout. In the United Kingdom between 1995 and 2002, for example, while the consumer paid less for beef (from 396.5 pence/kg to 381.0 pence/

kg) the amounts paid to beef farmers also declined (from 227.7 pence/kg to 170.2 pence/kg) *(110)*. There are similar patterns for mutton, pork and milk. If food security is to be sustainable to protect public health, consumers must be prepared to pay the true costs to the primary producer.

Gains from positive environmental action

An important principle is that limited resources are more efficiently used to promote practices that do not damage the environment than to clean up after a problem has been created. Positive environmental action can save substantial resources, as has been shown in a project initiated by the US Environmental Protection Agency to prevent agricultural contamination of the 500 000-ha Catskill-Delaware watershed region, which supplies New York City with most of its drinking-water *(111)*. To meet new drinking-water standards in the late 1980s, New York City faced having to construct a filtration facility, which would cost US $5–8 billion, and paying another US $200–500 million in annual operating costs. Further, some 40% of the cropland in the watershed would have to be taken out of farming to reduce run-off of eroded soil, pesticides, nutrients and bacterial and protozoan pathogens *(112)*.

Instead, New York City chose to work with farmers. It funded a Watershed Agricultural Council, a partnership of farmers, government and private organizations, both to protect the city's drinking-water supply and to sustain the rural economy. It works on whole-farm planning with each farm, tailoring solutions to local conditions to maximize reductions in off-site costs. The first two phases of the programme, leading to the 85% target in pollution reduction, cost US $40–100 million, a fraction of the cost of the filtration plant. Taxpayers benefit, but so do farmers, the environment and rural economies *(112)*.

Similar schemes for rewarding farmers for reducing environmental impact are being tried in Europe. For example, in a plan to protect the water supply in Copenhagen, Denmark, farmers will reduce fertilizer or pesticide use and receive compensation for lower crop yields, matched with market support for their farms' products.

Local food production

As described earlier in this chapter, studies of food production during periods of national food insecurity show the importance of small-scale farming in sustaining food supplies when large-scale enterprises are failing. Access to food in these circumstances depends on human capital – skills, techniques and experience – being available when commercial food supplies are insecure.

Food crises may not be limited to vulnerable economies such as those in transition. All countries that rely on long-distance imports of basic commodities must assume that their food supplies are vulnerable to shock. To defend themselves from unexpected food crises, countries should seek to develop farming systems that are "resilient, environmentally responsible and capable of sustaining production in the face of unforeseen developments" according to the US Center for Rural Affairs *(113)*. Food companies demand reduced biodiversity and greater crop and livestock uniformity as part of their management strategies for risk reduction, but this makes food production more vulnerable to unexpected shocks, such as weather and climate change, new pests and diseases or political interference.

Increasing global food trade may jeopardize local food supplies. For example, if vegetables are exported from California or Chile to Europe, they take the place of vegetables that could have been grown locally and require considerably more transport. As shown in Chapter 1, the consumption of plenty of fruit and vegetables is linked to good health and protection from degenerative disease, but increased imports of these commodities may undercut production by European farmers. If so, they will be under pressure to diversify out of fruit and vegetable production or out of food production entirely.

The quest for greater food production has progressively simplified landscapes, rural livelihoods and farming systems. During the last century, the number of farms declined and farm unit size increased in every country in the EU. When CAP was established in 1957, the 6 member countries had 22 million farms. By 1997, the 15 EU countries had less than 7 million *(114)*.

The number of people working on farms for their main employment fell to 7.1 million in the EU in 1998. Younger people are leaving rural employment, and the remaining workers may not be able to hand on their skills and knowledge: over half the farmers in the EU in 1993 were older than 55 years *(103)*. Similar trends are found in eastern countries: more than 50% of Lithuania's farmers are older than 60 years, and only 2% are younger than 30 *(115)*.

In terms of crude productivity, yields have increased while the population employed on farms has decreased. This has greatly enhanced the per-capita productivity of farm labour, although considerable capital investment and consumption of nonrenewable resources are required to achieve this degree of mechanization. This chapter has already considered the hidden costs of forms of intensive farming that offset the increases in productivity. There are also costs to social cohesion.

Small farms are recognized as providing other benefits to rural society than crude productivity. Perceiving these advantages requires stepping outside the orthodox economic mode that focuses primarily on financial capital and its returns and looking at the other forms of capital used in producing food (see Table 3.15). Small farms can contribute to both rural social capital (maintaining and improving skills, knowledge and social cohesion) and natural capital (maintaining and improving the fertility of the farm's ecology and the surrounding environment). In principle, small farms are better able to maintain both plant and animal biodiversity, to use energy more efficiently, and to preserve landscape and wildlife. They also tend to have a better record with animal welfare *(84)*.

Forms of capital needed for sustainable farming

A successful economy needs to be able to make use of various forms of accumulated assets. All agricultural and rural economies rely for their success on the total stock of natural, social, human, physical and financial capital, as shown in Table 3.15.

Table 3.15. Five assets for sustainable agriculture and sustainable livelihoods

Assets	Components
Natural capital	Nature's goods and services: food (both farmed and from the wild), wood and fibre; water regulation and supply; waste assimilation, decomposition and treatment; nutrient cycling and fixation; soil formation; biological control of pests; climate regulation; wildlife habitats; storm protection and flood control; carbon sequestration; pollination; and recreation and leisure
Social capital	Cohesiveness of people in their societies: relations of trust, reciprocity and exchanges between individuals that facilitate cooperation; the bundles of common rules, norms and sanctions mutually agreed or handed down within societies; the connectedness of networks and groups that may be formal or informal, horizontal or vertical, and between individuals or organizations; and access to social institutions beyond the immediate household or community
Human capital	Status of individuals: the stock of health, nutrition, education, skills and knowledge of individuals; access to services that provide these, such as schools, health care and adult training; the ways individuals and their knowledge interact with productive technology; and individuals' leadership ability
Physical capital	Nonrenewable resources and infrastructure: technology; housing and other buildings; roads and bridges; energy supplies; communication; markets; and air, road, water and rail transport
Financial capital	Stocks of money: savings; access to affordable credit; pensions; remittances; welfare payments; and grants and subsidies

Source: adapted from *Participatory appraisal for community assessment: principles and methods (116).*

The falling numbers of farms and jobs and the increasing scale of farming operations have reduced the accumulated assets in rural areas and have played a role in the rise of rural poverty and lack of services. About 30% of rural households in the United Kingdom have experienced poverty in the past decade *(117)*. People in outlying areas have to travel to larger towns for key services, such as schools, health care, pharmacies and shops, which are concentrated there. In 1997, 28% of parishes in rural England had no village hall or community centre; 29% no public house or inn; 42% no shop or post office; 70% no general store; 60% no primary school; 75% no bus service; 83% no physician's practice; and 91% no bank or building society *(117,118)*.

The result of this deprivation and decline in services is the gradual unravelling of communities, and in particular a decreased capacity among local people to cope with environmental and economic change. Social cohesion is destroyed *(117)*.

These trends towards reduced social cohesion are powerful but not inevitable. A commitment under Agenda 21 to encourage farming methods that are sustainable for future generations has nevertheless helped a wide range of more sustainable forms of agriculture to develop. Many different terms are now used, including organic, *biologique*, sustainable, alternative, integrated, regenerative, low-external-input, balanced-input, precision farming, targeted inputs, wise use of inputs, resource-conserving, natural, eco-agriculture, agro-ecological, biodynamic and permaculture. Some contribute substantially to natural capital and rural people's livelihoods and others, less *(119)*.

Sustainable food production and workers' rights

The international trade union movement *(120)* considered the need for secure, sustainable food supplies and concluded that much of the world's food supply is produced under: "unacceptable and unsustainable conditions, particularly for waged agricultural workers … many of the unsustainable features of the world's food and agriculture industry can be attributed to its increasing domination by a few large multinational corporations". It added that current patterns of production are unsustainable in a number of ways, including:

- effects on the natural environment
- food distribution patterns
- effects on producers and their communities
- public and occupational health effects
- effects on nutrition and food safety.

As noted earlier, in 30 years the agricultural workforce in the EU dramatically declined, from over 18 million to 7.1 million. Younger people have left, and more than half of farmers are older than 55 years. The human capital bound up in the farm workforce is being lost, especially that most useful in developing ecologically sensitive forms of food production: the local knowledge of the climate, soil, biodiversity and optimum crops and production methods that has been accumulated over centuries. As mentioned (see Fig 3.4), poverty can be as high among agricultural workers as among unemployed households in some EU countries.

Policies that can help to prevent the loss of skills and knowledge and to maintain a healthy rural economy need to be considered. Agricultural policies that continue to focus on yields and returns on financial capital will continue the concentration of intensive farming. Current moves to improve payment systems for environmental protection activities and to encourage rural regeneration programmes may improve the prospects for rural employment and reduce rural poverty, but this is not guaranteed. National policy-makers aiming to promote and protect public health in rural areas face many tough challenges.

Increasing interest in environmentally sensitive farming

While conventional farming methods have received substantial long-term public support, a small but increasing number of farmers have chosen to convert their farming methods to qualify for organic status. The EU provides support for conversion, although the amounts are small as a proportion of CAP expenditure.

The standards for certification are negotiated through various nongovernmental inspection agencies, coordinated through the International Federation of Organic Agriculture Movements (IFOAM). The numbers of farms and the proportion of agricultural land certified as organic are rapidly increasing (Table 3.16).

Sustainability and productivity

Few research projects have examined the productivity of sustainable farming methods. Conventional agriculture, using standard input–output measures and ignoring hidden and externalized costs, is usually assumed to be more productive than sustainable or organic systems.

An already mentioned report on apple production using management practices that combine environmentally sensitive farming methods with modern technology, however, shows that yields can be as high as those obtained using orthodox, high-input methods. A five-year study of three methods of apple production – conventional, organic and an intermediary (integrated) system –indicates that organic methods can give yields as high as other methods *(56)*. The organic and integrated systems had higher soil quality and potentially lower negative environmental impact than conventional farming. The organic system also produced sweeter apples, higher profitability and greater energy efficiency.

Urban food supplies

About 80% of the population of the EU lives in urban areas, compared with 66% of people in the CCEE. The figure is predicted to keep rising in the European Region *(122)* (see Chapter 4, p. 272).

Urban populations typically require large non-urban areas to support their food, water and other environmental needs. Reducing the environmental footprint of cities – the area of land and water required to support the population – requires focusing increasingly on providing foods from within the urban

Table 3.16. Certified organic farming in European countries, about 1993 and 2001

Country	Number of organic farms		Organic land as a share of all agricultural land about 2001 (%)
	About 1993	About 2001	
Austria	13 321	18 292	11.3
Belgium	158	694	1.6
Bulgaria	–[a]	50	< 0.1
Cyprus[b]	2 (1988)	15	< 0.1
Czech Republic	About 75 (1991)	563	3.8
Denmark	640	3525	6.5
Estonia	–	231	0.7
Finland	1599	4983	6.6
France	–	10 400	1.4
Germany	5866 (1994)	14 703	3.7
Greece	250	5270	0.5
Hungary	67	471	0.8
Iceland	7 (1995)	30	3.4
Ireland	238	1014	0.7
Italy	4189	56 440	7.9
Latvia	–	225	0.8
Liechtenstein	6	44	17
Lithuania	–	230	0.1
Luxembourg	About 15	51	0.8
Netherlands	About 500	1510	1.9
Norway	946 (1996)	2099	2.6 (1999)
Poland	174	1419	0.1
Portugal	73	917	1.8
Romania	–	100 (1999)	< 0.1 (1999)
Slovakia	–	100 (1999)	2.5 (1999)
Slovenia	44 (1998)	620	0.7
Spain	about 4 000	15 607	1.7
Sweden	1507	3589	6.3
Switzerland	3668 (1996)	6169	9.7
United Kingdom	476 (1995)	3981	4.0
EU 15[c]	–	140 976	3.2

[a] –: data not available.
[b] Cyprus became a WHO European Member State in 2003, but is included for the sake of completeness.
[c] EU 15: the 15 current members of the EU.

Note: Definitions of "organic" differ between countries. In most countries, the statistics for organic farms include farms in conversion.

Source: Forschungsinstitut für biologischen Landbau (FiBL) & Stiftung Oekologie & Landbau (SOEL) (121).

area. As a contribution, the WHO Regional Office for Europe has prepared the Urban and Peri-urban Food and Nutrition Action Plan, which looks at the current policies and initiatives in the European Region *(26)*.

Local and urban food policies seek to increase the availability of and access to locally produced food, and to improve the local economy, create more jobs and promote social cohesion by linking urban dwellers more closely to food producers. The opportunities for food production in cities may be exploited, especially where household food insecurity is high, as the following examples show *(26)*.

1. In the Russian Federation, town dwellers produce 88% of their potatoes, 43% of their meat, 39% of their milk and 28% of their eggs on household plots of 0.2–0.5 ha.
2. In Poland, one sixth of the national consumption of fruit and vegetables – 500 000 tonnes – was produced on 8000 council gardens in 1997.
3. In Georgia, home-produced food made up 28% of the income of city dwellers.
4. In Romania, the share of home-produced food rose from 25% to 37% from 1989 to 1994.
5. In Bulgaria, 47% of the urban population was self-sufficient in fruit and vegetables in 1997.
6. The City Harvest project estimates that about 18% of the WHO-recommended intake of fruit and vegetables could be produced in London.

With food retailing increasingly concentrated into large superstores, which may be located on peri-urban sites that can be reached only by private transport, local authorities may need to encourage alternative means of supplying food, such as street markets and community shops. Moreover, incentives may be given to produce foods in or near cities, using environmentally sound and sustainable methods.

Production closer to cities helps to ensure that the produce is fresh and likely to have a higher nutrient content than produce that has been stored or transported for long periods. Easy access and fresh supplies can be expected to encourage consumption. In Athens, for example, farmers, market gardeners and even householders sell their fresh fruits and vegetables in traditional street markets in almost every neighbourhood. Household budget surveys show that 600 g fruit and vegetables per person per day is available at the household level in Greece, but only half this amount in the Russian Federation. Restricted supplies are likely to lead to inequality and low intake for poorer families living, for example, in St Petersburg *(122,123)*.

Local food production in cities offers both potential benefits and potential problems (Table 3.17). The main health risks can be mitigated through adequate quality standards and their enforcement. Similar risks apply to rural agricultural production, and one might argue that urban production is easier to inspect and that authorities are better placed to ensure that high standards are met. Numerous measures are recommended for developing urban and peri-urban agriculture *(124,125)*.

Table 3.17. Potential benefits and problems of local food production

Benefits	Problems
Increased food security	Poor sanitation and crop contamination with pathogens
Improved nutrition	Crops take up heavy metals from contaminated soil
Income generation and poverty reduction	Contamination of crops, water and the environment by agricultural chemicals
Improved sanitation and recycling	Occupational health risks from agricultural chemicals and machinery
Increased physical exercise	Zoonoses from livestock and meat processing
Improved physical and mental health	Human disease transfer (such as malaria) from agricultural activities (such as irrigation)
Unusual plant varieties, biodiversity and nutrient diversity	Theft and vandalism of produce and equipment

Source: adapted from Birley & Lock *(124)*.

Farming in the 21st century

Calls for sustainable farming methods tend to be considered calls for a return to 19th-century peasant farming. Such a view is misguided. A form of sustainable farming can be foreseen that does not require the re-creation or preservation of a farming underclass.

Major changes are taking place in the economic relationships between countries in the European Region, for example, with the accession of 10 new countries to the EU, and between Europe and other regions, through bodies such as the WTO and the accession of China to trade agreements. Thus, the future of farming is inevitably difficult to predict. At present, two types of farming are emerging. The first consists of farms that produce on a large scale, using capital-intensive systems, growing crops genetically engineered for high yields and concentrating on mass commodity markets, and may dominate the world market. The second consists of farms that produce craft products on a small scale, are less reliant on financial capital and more environmentally sustainable, may serve more specialized and affluent markets and may receive support for their environmentally sympathetic activities. Farmers may work part-time on these smaller farms, and on other income-earning activities.

Both forms of farming need to be assessed for their real sustainability if they are to provide a secure food supply. The external costs of both need examination, so that the true costs of their methods are apparent and compared. Such research is already underway, with attempts to look at the details of the environmental effects of farming methods being developed in several countries.

Sustainable Food Production FOOD 21, funded by the Foundation for Strategic Environmental Research (MISTRA), is a pioneering project that involves agricultural research departments in Sweden working with several international institutions. It has developed methods for analysing indicators of sustainable farming. Research projects include farming input and output, soil nutrient and sustainable cropping, animal welfare and production intensity, food safety and food quality.

Farmers in Sweden are developing new projects to make their foods more consumer friendly. These include using food label codes to lead consumers to Internet sites where the farm, the farm suppliers, the abattoirs and food manufacturers can supply details on their policies and relevant statistical data. Through projects such as these, a more truly 21st-century form of farming might emerge in which rural development and environmental issues are integrated into modern farming systems using modern technology. This would make the systems more accountable to consumers.

Policies are needed that encourage more sustainable diets. As this chapter has suggested, there is some concordance between healthy dietary patterns and more sustainable food production methods.

WHO is increasingly committed to promoting: "healthy environments, social equity and sustainable development – essential ingredients for the improvement and maintenance of population health" *(2)*.

Achieving social and ecological sustainability without further depletion of energy reserves requires reducing global energy use by 50% and use by high-income countries by 90% by the year 2040 *(126)*. The alternative is to purchase short-term gains at the expense of long-term loss of the integrity of the ecosphere and biophysical life support – an unsustainable process. The health effects of failing to deal with such problems as depletion of the ozone layer, ocean pollution, declining fisheries, desertification, loss of biodiversity and increasing social injustice can all too easily be predicted.

Food production plays a role in this process. The methods of production, the types of food produced, its transport, the globalization of supplies and the concentration of ownership of food production and distribution both benefit and potentially threaten food and nutrition security and thus health.

The carrying capacity of the planet is likely to become a central issue in global development in this century. Trade globalization increases the separation of consuming populations from the ecological impact of their lifestyles, making continued growth and consumption appear sustainable when they are not. The ecological footprint of an industrialized population is typically several times larger than the area in which it lives *(127)*. For example, Italy's ecological footprint is estimated to be about eight times larger than the country. A global population of 9–10 billion living affluent lifestyles might need 2 or 3 extra earth-like planets *(127)*.

Reducing food transport and changing farming methods may further reduce the demands on natural resources. Less reliance on fossil fuels implies the need for alternative, sustainable forms of energy, including human labour. Combined with rural development policies to increase the standards of living in rural areas, improving food production policies can substantially improve the prospects for health.

References

1. *Earth Summit Agenda 21 – The United Nations programme of action from Rio* (http://www.un.org/esa/sustdev/agenda21text.htm). New York, United Nations Publications, 1993 (accessed 29 October 2002).
2. SOSKOLNE, C.L. & BERTOLLINI, R., ED. *Global ecological integrity and "sustainable development": cornerstones of public health* (http://www.euro.who.int/globalchange/Publications/20020627_4). Copenhagen, WHO Regional Office for Europe, 1999 (accessed 22 October 2002).
3. LANG, T. The public health impact of globalisation of food trade. *In*: Shetty, P.S. & McPherson, K., ed. *Diet, nutrition and chronic disease: lessons from contrasting worlds.* Chichester, Wiley, 1997, pp. 173–187.
4. MCMICHAEL, A. Impact of climatic and other environmental changes on food production and population health in coming decades. *Proceedings of the Nutrition Society,* **60**: 195–201 (2001).
5. MCMICHAEL, P. The impact of globalisation, free trade and technology on food and nutrition in the new millennium. *Proceedings of the Nutrition Society,* **60**: 215–220 (2001).
6. *FAO: large gap in food availability between rich and poor countries – New map on nutrition released* (http://www.fao.org/WAICENT/OIS/PRESS_NE/PRESSENG/1998/pren9870.htm). Rome, Food and Agriculture Organization of the United Nations, 1998 (Press release 98/70) (accessed 22 October 2002).
7. MAY, J. An elusive consensus: definitions, measurement and analysis of poverty. *In*: *Choices for the poor* (http://www.undp.org/dpa/publications/choicesforpoor/ENGLISH/index.html). New York, United Nations Development Programme, 2001 (accessed 29 October 2002).

8. CARTER, R. *The silent crisis: the impact of poverty on children in eastern Europe and the former Soviet Union.* London, European Children's Trust, 2000.

9. *Human development report 2000.* New York, United Nations Development Programme, 2000.

10. *Human development report 2001.* New York, United Nations Development Programme, 2001.

11. *World development report 2000–2001.* Washington, DC, World Bank, 2001.

12. 12.FALKINGHAM, J. *A profile of poverty in Tajikistan.* London, Centre for Analysis of Social Exclusion, London School of Economics, 2000 (CASE Paper 39).

13. *Making transition work for everyone.* Washington, DC, World Bank, 2000.

14. *The state of food insecurity in the world 2000.* Rome, Food and Agriculture Organization of the United Nations, 2000.

15. *Social portrait of Europe.* Luxembourg, Eurostat – Statistical Office of the European Commission, 1996.

16. *Poverty in Europe.* Brussels, European Anti-Poverty Network, 1998.

17. *Encyclopaedia britannica.* Chicago, Encyclopaedia Britannica, 2000.

18. *World resources 2000–2001.* Washington, DC, World Resources Institute, 2001.

19. THEUBET, M.-P. How much for a balanced diet? Low-income families and low-cost food. *In: Health inequalities in Europe.* Paris, Société Française de Santé Publique, 2000, p. 274.

20. DALLISON, J. & LOBSTEIN, T. *Poor expectations: poverty and diet in pregnancy.* London, Maternity Alliance and NCH Action for Children, 1995.

21. COLE-HAMILTON, I. & LOBSTEIN, T. *Poverty and nutrition survey 1990.* London, NCH Action for Children, 1991.

22. NELSON, M. Nutrition and health inequalities. *In:* Gordon, D. et al., ed. *Inequalities in health: studies in poverty, inequality and social exclusion.* Bristol, Policy Press, University of Bristol, 1999.

23. DEPARTMENT FOR FOOD, ENVIRONMENT AND RURAL AFFAIRS. *National food survey 2000.* London, The Stationery Office, 2001.

24. FOOD COMMISSION. The cost of food. *The food magazine,* **49**: 21 (2000).

25. ROKX, C. ET AL. *Prospects for improving nutrition in eastern Europe and central Asia.* Washington, DC, World Bank, 2001.

26. *Urban and Peri-urban Food and Nutrition Action Plan: elements for community action to promote social cohesion and reduce inequalities through local production for local consumption* (http://www.euro.who.int/Document/e72949.pdf). Copenhagen, WHO Regional Office for Europe, 2000 (accessed 29 October 2002).

27. McGLONE, P. ET AL. *Food projects and how they work.* York, York Publishing for Joseph Rowntree Foundation, 1999.

28. HAWKES, C. & WEBSTER, J. *Too much and too little? Debates on surplus food redistribution.* London, Sustain: the alliance for better food and farming, 2000.

29. RICHES, G. Hunger, food security and welfare politics. *Proceedings of the Nutrition Society,* 56: 63–74 (1997).

30. *Low income, food, nutrition and health: strategies for improvement.* London, Department of Health, 1996.

31. DOWLER, E. Inequalities in diet and physical activity in Europe. *Public health nutrition,* 4(2B): 701–709 (2001).

32. MORRIS, J. ET AL. A minimum income for healthy living? *European journal of epidemiology and community health,* 54: 885–889 (2000).

33. VEIT-WILSON, J. *Setting adequacy standards: how governments define minimum incomes.* Bristol, Policy Press, 1998.

34. ROBERTS, K. & FIELD, A. Physical activity: patterns and policy options. *In*: Sharp, I., ed. *Social inequalities in coronary heart disease: opportunities for action.* London, The Stationery Office for the National Heart Forum, 1998, pp. 99–105.

35. MATHIJS, E. & VRANKEN, L. *Farm restructuring and efficiency in transition: evidence from Bulgaria and Hungary.* Louvain, Catholic University of Louvain, 2000.

36. RIZOV, M. ET AL. *Post-communist agricultural transformation and the role of human capital: evidence from Romania.* Louvain, Catholic University of Louvain, 2000.

37. VON BRAUN, J. ET AL. *Russia's food economy in transition: what do reforms mean for the long-term outlook?* Washington, DC, International Food Policy Research Institute, 1996 (2020 Brief 36).

38. ARDY, B. *Agriculture and the food industry in central and eastern Europe and EU enlargement.* London, South Bank University, 2000.

39. PINSTRUP-ANDERSEN, P. & PANDYA-LORCH, R. Securing and sustaining adequate world food production for the third millennium. *In*: Weeks, D.P. et al., ed. *World food security and sustainability: the impacts of biotechnology and industrial consolidation.* New York, National Agricultural Biotechnology Council, 1999 (Report 11).

40. *Agriculture and food economy in Poland.* Warsaw, Ministry of Agriculture and Food Economy, 1999.

41. *International trade statistics.* Geneva, World Trade Organization, 2000.

42. *EU energy and transport in figures. Statistical pocketbook 2001* (http://europa.eu.int/comm/energy_transport/etif/index.html). Brussels, European Commission, 2001 (accessed 29 October 2002).

43. HEDBRAND, A. *Trends in road freight transport 1990–1998.* Luxembourg, Eurostat – Statistical Office of the European Commission, 2001.

44. *European retail handbook 1999.* London, Corporate Intelligence Group, 1999.

45. DOBSON CONSULTING. *Buyer power and its impact on competition in the food retail distribution sector of the European Union* (http://europa.eu.int/comm/competition/publications/studies/bpifrs). Brussels, European Commission, 1999 (accessed 29 October 2002).

46. *Combined food market share of the top five grocery retailers in selected European countries* (http://www.planetretail.net). Frankfurt, M+M Planet retail, 2003 (accessed 3 September 2003).

47. FOOD COMMISSION. The increasing cost of a healthy diet. *The food magazine,* **31**: 17 (1995).

48. *Commerce 2000: best European practice regarding local shops in disadvantaged rural areas* (http://europa.eu.int/comm/enterprise/library/lib-distributive_trade/doc/ruralb-pratiques-en.pdf). Brussels, Commerce Unit, European Commission Directorate for Enterprise Policy, Distributive Trades, Tourism and Social Economy, 2000 (accessed 29 October 2002).

49. PRETTY, J. ET AL. An assessment of the total external costs of UK agriculture. *Agricultural systems,* **65**: 113–136 (2000).

50. PRETTY, J. ET AL. Policy challenges and priorities for internalising the externalities of agriculture. *Journal of environmental planning and management,* **44**: 263–283 (2001).

51. FLEISCHER, G. & WAIBEL, H. Consequences for agricultural policies from analysing economic and political factors of pesticide use in developing countries. *In*: Wossink, G.A.A. et al., ed. *Economics of agro-chemicals – an international overview of use patterns, technical and institutional determinants, policies and perspectives. Selected papers of the conference of the International Association of Agricultural Economists held at Wageningen, the Netherlands, 24–28 April 1996.* Ashgate, Aldershot, 1998.

52. *Directions towards sustainable agriculture* (http://europa.eu.int/comm/agriculture/envir/9922/9922_en.pdf). European Commission, Brussels, 1999 (COM (1999) 22, accessed 29 October 2002).

53. *Proceedings of the First Workshop of the Central and Eastern Europe Sustainable Agriculture Network, FAO, Godollo, Hungary, 2–7 March 1999* (http://www.fao.org/Regional/SEUR/ceesa/contents.htm). Rome, Food and Agriculture Organization of the United Nations, 1999 (accessed 29 October 2002).

54. *The environmental impact of food from origin to waste: interim report.* Stockholm, Federation of Swedish Farmers, 2000.

55. KOOIJMAN, J.M. Environmental assessment of packaging: sense and sensibility. *Environmental management,* **17**: 575–586 (1993).

56. REGANOLD, J.P. ET AL. Sustainability of three apple production systems. *Nature*, **410**: 926–930 (2000).

57. AGRICULTURAL DEVELOPMENT AND ADVISORY SERVICE. *Energy use in organic farming systems*. London, Department for Environment, Food and Rural Affairs, 2001 (MAFF Consultancy Project OF0182).

58. PIMENTEL, D. ET AL., ED. *Ecological integrity: integrating environment, conservation and health*. Washington, DC, Island Press, 2000.

59. COSGROVE, W.J. & RIJSBERMAN, F.R. *World water vision: making water everybody's business*. London, Earthscan Publications, 2000.

60. KOVATS, S. ET AL., ED. *Climate change and stratospheric ozone depletion: early effects on our health in Europe*. Copenhagen, WHO Regional Office for Europe, 2000 (WHO Regional Publications, European Series, No. 88).

61. *Milk and the environment* (http://www.enheldelom.svenskmjolk.se/english/pdf/Milk_and_the_Environment_booklet.pdf). Stockholm, Swedish Dairy Association 2000 (accessed 29 October 2002).

62. *REDEFINE summary report. Relationship between demand for freight-transport and industrial effects* (http://www.cordis.lu/transport/src/redefinerep.htm). Luxembourg, CORDIS Transport RTD Programme, 1999 (accessed 29 October 2002).

63. KUNZLI, N. ET AL. Public-health impact of outdoor and traffic-related pollution: a European assessment. *Lancet*, **356**: 795–801 (2000).

64. WORLD HEALTH ORGANIZATION & UNITED NATIONS ECONOMIC COMMISSION FOR EUROPE. *Overview of instruments relevant to transport, environment and health and recommendations for further steps* (http://www.unece.org/doc/ece/ac/ece.ac.21.2001.1.e.pdf). Geneva, United Nations Economic Commission for Europe, 17 January 2001 (accessed 29 October 2002).

65. DORA, C. & PHILLIPS, M., ED. *Transport, environment and health*. Copenhagen, WHO Regional Office for Europe, 2000 (WHO Regional Publications, European Series, No. 89).

66. DEPARTMENT FOR TRANSPORT, LOCAL GOVERNMENT AND THE REGIONS. *Transport statistics Great Britain*. London, The Stationery Office, 1997.

67. LUCAS, C. *Stopping the great food swap: relocalising Europe's food supply*. Brussels, European Parliament, 2001.

68. CARLSSON-KANYAMA, A. Food consumption patterns and their influence on climate change. *Ambio (Royal Swedish Academy of Sciences)*, **27**: 528–534 (1998).

69. *Scotland's health: the Scottish diet*. Edinburgh, Scottish Office, 1993.

70. *31st financial report on the European Agricultural Guidance and Guarantee Fund EAGGF, Guarantee Section – 2001 financial year* (http://europa.eu.int/comm/agriculture/fin/finrep01/en.pdf). Brussels, Directorate General for Agriculture, European Commission, pp. 20–21 (COM(2002) 594 final, accessed 28 January 2003).

71. *Agriculture in the European Union. Statistical and economic information 1999* (http://europa.eu.int/comm/agriculture/agrista/table_en/index.htm). Brussels, European Commission, 2000 (accessed 20 January 2003).

72. EUROPEAN COURT OF AUDITORS. Special report No 8/2000 on the Community measures for the disposal of butterfat accompanied by the Commission's replies (http://www.eca.eu.int/EN/rs/2000/c_132en.pdf). *Official journal of the European Communities*, **43**(C132): 1–32 (2000) (accessed 29 October 2002).

73. EUROPEAN COURT OF AUDITORS. Special report No 20/2000 concerning the management of the common organisation of the market for sugar (pursuant to article 248, paragraph 4 (2), EC) (http://www.eca.eu.int/EN/rs/2000/rs20_00en.pdf). *Official journal of the European Communities*, **44**(C50): 1–30 (2001) (accessed 29 October 2002).

74. EUROPEAN COURT OF AUDITORS. Special report No 6/2001 on milk quotas (pursuant to Article 248, paragraph 4 (2), EC Treaty) (http://www.eca.eu.int/EN/rs/2001/rs06_01en.pdf). *Official journal of the European Communities*, **44**(C305): 1–34 (2001) (accessed 29 October 2002).

75. *Public health aspects of the EU CAP – developments and recommendations for change in four sectors: fruit and vegetables, dairy, wine and tobacco* (http://www.fhi.se/shop/material_pdf/eu_inlaga.pdf). Stockholm, National Institute of Public Health, 2003 (accessed 3 September 2003).

76. LOBSTEIN, T. & LONGFIELD, J. *Improving diet and health through European Union food policies.* London, Health Education Authority, 1999.

77. *The agricultural situation in the European Union – Agricultural production: crop products 1996.* Brussels, Directorate General for Agriculture, European Commission, 1997.

78. *Diet, nutrition and the prevention of chronic diseases. Report of a joint WHO/FAO expert consultation* (http://whqlibdoc.who.int/trs/WHO_TRS_916.pdf). Geneva, World Health Organization, 2003 (WHO Technical Series, No. 916) (accessed 3 September 2003).

79. WILLIAMS, C. ET AL., ED. Food-based dietary guidelines – A staged approach. *British journal of nutrition*, **81**(Suppl. 2): S29–S153 (1999).

80. TUDGE, C. *Functional foods and pharmacological impoverishment.* London, Caroline Walker Trust, 1999.

81. KANT, A.K. ET AL. A prospective study of diet quality and mortality in women. *Journal of the American Medical Association*, **283**: 2109–2115 (2000).

82. KANT, A.K. ET AL. Dietary diversity and subsequent cause-specific mortality in the NHANES I epidemiologic follow-up study. *Journal of the American College of Nutrition*, 14: 233–238 (1995).

83. WAHLQVIST, M. *Prospects for the future: nutrition, environment and sustainable food production. In: Conference on International Food Trade Beyond 2000: Science-Based Decisions, Harmonization, Equivalence and Mutual Recognition, Melbourne, Australia, 11–15 October 1999* (http://www.fao.org/docrep/meeting/X2638e.htm). Rome, Food and Agricultural Organization of the United Nations, 1999 (accessed 29 October 2002).

84. PRETTY, J. *Regenerating agriculture.* Washington, DC, Joseph Henry Press, 1995.

85. BROUGH, D. *Biodiversity shrinks as farm breeds die out* (http://www.news24.com/News24/Technology/Science_Nature/0,1113,2-13-46_1084537,00.html). Rome, Reuters, 25 September 2001 (accessed 29 October 2002).

86. TRICHOPOULOU, A. ET AL. Nutritional composition and flavonoid content of edible wild greens and green pies: a potential rich source of antioxidant nutrients in the Mediterranean diet. *Food chemistry*, 703: 319–323 (2000).

87. DELONG, G.R. ET AL. Effect on infant mortality of iodination of irrigation water in a severely iodine-deficient area of China. *Lancet*, 350: 771–773 (1997).

88. MAYER, A.-M. Historical changes in the mineral content of fruits and vegetables. *British food journal*, 99: 207–211 (1997).

89. BLYTHMAN, J. *The food we eat.* London, Michael Joseph, 1996.

90. ANDERSEN, J.-O. *Farming, plant nutrition and food quality* (http://www.pmac.net/farming_nutrition.html). Copenhagen, University of Copenhagen, 1999 (accessed 29 October 2002).

91. MAIANI, G. ET AL. Factors of change, technological process and the uncertain future of the Mediterranean diet. *Public health nutrition*, 4(2A): 415 (2001).

92. *Organic farming, food quality and human health. A review of the evidence.* Bristol, United Kingdom Soil Association, 2002.

93. CRAWFORD, M.A. Fatty acid ratios in free-living and domesticated animals. Possible implications for atheroma. *Lancet*, 1(7556): 1329–1333 (1968).

94. CRAWFORD, M.A. & MARSH, D. *The driving force.* London, Heinemann, 1989.

95. CRAWFORD, M.A. ET AL. Comparative studies on fatty acid composition of wild and domestic meats. *International journal of biochemistry*, 1: 295–305 (1970).

96. ENSER, M. ET AL. Manipulating meat quality and consumption. Animal Nutrition and Metabolism Group Symposium on 'Improving meat production for future needs'. *Proceedings of the Nutrition Society*, 58: 363–370 (1999)

97. SARGENT, J.R. & TACON, A.G.J. Development of farmed fish: a nutritionally necessary alternative to meat. *Proceedings of the Nutrition Society*, 58: 377–383 (1999).

98. HOLLAND, B. ET AL. *McCance and Widdowson's the composition of foods*, 5th ed. Cambridge, Royal Society of Chemistry, 1991.

99. CODEX ALIMENTARIUS COMMITTEE ON FOOD LABELLING. *ALINORM 01/22A Ottawa, Canada, May 2001* (http://www.fao.org/docrep/meeting/005/y0651e/y0651e00.htm). Rome, Food and Agricultural Organization of the United Nations, 2001 (accessed 29 October 2002).

100. *Our food: information on all aspects of our food – Food facts and figures.* London, McDonald's Restaurants Ltd, 2001.

101. LANG, T. & HEASMAN, M. *Food wars – public health and the battle for mouths, minds and markets.* London, Earthscan, 2003.

102. MILLSTONE, E. & LANG, T. *The atlas of food: who eats what, where and why.* London, Earthscan, 2003.

103. AGRICULTURAL COUNCIL OF THE EUROPEAN UNION. *Council strategy on environmental integration and sustainable development in the Common Agricultural Policy.* Press Release, 17/11/1999, No 13078/99 (http://ue.eu.int/Newsroom/loadDoc.asp?max=21&bid=75&did=59800&grp=2209&lang=1). Brussels, European Union, 1999 (accessed 5 November 2002).

104. *A sustainable food supply chain.* Stockholm, Swedish Environmental Protection Agency, 1999 (Report 4966).

105. BARNEY, G.O. *Global 2000 revisited: what shall we do?* Arlington, VA, Millennium Institute, 1993.

106. CENTRE FOR EUROPEAN AGRICULTURAL STUDIES, WYE & EUROPEAN FORUM ON NATURE CONSERVATION AND PASTORALISM. *The environmental impact of dairy production in the EU – Practical options for the improvement of the environmental impact* (http://europa.eu.int/comm/environment/agriculture/studies.htm). Brussels, European Commission, 2001 (accessed 29 October 2002).

107. GARDENER, B. *European agriculture in the new millennium.* London, Agra Europe, 1999.

108. DELGADO, C. ET AL. *Livestock to 2020: the next food revolution.* Washington, DC, International Food Policy Research Institute, 1999 (Food, Agriculture and Environment Discussion Paper 28).

109. GOODLAND, R. *The case against financing dairy projects in developing countries.* Washington, DC, Environment Department, World Bank, 2000.

110. *The Scottish farmer,* 111(5782): 32 (2003).

111. *Watershed progress: New York City watershed agreement* (http://www.epa.gov/OWOW/watershed/ny/nycityfi.html). Washington, DC, Office of Water, US Environmental Protection Agency, 1996 (accessed 29 October 2002).

112. PRETTY, J. *Changing agricultural practices and their impact on biodiversity.* Cambridge, University of Cambridge Committee for Interdisciplinary Environmental Studies, 2000.

113. HASSEBRUCK, C. Meeting food needs through sustainable production systems and family farms. *In*: Weeks, D.P. et al., ed. *World food security and sustainability: the impacts of biotechnology and industrial consolidation.* New York, National Agricultural Biotechnology Council, 1999 (Report 11).

114. *The agricultural situation in the European Union 1999.* Brussels, European Commission, 2000.

115. *Agriculture in Lithuania 2000.* Vilnius, Lithuanian Institute of Agrarian Economics, 2001.

116. *Participatory appraisal for community assessment: principles and methods. 2. Five assets for local communities and economies* (http://www2.essex.ac.uk/ces/ResearchProgrammes/pa&caover2.htm). Essex, Centre for Environment and Society, University of Essex, 1999 (accessed 29 October 2002).

117. POLICY AND INNOVATION UNIT. *Rural economics.* London, Cabinet Office, 1999.

118. *Rural services and social housing 1997–98.* London, Countryside Agency, 1999.

119. PRETTY, J. *The living land.* London, Earthscan, 1998.

120. INTERNATIONAL CONFEDERATION OF FREE TRADE UNIONS, TRADE UNION ADVISORY COMMITTEE TO THE OECD & INTERNATIONAL UNION OF FOOD, AGRICULTURAL, HOTEL, RESTAURANT, CATERING, TOBACCO AND ALLIED WORKERS' ASSOCIATIONS. *"Plough to plate" approaches to food and agriculture* (http://www.un.org/documents/ecosoc/cn17/2000/ecn172000-3add3.pdf). New York, United Nations Commission on Sustainable Development, 2000 (accessed 29 October 2002).

121. FORSCHUNGSINSTITUT FÜR BIOLOGISCHEN LANDBAU (FiBL) & STIFTUNG OEKOLOGIE & LANDBAU (SOEL). *Organic farming in Europe – provisional statistics 2001* (http://www.organic-europe.net/europe_eu/statistics.asp). Bad Dürkheim, Stiftung Oekologie & Landbau (SOEL), 2001 (accessed 29 October 2002).

122. PEDERSON, R.M. & ROBERTSON, A. Food policies are essential for healthy cities. *Urban agriculture magazine*, 1: 9–11 (2001).
123. BIRLEY, M.H. & LOCK, K. *The health impacts of peri-urban natural resource development.* Liverpool, Liverpool School of Tropical Medicine, 1999.
124. ZIGLIO, E. ET AL., ED. *Health systems confront poverty* (http://www.euro.who.int/InformationSources/Publications/Catalogue/20030814_1). Copenhagen, WHO Regional Office for Europe, 2003 (Public Health Case Studies No. 1) (accessed 3 September 2003).
125. LOCK, K. & DE ZEEUW, H. Mitigating the health risks associated with urban and periurban agriculture. *Urban agriculture magazine*, 1: 6–8 (2001).
126. *Getting eco-efficient.* Geneva, Business Council for Sustainable Development, 1993.
127. REES, W. Global change and ecological integrity: quantifying the limits to growth. *In*: Soskolne, C.L. & Bertollini, R, ed. *Global ecological integrity and "sustainable development": cornerstones of public health* (http://www.euro.who.int/globalchange/Publications/20020627_4). Copenhagen, WHO Regional Office for Europe, 1999, pp. 32–36 (accessed 22 October 2002).

4. Policies and strategies

WHO Action Plan on Food and Nutrition Policy

In September 2000, the WHO Regional Committee for Europe, representing the 51 Member States in the European Region, unanimously endorsed a resolution to implement The First Action Plan for Food and Nutrition Policy (Annex 1). The Action Plan makes the case for combining nutrition, food safety and food security and sustainable development into an overarching, intersectoral policy and offers support to governments in developing, implementing and evaluating such policies.

Progress with its implementation, by both WHO and Member States, will be regularly reported to the Regional Committee. In addition, a ministerial conference on food and nutrition will review more comprehensive evaluations of its impact.

This political commitment gives public health experts an extraordinary and important opportunity to advocate, at both the national and European levels, a food and nutrition policy that explicitly promotes health.

The Action Plan stresses the need to develop food and nutrition policies that protect and promote health and reduce the burden of food-related disease, while contributing to socioeconomic development and a sustainable environment. It insists on the complementary roles played by different sectors in formulating and implementing such policies. It provides a framework within which Member States can begin to address the issue. The framework consists of three interrelated strategies (Fig. 4.1):

- a nutrition strategy, geared to ensuring optimum health, especially among low-income groups and during critical periods throughout life, such as infancy, childhood, pregnancy and lactation and older age;
- a food safety strategy, highlighting the need to prevent both chemical and biological contamination at all stages of the food chain (new food safety systems that take a farm-to-fork perspective are being developed); and
- a strategy on a sustainable food supply (food security), aiming to ensure that enough food of high quality is available while helping to stimulate rural economies and to promote the social and environmental aspects of sustainable development.

Fig. 4.1. Framework of The First Action Plan for Food
and Nutrition Policy, WHO European Region, 2000–2005

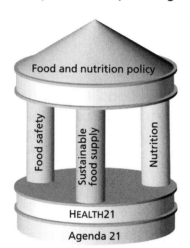

Nutritional imbalances have subtle and long-term effects, as shown in Chapter 1, and place a heavy burden on health and economic progress. The effects of nutrition are not as newsworthy as high-profile food safety crises, and in theory individuals have substantial control over their longer-term nutritional health. Thus, most policy-makers mistakenly consider that individual food choice, stimulated by appropriate educational initiatives, is the key to nutritional wellbeing.

Food safety usually concerns immediate effects on health that often have tremendous political, economic and strategic significance. Health ministers in Europe were heavily involved in reassessing food safety strategies in the 1990s (see Chapter 2, pp. 103–104).

Food and nutrition security has traditionally been important only when food supplies are threatened, for example, by war or drought. As a result of the increased recognition of the importance of environmental conditions, however, environmental policies relating to land use and food supply have a profound long-term impact on both the availability and quality of food.

This chapter considers how best to address all three issues and how to ensure that policies relating to one sector do not conflict with, but support, the needs of the others.

Need for integrated and comprehensive food and nutrition policies

A strong case can be made for developing national food and nutrition policies that address all three areas – nutrition, food safety and food security – since these political commitments overlap and since such an integrated approach can help to prevent the inadvertent development of potentially damaging policies. A written policy brings the following benefits *(1)*; it:

- sets out a clear statement of intent, legitimizes action and provides a firm foundation for food and nutrition initiatives;
- creates a framework for action for the health ministry and other sectors;
- removes any possibility of misinterpretation or misunderstanding of the government position on food and nutrition and any differences in interpretation between the sectors involved;
- provides a corporate document to which individuals and organizations can refer;
- demonstrates commitment to the public health of all citizens;
- justifies the allocation of resources to national plans and programmes on food and nutrition.

Discordant agricultural, industrial and food policies can harm health, the environment and the economy, but harmful effects can be reduced and health promoted if all sectors are aware of the policy options. The following sections give examples of the disadvantages of discordant policies and the advantages of concordant ones.

Policy discordance
CAP – multiple health effects
EU regulations on agriculture, industrial practice and taxation significantly affect the pricing of and policies on food throughout the world. The EU is the biggest importer and exporter of food in the world. Its criteria for food safety and the nutritional quality of different products and the policies relating to any selective promotion of specific foods therefore profoundly affect not only the EU itself but any country that exports or imports an appreciable part of its food supply. Owing to the expansion of the EU, its policies also profoundly affect the accession countries. The directives relating to food labelling, food safety, demands for specific agricultural and slaughtering practices in the animal food chain and the taxation systems relating to the support of less economically advanced areas within the EU affect the nature of the food supply and ultimately people's health.

An analysis by Sweden's National Institute of Public Health *(2)* concludes that the regulations and systems involved in CAP have led to effects on consumption that can harm health. Consumer groups have performed similar analyses and reached similar conclusions *(3)* (see Chapter 2, pp. 169 and 183–184).

For instance, CAP rules on fruit and vegetables raise the price of fresh fruit and vegetables, preventing low-income people from affording healthy food. In addition, subsidies of products containing milk fat and the promotion of full-fat milk conflict with the health aim of reducing saturated fat intake. CAP therefore does little to reduce the high rates of CVD within the EU. The "yellow fat regime" has kept the retail price of butter well above the world market price, however, so this could help to reduce saturated fat intake. Further, regulation of the wine market removes surplus production and keeps prices higher than the world market. This tends to limit the consumption of wine, although there is major pressure for allowing greater wine consumption, which would not be beneficial. The report from the National Institute of Public Health, Sweden, puts forward a number of specific recommendations that would lead to substantial improvements in the CAP from a public health point of view. Some important ones are (2):

- Phase out all consumption aid to dairy products with a high fat content.
- Limit the School Milk Measure to include only milk products with a low fat content.
- Introduce a similar school measure for fruits and vegetables.
- Redistribute agriculture support so that it favours the fruit and vegetable sector and increased consumption.
- Phase out support for the promotion of wine consumption.
- Improve and put a time limit on the support to farmers who wish to cease wine production.
- Develop a plan to phase out tobacco subsidies within a reasonable time.

BSE crisis: driven by cost-cutting feeding practices

The BSE crisis in the European Region (see Chapter 2, pp. 125–127) illustrates the importance of considering any potential health effects of agricultural and industrial practices. The advantage of including recycled animal protein in ruminant diets is that cattle and sheep respond especially well in production terms. The resulting widespread use of animal protein, whether from fish or recycled meat and bone meal, led to marked increases in productivity and increasingly inexpensive meat and milk supplies. This was considered important for health after the Second World War, as the nutritional wellbeing of the poor would be improved at that time if children and nursing mothers had access to inexpensive meat and milk.

The crisis in the United Kingdom, which began with the discovery of BSE in cattle in 1986, escalated when BSE was linked to vCJD. BSE has now affected all EU countries, and many others, such as Switzerland and Japan, with profound economic implications and the demand for ever more rigorous food safety measures. Based on a recent classification of the risk of BSE in many countries throughout the world, the EU now requires a substantial number of countries to institute slaughtering policies that specify the removal of the brain, spinal cord and often the vertebral column of animals. This is to exclude from the food chain as much as possible any potential infectivity with transmissible spongiform encephalopathies. The crisis has also necessitated changes in policies relating to the use of vaccines, medical implants and a range of other surgical procedures. It is still uncertain whether the disproportional impact of vCJD on young people is a feature of their age-related biological sensitivity or the incubation period of the disease is shorter in young people *(4)*.

Labelling of meat

An EU directive from 2000 *(5)* contains a set of new provisions to improve consumer information on prepacked meat products such as cooked meats, prepared dishes and canned meat. The previous EU definition of meat made no distinction between muscle-meat, fat and offal, while consumers usually perceive meat to mean muscle-meat. The existing system was therefore unsatisfactory, and several EU countries had already adopted their own definitions of meat for labelling. The new EU directive restricts the definition of meat to muscle-meat. Other parts – such as offal, heart, intestine, liver and fat – will now have to be labelled as such.

Nevertheless, a nutrition policy concern remains because this directive permits fat adhering to the muscle and comprising 25% or less of total weight to be called meat. This figure rises to 30% for pork products *(5)*. To help consumers reduce saturated fat intake, public health experts should therefore take the necessary intersectoral steps to ensure that meat has a much lower fat content. Without both clear labelling and more stringent definitions of meat, consumers cannot make informed choices on how to eat a healthier diet.

Promotion of olive oil

Olive oil has been advocated as beneficial to health because it is relatively high in monounsaturated fatty acids and has limited saturated fat. It is traditionally linked to the Mediterranean diet, with its beneficial health effects. Industrial and farming groups in Mediterranean regions that need economic development are therefore heavily promoting olive oil. Olive oil may indeed be conducive to health, especially if it replaces other saturated fat. Alternative plant oils such as rapeseed oil are also being produced, so there is no intrinsic need to promote olive oil alone.

Current EU policies to promote olive oil production and consumption, however, have led to much of the global supply being produced in Greece, Italy, Portugal and Spain. This in turn has led to intensification of production, resulting in severe soil erosion and a remarkable decline in water availability. Thus, intensive agriculture, geared to increasing olive oil production subsidized by the EU, is threatening the long-term viability of these olive-producing areas *(6–9)*. Statistics from FAO show that olive oil production doubled in the EU (the current 15 EU countries) from 1990 to 2001: from 1 025 572 metric tonnes to 2 045 300 tonnes (http://apps.fao.org/page/collections?subset= agriculture, accessed 22 January 2003). The recommendations of food and nutrition policy should ensure the sustainability of these food-growing regions.

Fish

The consumption of fish is advocated for its health-beneficial fatty acids. The very-long-chain omega-3 polyunsaturated fatty acids derived mainly from fish are now recognized to have marked favourable effects on CHD and other positive effects on health (see Chapter 1, p. 10). Although eating more fish has clear benefits, European stocks of fish are rapidly declining, a decline accelerated by the escalating world demand. This demand has led to a major drive to increase fish farming. This should be developed further, with a limitation on the use of fish meal as feed, and aquacultural methods should be improved, including limiting the accumulation of toxins such as dioxin (see Chapter 2, p. 113), a fat-soluble carcinogenic compound, contained in omega-3 fatty acids.

Integrated intervention by the nutrition, food safety and environmental sectors is thus warranted. Nutritionists' advocacy of greater consumption of fish must be backed by food safety measures to control dioxin contamination and environmental measures to promote the management of clean bodies of water. A similar dilemma occurs when, on the one hand, low-fat chicken meat is recommended and, on the other, there are food safety concerns about *Salmonella* (see Chapter 2, pp. 121–124).

Food fortification: the case of universal salt iodization

The international policy recommendation for eliminating iodine deficiency is universal salt iodization: depending on salt consumption patterns, all salt used at the table, for cooking and by food manufacturers and all salt fed as fodder to animals should be iodized. In some countries, only table salt is iodized. This may lead to the unintentional promotion of salt, and excessive salt intake can adversely affect blood pressure *(10)*. If consumers reduce their salt intake, as recommended in most dietary guidelines, and if only table salt is iodized, they may become deficient in iodine. Iodine deficiency disorders can be more sustainably eradicated if all salt is iodized. The iodization of animal fodder needs to be explored further because the various approaches to correct iodine deficiency have underestimated it as a component of universal salt iodization.

Universal salt iodization is another example of a policy warranting integrated intervention by nutritionists, food safety experts, the food industry and farmers. Nutritionists should ensure sufficient iodine intake; food safety experts should monitor the fortification levels of iodine in line with national regulations; the food industry should ensure all salt is iodized, and farmers should ensure implementation of the regulations on iodized fodder in animal husbandry. Consumers should automatically get sufficient iodine from manufactured foods such as bread, without having to add extra salt to their food. In western Europe, about 75% of salt intake comes from salt added to processed foods and only 25% from cooking or table use. Studies show that bread accounts for nearly 25% of the salt in diets in the United Kingdom, although sodium levels in bread were reduced by up to 21% between 1998 and 2001. The Department of Health now wants to see all food industries follow the example set by the bread industry. Sir John Krebs, Chair of the United Kingdom Food Standards Agency, stated: "This change is of real importance for the health of our bread eating nation – particularly for those who have been advised to reduce their salt intake. In the [United Kingdom], people eat on average three slices of bread per day, so this is key to lowering their overall dietary intake of salt." *(11)*.

Pesticide residues in fruits and vegetables

Consumers' exposure to pesticides should be minimized for safety reasons. In the United Kingdom, more than 450 active pesticide ingredients are licensed for use in agriculture *(12)*, and about 25 000 tonnes of pesticides were applied to crops in 2000 (http://apps.fao.org/page/collections? subset=agriculture, accessed 22 January 2003). Because many pesticides are persistent, they contaminate air, water and soil. Nearly half (48%) of all fruit and vegetables tested in the United Kingdom in 1999 contained detectable pesticide residues. The maximum acceptable residue limit was exceeded in 1.6% of samples. Although the Working Party on Pesticide Residues *(13)* reported that most of these residues above maximum limits posed no threat to human health, it found potentially harmful levels in pears and peppers. The threat of accumulation of pesticide residues in the body could discourage consumers from increasing their intake of fruits and vegetables. As discussed in Chapter 1 and in this chapter, nutrition recommendations promote increased intake of fruits and vegetables, to at least 400 g per day *(10)*. Convincing consumers to do this may be difficult if they are concerned about ingesting pesticide residues (see Chapter 2, pp. 129–135).

Policy concordance
Health-driven changes in the food chain: Finland

Finland has managed to decrease CVD dramatically by taking into consideration environmental, industry and dietary concerns (see Chapter 1, Fig. 1.6, p. 15). In the early 1970s, Finland had the highest recorded coronary mortality in the world. A government-led project targeted smoking, blood pressure control and diet, and started preventive activities throughout the country involving the health education and industrial sectors, with changes in the availability and nutritional quality of foods provided in schools, canteens, restaurants and the marketplace. Simultaneously, a market was created for locally produced rapeseed oil to counter the culture of consuming butter and fatty dairy products. The development of a local product ensured its accept-ability throughout society and linked to the development of a health-con-scious and environment-friendly branch of the food industry.

Consumption of fruit and berries – the latter culturally important in Fin-land – was also successfully promoted. In addition, vegetable consumption doubled, the proportion of saturated fat in total fat consumption declined and fish consumption rose. This concerted effort to change the whole pattern of eating resulted in a substantial improvement in the health of the whole popu-lation. The secret was close integration between health and other agencies. For example, dietary guidelines were designed for schools, other mass-catering in-stitutions and other social groups, including elderly people and the armed forces *(14,15)*.

Industrial and fiscal policies leading to health benefits: Poland
While the initiative in Finland arose from health considerations, in Poland the primary concern was to liberate food producers from economic constraints (see Chapter 1, p. 28). Small private farmers were given greater freedom to market their abundant production of fruits and vegetables in Poland, and the selective taxes on different types of fat were changed. This meant that butter and lard were no longer promoted in preference to other types of fat.

A dramatic reduction in saturated fat intake followed. Freeing the agricul-tural markets allowed fruits and vegetables to be far more readily available throughout the year. A decline in heart disease in association with these changes was evident within two years. This illustrates the profound effect of nutritional change induced by multisectoral policies on disease rates in Po-land.

Local agricultural initiatives: St Petersburg, Russian Federation
As a response to the shortages of basic foodstuffs and environmental problems experienced by people in St Petersburg, the Urban Gardening Club started rooftop gardening initiatives to produce vegetables for people with no access to land outside the city *(16)*. Just one district in St Petersburg can now grow 2000 tonnes of vegetables. Despite growing in a city environment, the veg-etables from rooftop gardens proved to have lower levels of contaminants than the usual vegetables sold in the market.

A special feature of the Club is the associated research into techniques for rooftop gardening in urban conditions, such as in residential buildings, schools, hospitals and other institutions. In addition, the project provides employment training and rehabilitation, providing new skills for people with reduced ability to work.

Such initiatives have many benefits. They promote local economic growth, encourage the production of healthy and safe foods, make environmentally friendly use of otherwise unexploited urban spaces and help to promote social cohesion.

Food safety and the environment: Sweden

Sweden's development of an integrated policy on food and health stemmed from a food crisis. A proactive food hygiene policy (see Chapter 2, pp. 106–107) was introduced following the deaths of about 100 people from salmonellosis in the early 1950s. Sweden set up the National Food Administration and made more effort to link good, safe production with high health standards. The progressive stance of farming organizations in Sweden, as well as pressure for change from consumers and other interests outside the food and agricultural sectors, helped such integration *(17)*.

Sweden's Ministry of Agriculture, Food and Fisheries and its Ministry of the Environment are developing programmes to reduce the use of fossil fuels and meet food safety and environmental targets *(18)*. Sweden is also exploring methods to reduce the amount of greenhouse gases produced during food production, as recommended by WHO, the World Meteorological Organization and the United Nations Environment Programme *(19)*. The country aims to halve resource use by 2021, but current evidence indicated that it is unlikely to meet this target. A comprehensive audit of the consequences of eating and travelling in Sweden has shown that far more energy is used than fits the proposed energy quota. This implies "substantial lifestyle changes" *(20)*. New methods are being developed to improve energy auditing in food systems.

Urban food security: food charter in Toronto, Canada

The Toronto City Council formed the Food and Hunger Action Committee in 1999 following a recommendation made by Hunger Watch (a coalition of emergency food organizations) and endorsed by the city's Millennium Task Force. In July 2000, the Action Committee presented a report to the Council *(21)* that identified serious food security issues in Toronto:

- 120 000 people (40% of them children) in the greater Toronto area relied on food banks;
- elderly people and families relied on 1 250 000 hot meals served every year;
- half of food bank users ran out of food at least once each week; and
- 20% of residents had too little money to meet their basic food needs.

The City Council unanimously endorsed the report, adopted its recommendations and asked the Action Committee to create a food charter for the city and to present an action plan to improve Toronto residents' access to safe, affordable and nutritious food and to enhance the coordination and delivery of related services.

The Food and Hunger Action Committee developed the action plan, in consultation with a community reference group, based on the following *(22)*.

1. High rents and low incomes imposed hunger on Toronto's poorest residents.
2. Food programmes provided by city and community groups were effective and merited continued support.
3. Existing programmes were not available in all areas of the city. The former suburbs were less likely to have programmes that met local needs, although they had problems as severe as those downtown.
4. Food security initiatives offered the city an opportunity to save money, create jobs, strengthen local communities and stimulate the economy.
5. The volunteer and charitable sector currently provided most of the food relief services, but could not handle the ever-increasing demands for assistance resulting from cutbacks to federal and provincial social programmes.
6. Food security measures could help Toronto to reduce the amount of food and organic material it sent to landfill.
7. Food security measures could be revenue neutral, because food security was both a motivation and a vehicle for the productive use of previously wasted resources, and because it offers the city the opportunity to get full value from underused existing assets.

The action plan is organized according to the roles that the City can play as an advocate to other levels of government, a coordinator of community initiatives, a supporter of access to food through its own programmes and an innovator in using food security initiatives to meet the City's economic and environmental goals *(22)*.

Food and nutrition policies in the European Region

The following sections of this chapter consider policies in the three interrelated parts of food an nutrition policy: nutrition, food safety and food security. Each discusses both existing policies and considerations for the future. Information on existing policies comes from surveys of European Member States' main policies and practices on nutrition, food safety and food security, performed by the nutrition programme of the WHO Regional Office for Europe during 1999–2000 *(23–25)*.

Nutrition policy
Existing policies
In summary, the survey *(23)*, showed that:

- 16 Member States have administrative structures for implementing food and nutrition strategies;
- 28 have a nutrition council or equivalent technical advisory body;
- 36 have national recommended nutrient intake or equivalent tables;
- 27 have national dietary guidelines; and
- 17 collect national data on dietary intake using a variety of methods.

Countries with national coordination bodies for food and nutrition appear to be the most effective in developing and implementing policies. Such a body advises the government on developing, implementing, monitoring and evaluating intersectoral policies and their associated guidelines and action plans. It can also be responsible for ensuring the consistency of information given by different sectors to the public, encourage and respond to public interest about food issues and advise the government on how to meet its international commitments.

Table 4.1 shows the numbers of countries in each subregion that take various types of action on nutrition. Over half the countries in the Region have nutrition councils or bodies that can provide scientific advice to politicians and policy-makers, with the Nordic countries being most fully developed. Less than one third reported having administrative structures to ensure that policy is implemented. Thus, capacity in this area clearly needs to be strengthened.

Two tools a health ministry must have to support nutrition policy development are a set of recommended nutrient intakes and food-based dietary guidelines *(23)*:

Subregion (responding countries/total countries)	Number with recommended nutrient intake values
South-eastern Europe (5/5)	5
Baltic countries (3/3)	2
Central Asian republics (3/5)	3
CCEE (5/6)	4
CIS (4/7)	4
Nordic countries (5/5)	5
Southern Europe (6/10)	5
Western Europe (9/9)	8
Total (40/50)	36

Table 4.1. Number of countries taking government-initiated action to implement and monitor nutrition policy according to subregion, 1999

Subregion (responding countries/total countries)	Number of countries				
	Policy document	Adminis-trative structure to implement policy	Advisory body on technical issues	Regular initiated inter-sectoral collabora-tion	Regular collabora-tion between health and agricul-ture ministries
South-eastern Europe (5/5)	4	2	2	4	5
Baltic countries (3/3)	2	1	2	1	1
Central Asian republics (3/5)	3	2	2	3	3
CCEE (5/6)	4	3	2	4	4
Commonwealth of Inde-pendent States (CIS) (4/7)	3	1	2	2	3
Nordic countries (5/5)	4	1	5	3	2
Southern Europe (6/10)	4	4	6	4	4
Western Europe (9/9)	5	2	7	5	6
Total (40/50)	29	16	28	26	28

Source: Comparative analysis of food and nutrition policies in the WHO European Region 1994–1999. Summary report (23).

About half of Member States have developed food-based dietary guidelines (Table 4.2). These can be used to disseminate information to the public and to form the basis of other programmes and policies.

Table 4.2. Number of European countries with national food-based dietary guidelines, according to subregion, 2002

Subregion (countries)	Guidelines?			
	Yes	In progress[a]	No	No answer
Nordic countries (5/5)	5	0	0	0
Western Europe (9/9)	5	1	2	1
Southern Europe (8/10)	6	1	0	1
CCEE (6/6)	5	1	0	0
Baltic countries (3/3)	2	1	0	0
South-eastern Europe (5/5)	2	1	2	0
CIS (7/7)	1	0	1	5
Central Asian republics (5/5)	0	0	1	4
Total (48/50)	26	5	6	11

[a] Food-based dietary guidelines being developed or await endorsement by the government.

Source: Food-based dietary guidelines in WHO European Member States (25).

Policy-makers can use dietary targets or goals to monitor and evaluate the population's nutritional health. In addition to considering the results of surveys on dietary intake, health ministries may decide to compare dietary targets with national statistics on agriculture and food supply (see Chapter 3, Table 3.10, p. 187). Table 4.3 summarizes the national population targets for nutrition of governments throughout the European Region. The figures used reflect the range reported by different countries.

Table 4.3. Population goals for dietary recommendations in different countries of the European Region, 2002

Component	Goals
Proportion of total energy intake from:	
• total fatty acids	< 30–35%
• saturated fatty acids	< 10%
• sugar	< 10%
Fruits and vegetables	> 400–600 g per day
Salt	< 5–8 g per day
Body weight	BMI of 18–27
Physical activity	30 min moderate exercise per day
Breastfeeding	4–6 months[a]

[a] Many countries are revising their breastfeeding recommendations to 6 months, in accordance with World Health Assembly resolution WHA54.2 (26).

Source: Food-based dietary guidelines in WHO European Member States (25).

Considerations for the future

The following sections discuss some of the most important considerations for the future.

Elements of successful policy

A review of WHO food and nutrition policies throughout the world, according to the WHO Global Database on National Nutrition Policies and Programmes (http://www.who.int/nut/db_pol.htm, accessed 8 July 2003), outlined key elements for success and obstacles to development and implementation. Three key elements for successful development of policies are:

1. political commitment (with an influential ministry to lead the process and a high-profile advocate);
2. strong human capacity in nutrition (skills, knowledge, numbers of staff); and
3. availability of reliable national data on food, nutrition and health.

Common obstacles to developing national nutrition plans are:

1. low priority given to nutrition by governments;
2. lack of intersectoral coordination;
3. lack of local experts;
4. political instability; and
5. lack of reliable data on food and nutrition.

Five key elements for successful implementation of national food and nutrition plans and policies are:

1. official government adoption and political support, including government funds specifically allocated to nutrition;
2. an intersectoral coordination mechanism, located in the government and allocated a budget;
3. priorities set for activities and responsible sectors or ministries designated;
4. ability to translate plans into action, including strengthening human capacity in designing and planning programmes for nutritional improvements;
5. a mechanism for monitoring and evaluation.

Obstacles to policy implementation are the lack of: political commitment, at both the national and local levels; technical expertise; and funding.

Recommendations, goals and guidelines

In addition to political commitment and a focused approach, specific recommendations are required to achieve active consultation with stakeholders. As mentioned above, national recommended nutrient intakes, developed by health ministries, are essential; Annex 2 lists international and selected national recommendations. Fourteen European Member States, especially NIS, did not report having national recommended nutrient intakes (24). These countries may wish to compare or update their existing recommendations with those presented in Annex 2.

Establishing recommended nutrient intakes is a difficult scientific process because many issues should be considered. For example, how much of each nutrient is needed to maintain optimal health, and is it sufficient to prevent signs of clinical deficiency, such as prevention of anaemia in the case of iron intake. Moreover, the fact that excessive consumption of some nutrients may be harmful needs to be considered. How can policy-makers ensure that single values cover the wide range of individual variation in, for example, energy needs? Other factors, such as the bioavailability of nutrients, affect the difference between what a specific person needs and the value adopted to safeguard most of the population against nutrient deficiency.

Owing to these complex scientific issues, most countries are unable to establish their own national norms and standards. WHO and FAO therefore develop international standards that countries can adopt. These standards are relevant to healthy populations, not to sick people or to individuals. The recommendations can be used as a planning tool, to decide on the quantities of foodstuffs needed for national populations and for nutrition labelling. Different countries use different names for recommended nutrient intake – such as reference nutrient intake, population reference intake, physiological norms or recommended daily allowance – but they all have the same role.

After establishing national recommended nutrient intakes, health ministries should establish nutrient goals for their population. Table 4.4 outlines European nutrient goals that are in line with the outcome of an expert consultation held by WHO and FAO in 2002 *(10)*. These goals are very important in establishing specific targets or benchmarks against which dietary intake can be assessed and monitored. They set a direction and display the extent of change necessary to achieve good health in the population. They also provide a lead for health promotion programmes and a focus for policy development. The sectors that should be involved can be more easily identified and responsibilities allocated to the appropriate change agent. Since health care resources are limited, priorities must always be set, and national goals can help to allocate resources to the areas identified as most important.

To be understood, nutrient population goals need to be translated into food-based dietary guidelines at the national level *(29)*. The health ministry should endorse dietary guidelines that are consistent and easily understood. Many primary care experts and other health specialists, such as paediatricians, obstetricians and cardiologists, have opportunities to give advice on healthy eating. There are at least 26 examples of national dietary guidelines in the Region (Table 4.2). Some examples are based on the *CINDI dietary guide* and its 12 steps to healthy eating *(30)*, developed by the WHO Regional Office for Europe:

1. Eat a nutritious diet based on a variety of foods originating mainly from plants, rather than animals.
2. Eat bread, grains, pasta, rice or potatoes several times a day.
3. Eat a variety of fruits and vegetables, preferably fresh and local, several times per day (at least 400 g per day).
4. Maintain a body weight between the recommended limits (a BMI of 20–25 [adapted from the global WHO recommendation of 18.5–24.9 as normal values]) by taking moderate levels of physical activity, preferably daily.
5. Control fat intake (not more than 30% of daily energy) and replace most saturated fats with unsaturated vegetable oils or soft margarines.

6. Replace fatty meat and meat products with beans, legumes, lentils, fish, poultry or lean meat.

7. Use milk and dairy products (kefir, sour milk, yoghurt and cheese) that are low in both fat and salt.

8. Select foods that are low in sugar, and eat refined sugar sparingly, limiting the frequency of sugary drinks and sweets.

9. Choose a low-salt diet. Total salt intake should not be more than one teaspoon (6 g) per day, including the salt in bread and processed, cured and preserved foods. (Salt iodization should be universal where iodine deficiency is endemic.)

10. If alcohol is consumed, limit intake to no more than two drinks (each containing 10 g of alcohol) per day.

11. Prepare food in a safe and hygienic way. Steam, bake, boil or microwave to help reduce the amount of added fat.

12. Promote exclusive breastfeeding and the introduction of safe and adequate complementary foods from the age of 6 months while breastfeeding continues during the first years of life.

Table 4.4. Population goals from recent international expert analyses and levels of evidence

Component[a]	Population goals	Levels of evidence[b]
Physical activity level	> 1.75[c]	A
Adult body weight	BMI of 21–22	A
Proportion of total energy intake from:		
• total fatty acids	< 30%	A
• saturated fatty acids	< 10%	C
• *trans*-fatty acids	< 2%	A
• polyunsaturated fatty acids:		
– omega-6	< 7–8%	A
– omega-3	2 g/day of linolenic + 200 mg/day of very-long-chain	A
• carbohydrates	> 55%	B
Sugary foods	4 occasions/day[d]	A
Fruits and vegetables	> 400 g/day	A
Folate from food	> 400 µg/day	B
Dietary fibre	> 25 g/day (or 3 g/MJ of energy intake)	A
Sodium as NaCl	< 6 g/day	B
Iodine	150 µg/day (infants: 50 µg/day; pregnant women: 200 µg/day)	B
Exclusive breastfeeding	About 6 months	B

[a] The source report includes goals for other important nutrients, such as iron, calcium, alcohol, water and vitamin D.

[b] Levels of evidence are based on those used in several guideline systems, such as the Cochrane system, the US National Academy of Sciences scheme and the systems used in assessing diet in relation to cancer by the World Cancer Research Fund and American Institute for Cancer Research (27) and expert bodies in Member States. These other systems

are included because undertaking double-blind placebo-controlled studies is often more difficult for dietary research than drug trials. Thus, the best evidence is considered as convincing by these expert groups when meta-analyses of different types of study are integrated but are nevertheless classified as either ecological analyses compatible with non-double-blind intervention and physiological studies or only integration of multiple levels of evidence by expert groups. These trials and other analyses do not prove that only the precise values in the table are correct, but that the evidence from dietary change or differences supports them.

[b] A = ecological analyses compatible with non-double-blind intervention and physiological studies; B = single study of double-blind analyses or, for breastfeeding, a series of non-double-blind analyses; C = multiple double-blind placebo-controlled trials.

[c] Ratio of total daily energy expenditure to basal metabolic rate.

[d] An occasion includes any episode of food and drink consumption during the day. This limited intake is compatible with many EU member states' limits on total sugar intake and the Nordic concern to limit the intake by children and those adults on low energy intakes to no more than 10% of total energy.

Source: adapted from EURODIET Working Party 1 *(28).*

Food-based dietary guidelines must be adapted to a country's needs, ensure that the nutrient needs of the population are covered and help to reduce the risk of CVD and cancer (see Chapter 1). They should also be in accordance with public policies that promote food safety and a healthy environment and a robust local food economy.

Recommendations vary between countries according to the availability and cultural acceptability of foods. For effective implementation, dietary guidelines must take account of dietary patterns and the prevalence of both deficiency disorders and noncommunicable diseases in each country. Health professionals should review the data on premature mortality, morbidity and diet and nutritional status before developing their own dietary guidelines. This will ensure that the recommendations are tailored to national conditions.

Posters or food selection guides should accompany dietary guidelines, to help people select a diet that is adequate in nutrients, contains a high level of complex starches, dietary fibre and fruits and vegetables and that avoids excessive intake of fat, salt and added sugar.

Food selection guides should promote food choices that are consistent with the conservation of national resources, which includes promoting local production for local consumption. A food guide should be culturally inclusive and incorporate foods that are generally available and accessible at a reasonable price. It should also be based on sound educational principles and be comprehensible to people with a wide range of educational levels in communities.

Promoting physical activity

National guidelines should include the promotion of physical activity (see Chapter 1, pp. 38–40), as stated in step 4 of the 12 steps to healthy eating *(30).* Because health professionals are a trusted source of information, they can promote healthy nutrition and physical activity to patients and the wider community. Governments and health professionals can promote physical activity to adults by:

- developing guidelines for counselling on exercise
- raising the awareness of health care staff
- developing specifications for health-related physical activity.

The physical activity level is the ratio of total daily energy expenditure to basal metabolic rate. A physical activity level of 1 would involve no physical activity, and the energy required would simply go to maintaining the basal metabolic rate. EURODIET's population goal of a physical activity level of at least 1.75 (Table 4.4) is equivalent to walking 60–80 minutes each day and is more than the 30 minutes recommended for heart health *(24)*. This is based on needing to be more physically active to avoid weight gain on high fat intake; sedentary societies probably need a lower fat intake, such as 20–25% of total energy, to avoid excessive weight gain. Moderate weekly exercise reduces morbidity rates by 30–50%.

Raising physical activity levels is one of the most important goals for public health in the European Region because it has such a strong effect on the risk of CVD and because activity levels in the population are so low. Inadequate physical activity is more common than any of the classic risk factors for chronic diseases: smoking, hypertension, high blood cholesterol and overweight. The proportion of CVD incidence that more physical activity in the European population could theoretically prevent – the population-attributable risk – is estimated to be about 30–40% *(31)*.

Health-enhancing physical activity *(32)* is any form of activity that benefits health and functional capacity without undue harm or risk. Physical activity does not need to be strenuous to be effective. At least 30 minutes a day of moderate-intensity activity is enough to benefit health. The choice of activities is ample and includes *(33)*: brisk walking, cycling, swimming, dancing, cross-country skiing, gardening, mowing the lawn, walking the dog, washing windows or a car, shovelling snow and walking to work or shops.

WHO has developed guidelines to encourage increased physical activity as part of regular daily living *(34)*. The aim is to make daily physical activity an easy choice and thus to prevent obesity, reduce the risk of diabetes and CVD, and promote good health and wellbeing.

In 1996, the EC created the European Network for the Promotion of Health-enhancing Physical Activity, which aimed to facilitate the development of national policies and strategies *(35)*. Major national initiatives, strategies or programmes promoting health-enhancing physical activity have been developed and are being implemented in the Scandinavian countries, the

Netherlands, Switzerland and the United Kingdom, and similar preparatory work is in progress in most other EU countries and in some non-EU countries. The European Commission has also published a review of its activities in nutrition *(36)*.

Preventing CVD and cancer

Eating a diet low in saturated fat and high in fruits and vegetables, taking regular exercise and not smoking can help to prevent premature mortality from CVD and cancer.

Significantly reducing dietary saturated fat, getting plenty of aerobic exercise and losing weight are also good ways of reducing serum cholesterol levels (see Chapter 1, p. 25–27). In addition, appropriate intake of salt is important in controlling blood pressure. Several diets have been developed specifically to control hypertension. For example, DASH *(37)* is a combination diet: low in saturated fat and rich in fruits and vegetables: high dietary fibre, potassium, calcium and magnesium (see Chapter 1, pp. 29–30).

DASH includes more than 600 g per day of fruits and vegetables, especially those high in potassium and magnesium. Low-fat dairy products contribute calcium and protein; whole grains from cereals, breads and crackers contribute fibre and energy. Intake of lean meat, poultry and fish is moderate: less than 150 g per day. To boost potassium, fibre, protein and energy even more, DASH recommends nuts, seeds, and cooked dried beans 4–5 times per week.

The original study, with 454 subjects, showed that the systolic blood pressure of hypertensive patients complying with DASH declined by an average of 11.4 mmHg and diastolic blood pressure by 5.5 mmHg. These results occurred without medication, from losing weight and reducing sodium intake *(37)*. The benefit of the DASH diet is that, in addition to reducing hypertension, it is the same as the diet recommended to prevent CVD, cancer, diabetes and overweight.

Preventing overweight and obesity

Comprehensive strategies have not yet been developed to address the problem of overweight and obesity among adults and children at a population level (see Chapter 1, pp. 35–38). Governments must develop stronger approaches to nutrition and physical activity that require coordinated intersectoral commitment at all levels, rather leaving the task to health policy alone. Too often policy-makers assume that personalized health education is the only way to help.

The huge interest in slimming, the vast market for slimming foods and other aids to weight reduction, alongside escalating rates of overweight and obesity, show that this approach is failing. WHO has launched a new Global

Strategy on Diet, Physical Activity and Health. Descriptions of the Strategy and the consultation process completed in 2003 are available on the Internet (www.who.int.hpr/gs.consultation.document.shtml, accessed 3 September 2003). The European Region needs to develop broader, more coherent policies to counteract similar pressures now affecting widespread populations (38). Obesity in children is causing particular concern and recommendations have been developed (39,40) (see pp. 248–249). BMI charts for children from birth up to 20 years for boys and girls have been developed in Germany, France and United Kingdom (http://www.healthforallchildren.co.uk/acatalog/HFAC_Catalogue_BMI_Charts_5.html, accessed 3 September 2003).

The CINDI dietary guide (30) provides advice on weight control, and the ideal adult body is accepted as having a body mass index (BMI) of between 18.5 and 24.9 (41) (Fig. 4.2). People who are underweight (BMI under 18.5) may need more food, which should be part of a well balanced and nutritious diet. Those with very low weight should consult a physician. People whose BMI is 18.5–24.9 are eating the right quantity of food to maintain weight in the desirable range for health, but should make sure there is a healthy balance in the diet. People at the lower end of the weight range should maintain their weight and not be tempted to aim for the underweight category. Some loss of weight would benefit the health of overweight people, and it is an important task for obese people, in view of the risk from further weight gain. Being very obese could seriously affect health and wellbeing. People with a BMI over 40 need to lose weight urgently, and should consider consulting a physician or dietitian (30).

Moreover, how fat is distributed within the body, measured by waist circumference, confers additional risk. The risk of developing type 2 diabetes, hypertension and CHD is much greater in people with excess fat in the abdominal area (upper-body obesity or an apple shape) compared with the hips and thighs (lower-body obesity or a pear shape). Waist measurement is therefore very useful for indicating who is most at risk of metabolic complications, and appears to be even more predictive than BMI.

The risk of metabolic complications associated with obesity increases with a waist circumference over 95 cm among men and 80 cm among women (corresponding approximately to overweight), and the risk increases substantially if the waist is over 100 cm among men and 90 cm among women (corresponding approximately to obesity) (41).

WHO has published detailed recommendations for preventing and managing obesity (38). These emphasize the need for early prevention to ensure lifelong healthy eating and physical activity patterns and the need for coordinated partnerships involving governments, communities, the mass media and the food industry to ensure that diet and everyday levels of physical activity can be changed effectively and sustainably.

Fig. 4.2. BMI chart

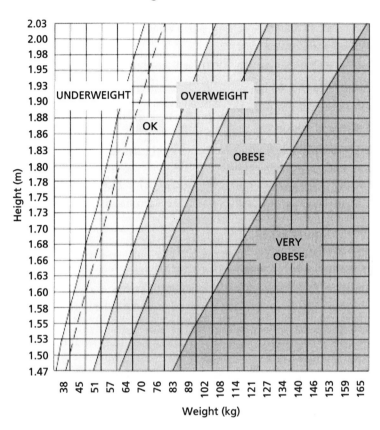

Source: adapted from *Eight guidelines for a healthy diet (42).*

At the end of 2001, the Surgeon General of the United States called for sweeping changes in schools, restaurants, workplaces and communities to help combat the growing epidemic of obesity in the country *(43).* In outlining the first national plan of action in the United States, he recommended improving school lunches, restricting the vending machines that provide students with ready access to energy-dense foods and soft drinks, and resuming daily physical activity classes for all children and adolescents. The report advises that restaurants and fast-food outlets, which account for 40% of food expenditure in the United States, should provide more nutrition information, for which consumer groups have long lobbied. It also outlines changes to improve healthy eating and exercise at work, and urges employers to include counselling on weight management and physical activity as part of health insurance coverage. In 2003, the National Board of Health of Denmark published recommendations to combat obesity and to increase levels of physical activity (http://www.sst.dk/publ/publ2003/National_action_plan.pdf, accessed 3 September 2003).

Preventing diabetes

Avoiding overweight can reduce the risk of developing type 2 diabetes. Appropriate lifestyle measures are especially important for those with a familial predisposition to diabetes. Regular moderate physical activity and a healthy diet (reducing saturated fat and increasing fruits and vegetables) facilitate weight and weight maintenance. Physical activity may have an independent beneficial effect by reducing resistance to the action of insulin (44).

Preventing undernutrition in hospital patients

A report from the Council of Europe (45) recommends five measures against undernutrition among people in hospitals.

First, responsibilities in planning and managing nutritional care should be clearly defined. Standards of practice for assessing and monitoring patients' nutritional risks and status should be developed at the national level, and the responsibility for these tasks clearly assigned. The hospital's responsibility for the nutritional care and support of patients should not be limited to their hospital stay.

Second, the educational level of all staff groups in general needs improvement. Specifically, a continuing education programme on general nutrition and techniques of nutritional support for all staff involved in the nutritional care of patients should be available, with a focus on training non-clinical staff members and defining their responsibilities.

Third, patients should have the chance to be more involved in decisions about their nutritional care. The provision of meals should be individualized and flexible, and all patients should be able to order food, including extra food, and be informed about this option. Patients should be involved in planning their meals and have some control over food selection. This should include the possibility of immediate feedback from their likes and dislikes of the food served, and the use of this feedback to develop appropriate menus for particular target groups. Patients should be informed about the importance of good nutrition for successful treatment before admission and at discharge.

Fourth, different staff groups should cooperate better. Hospital managers, physicians, nurses, dietitians and food service staff should work together towards the common goal of optimal nutritional patient care. Hospital managers should give priority to cooperation by, for example, initiating organizational research to optimize cooperation. In addition, organized contact between the hospital and the primary health care sector should be established.

Fifth, hospital managers should be involved. They should see the provision of meals as an essential part of treatment, not a hotel service. They should acknowledge responsibility for food service and the nutritional care of patients and give priority to food policy and management of the services. When assessing the cost of food services, they should take account of the costs of complications and prolonged hospital stay due to undernutrition.

In addition, further research is needed to improve nutritional care and support in hospitals:

- developing and validating simple screening methods for use in hospitals and primary health care, and simple food-recording methods;
- determining the effect of nutritional support on both nutritional status and clinical outcome (including physical and mental functioning: quality-of-life measures), and the effect of energy- and protein-dense menus on food intake and patient outcome;
- determining methods of ensuring patients' intake of ordinary hospital food and assessing patient satisfaction; and
- determining the influence of food service practice on food wastage.

In recent years, increasing numbers of successful initiatives to improve nutritional practices have been documented from all over the Region. It therefore seems the right time to combine the experience gained in a common struggle to ensure that patients have adequate food intake and to prevent disease-related undernutrition in hospitals.

Promoting nutritional health throughout life

Good nutrition in the first few years pays dividends throughout life. This starts with maternal nutrition, because of its importance to the fetus and the evidence that a poor fetal nutritional environment raises the risk of chronic disease in later life (see Chapter 1, pp. 48–50). The failure of pregnant women to obtain a safe and healthy variety of food has long-term social and economic effects. The WHO Regional Office for Europe and UNICEF have developed training materials to help health professionals (46), especially paediatricians, obstetricians and hygienists, to improve the health of women and children through safe food and good nutrition.

Breastfeeding

Exclusive breastfeeding for 6 months is a global health recommendation (26). Many maternity hospitals throughout the European Region have been active in implementing 10 steps to successful breastfeeding, which are the foundation of the baby-friendly hospital initiative, launched worldwide by UNICEF and WHO in 1992. The 10 steps summarize the maternity practices necessary to establish a supportive environment for women wishing to breastfeed and thereby bring about improvements in the incidence and duration of breastfeeding (http://www.euro.who.int/nutrition/Infant/20020808_1, acces-sed 9 July 2003):

1. Have a written breastfeeding policy that is routinely communicated to all health care staff.
2. Train all health care staff in skills necessary to implement this policy.
3. Inform all pregnant women about the benefits and management of breast-feeding.
4. Help mothers initiate breastfeeding within a half-hour of birth.
5. Show mothers how to breastfeed and how to maintain lactation even if they should be separated from their infants.
6. Give newborn infants no food and drink other than breast-milk, unless medically indicated.
7. Practise rooming-in – allow mothers and infants to remain together – 24 hours a day.
8. Encourage breastfeeding on demand.
9. Give no artificial teats or pacifiers (also called dummies or soothers) to breastfeeding infants.
10. Foster the establishment of breastfeeding support groups and refer mothers to them on discharge from the hospital or clinic.

The initiative also prohibits the supply of free and low-cost infant formula in hospitals and demands the elimination of advertising and promotional activities for infant formula or feeding by bottle. To become a baby-friendly hospital, every facility that contributes to maternity services and to the care of newborn infants must implement the 10 steps (47).

When a woman is HIV-positive, it is uncertain whether she should breast-feed, as HIV can be transmitted to the child through breast-milk. As a general principle and irrespective of HIV infection rates, breastfeeding should con-tinue to be protected, promoted and supported in all populations. WHO, UNICEF and UNAIDS guidelines for breastfeeding by HIV-positive women (48,49) vary according to local physical and cultural ecology.

When replacement feeding is acceptable, feasible, affordable, sustainable and safe, HIV-infected mothers should avoid all breastfeeding. If the water supply is in general unsafe without additional preparation steps, infant mor-tality is high and cultural norms foster breastfeeding, however, then exclusive breastfeeding is recommended, and weaning should occur as soon as feasible – taking into account local circumstances, such as the individual woman's situa-tion and the risks of replacement feeding, including infections other than HIV and malnutrition (49).

Strategies to reduce mother-to-child transmission of HIV must be multi-factorial. First, reducing the viral load of lactating women is essential to minimize the excess risk of infection to breastfeeding infants. This may be achieved by making highly active antiretroviral therapy and/or prophylactic antiretroviral regimens available to women *(49)*. In addition, women should be advised to use barrier contraceptives during lactation to prevent further viral infections and consequent enhanced viral loads in breast-milk. Moreover, lactating mothers should be counselled on proper breastfeeding practices to prevent HIV transmission through cracked nipples and mastitis. Further, mothers should restrict the weaning period involving mixed feeding, as this may pose excess risk of HIV transmission *(49)*.

Breastfeeding should be encouraged even where contamination of breast-milk is a concern. Mothers should be reassured that the risk from contamination is very small compared with the overall benefits of breastfeeding.

Introducing semi-solid foods

The age during which complementary foods are introduced is an especially sensitive time in infant development. This transition is associated not only with increasing and changing nutrient requirements but also with the rapid growth, physiological maturation and development of the infant. Poor nutrition and less than optimum feeding practices during this critical period may increase the risk of wasting and stunting and nutritional deficiencies, especially of iron, and may harm health and mental development in the long term. Thus, health ministries should give high priority to the timely introduction of appropriate complementary foods that promote good health and growth among infants and young children.

A WHO publication *(47)* provides information to help health ministries develop their own national guidelines for feeding infants and young children. It recommends that each country review, update, develop and implement national nutrition and feeding guidelines for infants and young children, using the following recommendations *(47)*:

Health and nutritional status and feeding practices

It is recommended that each country establish nutrition surveillance of infants and young children as an integral part of its health information system.

Breastfeeding practices, feeding patterns and the nutritional status of infants and young children should be monitored regularly to enable problems to be identified and strategies developed to prevent ill health and poor growth.

Recommended nutrient intakes

Each country should use recommended nutrient intakes for infants and young children, based on international scientific evidence, as the foundation of its nutrition and feeding guidelines.

Energy and macronutrients

Provision of adequate dietary energy is vital during the period of rapid growth in infancy and early childhood. Attention must be paid to feeding practices that maximize the intake of energy-dense foods without compromising micronutrient density.

An adequate protein intake with a balanced amino acid pattern is important for the growth and development of the infant and young child. If the child receives a varied diet, however, the quantity and quality of protein are seldom inadequate. Avoiding a high-protein diet is prudent because this can have adverse effects.

During complementary feeding and at least until 2 years of age, a child's diet should not be too low in fat (because this may diminish energy intake) or too high in fat (because this may reduce micronutrient density). A fat intake providing about 30–40% of total energy is thought to be prudent.

Consumption of added sugar should be limited to about 10% of total energy, because a high intake may compromise micronutrient status.

Vitamins

In countries with a high prevalence of childhood infectious disease, determining whether vitamin A deficiency is a public health problem is important.

In countries where rickets is a public health problem, all infants should receive a vitamin D supplement as well as adequate exposure to sunlight.

Minerals other than iron

In countries where iodine deficiency is a public health problem, legislation on universal salt iodization should be adopted and enforced.

Control of iron deficiency

Iron deficiency in infants and young children is widespread and has serious consequences for children's health. ...

When complementary foods are introduced at about 6 months of age, it is important that iron-rich foods such as liver, meat, fish and pulses or iron-fortified complementary foods are included.

The too-early introduction of unmodified cow's milk and milk products is an important nutritional risk factor for the development of iron deficiency anaemia. Unmodified cow's milk should not therefore be introduced as a drink until the age of 9 months and can be increased thereafter gradually.

Because of their inhibitory effect on iron absorption, all types of tea (black, green and herbal) and coffee should be avoided until 24 months of age. After this age, tea should be avoided at mealtimes.

Optimal iron stores at birth are important for preventing iron deficiency among infants and young children. To help ensure good iron stores in her children, the mother should eat an iron-rich diet during pregnancy.

At birth, the umbilical cord should not be clamped and ligated until it stops pulsating.

Breastfeeding and alternatives

All infants should be exclusively breastfed from birth to about 6 months of age.

Breastfeeding should preferably continue beyond the first year of life, and in populations with high rates of infection, continued breastfeeding throughout the second year and longer is likely to benefit the infant.

Each country should support, protect and promote breastfeeding by achieving the four targets outlined in the Innocenti Declaration [on Protection, Promotion and Support of Breastfeeding]: appointment of an appropriate national breastfeeding coordinator; universal practice of the Baby Friendly Hospital Initiative; implementation of the International Code of Marketing of Breast-milk Substitutes and subsequent relevant resolutions of the World Health Assembly; and legislation to protect the breastfeeding rights of working women.

Complementary feeding

Timely introduction of appropriate complementary foods promotes good health, nutritional status and growth among infants and young children during a period of rapid growth and should be a high priority for public health.

Throughout the period of complementary feeding breast-milk should continue to be the main type of milk consumed by the infant.

Complementary foods should be introduced at about 6 months of age. Some infants may need complementary foods earlier, but not before 4 months of age.

Unmodified cow's milk should not be used as a drink before the age of 9 months, but can be used in small quantities in the preparation of complementary foods from 6–9 months of age. From 9–12 months, cow's milk can be gradually introduced into the infant's diet as a drink.

Complementary foods with a low energy density can limit energy intake, and the average energy density should not usually be less than 4.2 kJ(1 kcal)/g. This energy density depends on meal frequency and can be lower if meals are offered often. Low-fat milk should not be given before the age of about 2 years.

Complementary feeding should be a process of introducing foods with an increasing variety of texture, flavour, aroma and appearance while maintaining breastfeeding.

Highly salted foods should not be given during the complementary feeding period nor should salt be added to food during this period.

Caring practices

Policy-makers and health professionals should recognize the need to support care-givers and the fact that caring practices and resources for care are fundamental determinants of good nutrition and feeding and thereby of child health and development.

Growth assessment

Regular monitoring of growth is an important tool for assessing the nutritional status of infants and young children and should be an integral part of the child health care system.

Dental health

It is recommended that the frequent intake of foods high in sugar, sugary drinks, sweets and refined sugar should be limited to improve dental health.

Teeth should be cleaned gently twice a day as soon as they appear.

An optimal fluoride intake should be secured through water fluoridation, fluoride supplements or the use of fluoride toothpaste.

Food safety

Safe food, clean water and good hygiene are essential to prevent diarrhoea and foodborne and waterborne diseases, which are major causes of poor nutrition, stunting and recurrent illness.

Developing good eating habits and preventing childhood obesity

A newborn baby shows innate preferences for sweet tastes and innate dislike for sour or bitter ones (50,51). The classic work of Clara Davis (52,53) showed that children self-selected a healthy diet without being influenced by adults. This points to the possibility that human infants possess a biological control system that enables nutritionally adequate food choice if a variety of wholesome and natural foods is available, but nobody knows whether this still holds when more energy-dense and processed foods become available. From the very beginning, these innate preferences are modified by learning processes, which in turn play a major role in the development of food preferences and food rejection (54,55). Three major processes have been described that modify the child's food acceptance patterns.

- Mere exposure to unknown food – the repeated experience of tasting and eating it – reduces the tendency to reject it. Consequently, children's preference for vegetables, for example, increases with exposure (56).
- Social influences modify food acceptance. Children learn to prefer food eaten by their peers; peer influence may be more influential than parental influence and has been shown to be effective in preschool children (57,58).
- Children learn to associate the physiological consequences of food intake with taste (59,60).

Childhood and adolescence are good times for health promotion interventions based on appropriate knowledge of the personal and environmental determinants of food choice (see Chapter 3, Fig. 3.5, p. 166). Some factors that can improve the eating behaviour and physical activity levels of adolescents include:

- active participation of adolescents in health promotion, such as learning how to grow, harvest and cook vegetables;
- services for adolescents that ensure confidentiality, such as counselling services;
- appropriate and convenient centres for adolescent health promotion, such as physical activity after school;
- a staged approach to changing behaviour, such as opportunities to experiment with eating fruits and vegetables;
- realistic objectives, such as gradually reducing the intake of sweets, snacks and sugar-containing drinks;
- specific information on the changes advocated and how to achieve them delivered through, for example, interactive internet programmes;
- delivery of the same message from different sources, or restricting conflicting messages *(61)*;
- information that allows reasoned choice, for example, using BMI charts (see pp. 240–241);
- utilization of social and community networks, for example, to create a trend towards healthy eating and increased physical activity;
- the association of desirable behaviour with self-satisfaction and reward, rather than rewarding children with sweets and other unhealthy foods.

The ultimate aim is to strengthen self-efficacy in children and adolescents (for more information, see pp. 239–242 and tables 4.7 and 4.8, pp. 284–287).

Preventing micronutrient deficiency

Micronutrient deficiency is mainly a consequence of poverty and affects a significant proportion of the population even in industrialized countries. Prevention strategies must therefore involve input and resources from a wide range of organizations and sectors, such as agriculture, health, commerce, industry, education and communication *(62)*. They should then work in concert with communities and local nongovernmental organizations (NGOs) to reduce poverty, to improve access to diversified diets, to improve health services and sanitation and to promote better care and feeding practices.

Food-based strategies are the most desirable and sustainable method of preventing micronutrient malnutrition and are designed to increase micronutrient intake through the diet. They can result in multiple nutritional benefits. These, in turn, can achieve short-term impact and long-term sustainability *(62)*. Food-based strategies should work to improve the year-round availability of micronutrient-rich foods, to ensure the access of households, especially those at risk, to these foods and to change feeding practices with respect to these foods.

Iodine

WHO published a review of iodine deficiency in Europe in 2003 *(63)*. As mentioned, universal salt iodization is the agreed strategy for preventing iodine deficiency disorders *(64)*. It can easily eliminate iodine deficiency globally, but this has not yet been achieved.

The European Region has one of the worst iodization records in the world, possibly because of lack of political will and enforcement of legislation, despite the reported presence of iodine deficiency disorders (see Chapter 1, pp. 40–41). Also, the successful universal salt iodization programmes in some eastern countries in the Region were interrupted and may be difficult to resume *(65)*.

A joint report by WHO, UNICEF and the International Council for Control of Iodine Deficiency Disorders *(66)* suggested the following action plan to eliminate iodine deficiency disorders in Europe:

- maintaining and even reinforcing advocacy and training on the disorders at the local, national, regional and global levels;
- continuing detailed evaluation and registration of their extent in the Region;
- contributing to implementing universal salt iodization, if not yet achieved, wherever iodine deficiency disorders are documented;
- if necessary, in hard-to-reach areas with severe iodine deficiency and persistent cretinism, administering iodized oil at least to women of childbearing age *(67)*;
- in areas with mild or moderate iodine deficiency, iodine supplementation for infants, children and women of childbearing age by tablets of potassium iodide at physiological levels during gestation *(68)*, lactation, infancy and early childhood;
- organizing quality control and monitoring the programmes of iodine supplementation from the producer to the consumer, including ensuring that the food industry continuously checks the level of fortificants added to food under the supervision of the health ministry and that the health ministry monitors the iodine status of the population *(69)*;
- evaluating the side effects of iodine: essentially the occurrence of iodine-induced hyperthyroidism; and
- monitoring salt intake.

In addition, a communication strategy should accompany iodization programmes and simultaneously promote a healthy diet.

Iron

Efforts to eliminate iron deficiency should first be directed towards promoting breastfeeding and the use of iron-rich complementary foods; then the availability of and access to iron-rich foods should be ensured. Complementary foods include meat and organs from cattle, fowl, fish and poultry and non-animal foods such as legumes and green leafy vegetables. The focus should also be on foods that enhance the absorption or utilization of iron, such as both animal and non-animal foods that are rich in vitamins A and C and folic acid *(62)* (Table 4.5).

Table 4.5. Enhancers and inhibitors of iron absorption

Enhancers	Inhibitors
Haem iron, present in meat, poultry, fish and seafood	Phytates, present in cereal bran, cereal grains, high-extraction flour, legumes, nuts and seeds
Ascorbic acid or vitamin C, present in fruits, juices, potatoes and some other tubers, and other vegetables such as green leaves, cauliflower and cabbage	Food with high inositol content
	Iron-binding phenolic compounds (tannins), foods containing the most potent inhibitors resistant to the influence of enhancers (including tea, coffee, cocoa, herbal infusions, certain spices, such as oregano, and some vegetables)
Some fermented or germinated food and condiments, such as sauerkraut and soy sauce[a]	
	Calcium, especially from milk and milk products

[a] Cooking, fermentation or germination of food reduces the amount of phytates.
Source: Michaelsen et al. *(47).*

As noted in Chapter 1 (see Fig. 1.24, p. 52), unfortunately tea is often introduced as early as 2 weeks in most central Asian republics and other countries *(46).* Exclusive breastfeeding should therefore be strongly promoted throughout the Region to reduce the risk of anaemia in both infants and young children.

General food fortification uses the existing food production and distribution system. Adding iron to foods does not necessarily mean that it will be absorbed or will help to prevent deficiency. Much iron added to cereal food today, especially reduced elemental iron, is poorly absorbed. For example, soluble iron fortificants such as ferrous sulphate are absorbed to the same degree as the intrinsic non-haem iron in the diet. Iron fortificants are therefore poorly absorbed when added to cereal-based diets. Fortifying basic foods such as wheat flour provides extra iron for adult men and post-menopausal women who often have no deficiency; this could lead to an increased risk of atherosclerosis and cancer because of increased oxidative stress from the pro-oxidant properties of iron *(70).*

The causes of iron deficiency in the target population must be established before fortification programmes are introduced. Fortifying a foodstuff is appropriate only if iron deficiency is related to low intake, low bioavailability or both, and not to the presence of gut parasites (71). Although flour is a suitable vehicle for iron fortification in programmes aimed at older children and adults, it is not suitable for infants and young children because they cannot eat enough.

Iron-only interventions cannot solve the problem of anaemia, as all anaemia is not related to iron deficiency (72).

Promoting healthy ageing

Healthy ageing is a major concern in the European Region (see Chapter 1, pp. 58–59). Decreasing levels of physical activity reduce energy needs, so older people should eat foods rich in micronutrients to compensate for the reduction in intake. Again, WHO recommends a daily intake of at least 400 g of fruits and vegetables for older people (10). Degeneration of eyesight, lower resistance to infection and other micronutrient-related deficiencies can coexist with obesity, making managing the health of older people difficult.

Although genetic and hormonal factors have a role in determining bone mass, environmental factors can also contribute. Nutrition and physical activity contribute both to attaining optimal peak bone mass in young adulthood and to the rate at which it is lost afterwards. People who experience bone loss may benefit from a programme of weight-bearing and endurance exercises. These include walking, climbing stairs, swimming and dancing. The principal benefit from an exercise programme, increasing muscle strength and endurance, should help prevent falls (73).

Fig. 4.3 (resembling Fig. 3.5) summarizes the risk factors for poor nutritional status among older people. Risk factors for malnutrition – including socioeconomic status, health, lifestyle, environment, mental and physical functioning and cultural and social situation – are the underlying reasons why people eat less or poorly. People with one or more risk factors are more likely to become malnourished. Various risk factors are often linked and may be more or less common in certain situations.

Marketing food

Advertising is one of the most powerful tools shaping food preferences (75). Experiments have shown that exposing children aged 2–6 years to 20-second commercials significantly influences their food preferences (76). "Exploiting kids, corrupting schools" (77) describes the creativity of marketing by the food industry, which extends beyond television, magazines, billboards, store displays and the Internet to schools.

In 1996, Consumers International found that candy, sweetened breakfast cereals and fast-food restaurants accounted for over half of all food advertisements in Australia, Austria, Belgium, Denmark, Finland, France, Germany,

Fig. 4.3. Risk factors for poor nutritional status in older people

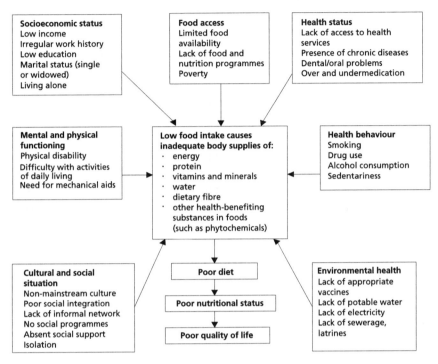

Socioeconomic status	Food access	Health status
Low income	Limited food	Lack of access to health
Irregular work history	availability	services
Low education	Lack of food and	Presence of chronic diseases
Marital status (single	nutrition programmes	Dental/oral problems
or widowed)	Poverty	Over and undermedication
Living alone		

Mental and physical functioning
Physical disability
Difficulty with activities of daily living
Need for mechanical aids

Low food intake causes inadequate body supplies of:
· energy
· protein
· vitamins and minerals
· water
· dietary fibre
· other health-benefiting substances in foods (such as phytochemicals)

Health behaviour
Smoking
Drug use
Alcohol consumption
Sedentariness

Cultural and social situation
Non-mainstream culture
Poor social integration
Lack of informal network
No social programmes
Absent social support
Isolation

Poor diet

Poor nutritional status

Poor quality of life

Environmental health
Lack of appropriate vaccines
Lack of potable water
Lack of electricity
Lack of sewerage, latrines

Source: adapted from Bermudez & Dwyer *(74).*

Greece, the Netherlands, Norway, Sweden, the United Kingdom and the United States *(75).* The study found that food advertising comprises the largest category of products advertised to children and adolescents in virtually all countries. Among the European countries, Sweden and Norway had the least advertising per hour and the United Kingdom the most.

Unfortunately, the most heavily advertised foods tended to be those high in fat and energy and low on micronutrients. A nutritional analysis of the advertised products found that 62% of advertisements were for products high in fat (> 30% energy), 50% for products high in sugar (> 20% energy) and 61% for products high in sodium. Most consumers probably do not know that salt and sugar are the ingredients most widely added to food, followed by fat and oil. The sugar and salt added during food processing, hidden from the consumer, account for three quarters of the total consumed *(75).* In the United Kingdom *(78)* and France *(79),* most advertisements are for food products, and the vast majority of these are for foods high in sugar and/or fat.

Whatever the marketing strategy, food advertising dwarfs efforts for health education in most countries. This imbalance in information and power between industry, consumers and government results in the unprecedented promotion of energy-dense food.

Health authorities should encourage companies' promotional messages to be consistent with national dietary guidelines. They may also develop partnerships to promote nutrient-dense foods such as fruits and vegetables. The aims of marketing strategies could also include stimulating or rebuilding local markets for regional food, especially by incorporating aspects of fair trade, environmental protection, traceability and safe food production.

Labelling and health claims

Food labelling is important for informing the consumer of the nature of processed food and forms an important part of food legislation *(80)*. A food label must by law inform the consumer about the product's weight, production and/or expiration date, ingredients, manufacturer's name and address, place of origin and nutrition information. Other details are optional. Nutritional labelling focuses on energy, protein, fat and carbohydrate and, increasingly, fat composition, dietary fibre, salt and sugar. Information on minerals and vitamins is required when nutritional claims are made *(81)*.

Claims

Claims – the producer's description of product characteristics – often receive a lot of label space *(82)*. These may be:

- nutrition and health claims, although whether health claims should be permitted is heavily discussed globally;
- environmental labels, which may result in the consumer being more concerned with the environmental friendliness of the food than the nutritional aspects;
- quality labelling schemes, although the meaning of quality varies considerably between producers; and
- negative declarations, stating ingredients the product does not contain or treatments to which it has not been subjected.

Many members of the Codex Committee on Food Labelling have expressed concern about health claims, as they would be misleading and confusing, especially if provided without appropriate consumer education programmes *(83)*.

Each country in the EU currently has its own regulations *(82)*. An overall labelling policy for the Region is needed based on factual knowledge, evaluation of all labelling elements and fundamental goals and objectives *(84)*. Consumer representatives should be closely involved in developing such a policy and the strategies and measures introduced for implementing it.

A survey by the British Heart Foundation Health Promotion Research Group in 1997 *(85)* found that consumers use the nutrition information panel on food packets in less than 1% of purchases and use nutrition claims such as "low fat" and "high fibre" for about 5%. If specifically shopping for a healthier diet, consumers were found to be nearly twice as likely to use the nutrition claims than the nutrition information table. Moreover, at least 40% of decisions involving the nutrition information table were incorrect.

In some countries symbols are used as an overall sign of low fat, low salt and sugar, such as "S" in Denmark and keyholes in Sweden *(86)*.

Food control policy
Existing food control policies
Agencies for food safety control
The 1999 WHO survey *(24)* reports food safety information for individual countries. A major component of an effective food safety strategy is the coordination and harmonization of national and international food safety control services. A WHO meeting in 2001 *(87)* aimed: to evaluate the advantages and disadvantages of using independent, scientific consumer protection agencies to coordinate food safety control at the national level; and to compare existing alternatives. Part of WHO's mission is to ensure that decisions on risk management consider consumer health first and foremost and to inform WHO Member States about developments in other countries and parts of the European Region (http://www.euro.who.int/foodsafety, accessed 3 September 2003).

In countries, several agencies and/or ministries have different roles and responsibilities in policy on and monitoring and control of food safety. Communication between and within them is therefore essential for effective coordination. A food agency should establish networks of experts and organizations within the country and internationally *(88)*.

A food authority needs a variety of resources to succeed. These include access to high-quality information, experts performing research, high-quality technical support to ensure that laboratory tests are correctly made and interpreted, and the transmission of information, including the results of surveillance *(88)*. In addition, an agency should have procedures for rapid response to emergencies *(88)*.

Example: the French Food Safety Agency
The French Food Safety Agency was established in 1999 under the triple supervision of the ministries of health, agriculture and consumer affairs, and against a background of growing consumer concern about HIV transmission through blood and a variety of other issues, including the BSE crisis and the heterogeneity of the scientific committees *(88)*.

The Agency's structure, objectives and responsibilities are more comprehensive than those of some other national food agencies. Its wide evaluation responsibilities cover the entire food chain, including food for human and animal consumption, animal welfare, water and genetically modified organisms (GMOs). Unlike agencies in some other countries, however, it has no authority to enforce the law, and is accountable to three ministries.

The Agency is a government institution, led by a board of directors with a president and 24 members, including representatives of the Government, of consumer associations and professional organizations, and Agency staff and scientists. The Agency draws on the knowledge of experts who are members of its steering committee, specialized committees and different working groups on specific issues.

It has a Science Council whose purpose is to "watch over the consistency of scientific policy". The Agency's laboratories carry out scientific research and provide knowledge and scientific and technical support.

The internal organization of the Agency comprises a General Management Division, headed by the Managing Director; the Secretary's Office; and four departments responsible for the scientific activities of the Agency: evaluation of nutrition and health risks, veterinary medicine, animal health and well-being, and food safety.

The Agency's role is to issue opinions, draw up recommendations, carry out research, provide technical and scientific expertise and carry out education and information activities. It monitors and evaluates risks within the framework of food safety in the country, but has no direct monitoring or enforcement powers. These are the responsibility of the ministries concerned.

In relation to food safety, the Agency is systematically consulted on all projects concerning the drafting of regulations or legislation or the authorization of a new product or process within its field of competence. In particular, it is responsible for:

• the nutritional and functional properties of food or dietary products, with the exception of medicines for human use; and
• health risks related to the consumption of food products composed of or resulting from GMOs.

The Agency's evaluation activities cover:

• the entire food chain (including drinking-water), from the production of raw materials to distribution to the final consumer;
• each of the stages of this chain as specified by law: production, transformation, preservation, transport, storage and distribution; and
• food products for both human and animal consumption.

The Agency supervises the National Agency for Veterinary Medicinal Products. Its independence is guaranteed by the appointment of experts solely on academic criteria, procedures to avoid conflicts of interest, autonomy to determine areas of work and the publication of all its opinions.

Food control systems

Growing concerns about food safety have led many countries to review the effectiveness of their food control systems. Throughout the European Region, countries show marked differences in approach, including the division of responsibilities for risk assessment, management and communication. They also differ on the question of whether local or central authorities or a mixture of the two should be responsible for enforcing food law. Food control systems are most effective when based on the best available scientific advice from all sectors concerned and using a transparent and open approach to decision-making. A food control agency must fit the cultural, economic and political needs and conditions of the country: there is no single model (88).

Chapter 2 discussed the proportion of foodborne disease that relates to each part of the food chain. Most problems come from the farming sector as a primary source of pathogens; slaughterhouses; and food handling and catering.

Each sector needs separate measures, and several reports have outlined these needs. Not only is an appropriate surveillance system needed for assessing the dominant organisms involved, the regional distribution of problems and their potential sources, but, more important, all countries should consider instituting the HACCP (hazard analysis and critical control point) approach to controlling hazards (89).

Countries often take different approaches to dealing with the same pathogen, and each needs to consider the best strategy. For example, Sweden has worked for many years to ensure that its poultry flocks are *Salmonella*-free without the routine use of antibiotics (see Chapter 2). The EU has established a wide range of regulations relating to the proper conduct of slaughterhouses, and criteria for limiting the risk of contamination of carcasses by *E. coli*, by such means as insisting that the animals entering the slaughterhouse be clean. The BSE regulations also demand very specific measures. Further, many countries require that transport systems comply with temperature regulations, and storage systems need to be developed to limit cross-contamination.

Given the complexity of these issues, it is necessary to assess the most hazardous part of the operation and to seek to reduce progressively the entry of pathogens into the food supply. Catering and other retail establishments demand a further range of regulations and, in many countries, specific groups, often attached to or part of local authorities, are responsible for registering and authorizing food outlets, with strict rules for compliance, food sourcing and food hygiene. The CCEE have a strong tradition for maintaining a public hygiene service, while in western Europe responsibility has shifted from the local authority and public health officers to supermarket chains and food manufacturers. Each country needs to ensure that a proper system is in place both to assess hazards and to handle them effectively, recognizing that the EU has explicit regulations and that countries seeking to export to the EU will have to comply with them.

The food control infrastructure in each country in the European Region is the result of development over more than a century and has been influenced by the need to cope with the various problems encountered during this period. In Scandinavian countries, for instance, food control systems have traditionally focused on animal foods and microbiology, and veterinarians have played a key role. The Netherlands and the United Kingdom have traditionally emphasized food contamination and composition, and chemists have had central positions. In the NIS, food control grew out of the medical profession and has been closely linked to epidemiology, medical investigation and a public hygiene service.

In most countries, several ministries, departments and branches have shared the responsibility for food control. Health, agriculture, environment, trade and industry ministries are normally involved. The responsibility may also be divided between national, regional and local governments.

Considerations for the future

Every country has its own food control infrastructure and social, economic and political environments. National food control strategies are therefore normally country specific. To modernize the food control infrastructure, government agencies may choose to seek assistance in the various guidelines given by international organizations. The WHO *Guidelines for strengthening a national food safety programme (90)*, gives guidance for strengthening food safety programmes. It recommends that the process start with the preparation of a country profile that assesses the problems and the food control infrastructure at the national level. It advises on preparing and implementing a national food safety programme and formulating food law and regulations, and gives recommendations on control activities, such as food inspection and risk analysis.

Risk analysis

The concept of risk has become central to the regulation of food safety. An objective basis is required for regulating food safety and for solving conflicts in food trade. Legislation traditionally protected national food production against competition from imports. Self-sufficiency in food and food security were important and legitimate objectives for most countries following food shortages caused by international conflicts, particularly following the Second World War. Protective barriers against imported food were crucial for the survival of certain food industries and are therefore often associated with commercial interests, although they may claim to be based on scientific evidence.

To address some of these problems – as well as to protect the consumer – the FAO/WHO Codex Alimentarius Commission was set up in 1962. Since then it has worked to develop international food standards, guidelines and recommendations to facilitate the free flow of food across borders.

During the negotiations on liberalization of the world trade in food in the General Agreement on Trade and Tariffs (GATT) in the early 1990s, the participating countries agreed to remove the technical barriers to trade. At the same time, they selected scientific risk assessment as the best tool to help harmonize food legislation. A country could only hinder or prohibit imports of certain foods if scientific analysis demonstrated that they presented risks to the population or the environment. The aim is to use risk assessment as an objective and universally accepted basis for food regulations and a tool to resolve trade disputes. These efforts have largely succeeded.

Nevertheless, the scientific concept of risk differs greatly from consumers' perceptions. The scientific evaluation of risk is typically expressed in terms of the numbers of expected additional cases from a well defined cause over a specified time period. In the mind of the individual consumer, however, other aspects of risk are equally important. Whether consumers run a risk voluntarily (such as smoking) or involuntarily (such as the risk of BSE) makes a large difference in individual reactions (92,92). They may also consider factors other than personal risk – such as the risk of damage to the natural environment. As a result, consumers may be unwilling to accept food regulations that conflict with their perception of risk or harm – as shown, for example, by reactions against GMOs in the Region. The risk may be small, but consumers perceive it as beyond their personal control and as bringing potential harm with no obvious benefit.

The internationally accepted concept of risk is technically and economically oriented and based on principles formulated by a FAO/WHO expert group in 1998 (93). The main conceptual tool is risk analysis, which consists of three elements: risk assessment (scientific advice and information analysis), risk management (regulation and control) and risk communication (see Fig. 4.4). Risk assessment is considered a scientific discipline in which researchers assess the nature of the hazard, the exposure of the population and the likely incidence of illness as a result.

There is great debate about how to ensure that the distinct needs of each of the three components of risk analysis are dealt with properly. In countries such as the United Kingdom, a quasi-independent national body undertakes all three, with an agreed limited remit in management and the need to report to Parliament and making the health minister ultimately responsible for management decisions. Other agencies, such as the new European Food Safety Authority, consider that risk assessment must be conducted independently and the analysis made public. Risk management is then a different responsibility because, although health may be seen to be paramount, other economic, political and societal issues may need to be taken into account in practice. Thus, the EC, with the Council of Ministers and the European Parliament, has the formal responsibility for deciding how to manage environmental, food safety and public health issues, and a scientific group is responsible for providing the best possible scientific assessment of the issues to be addressed and the attendant uncertainties.

Separating risk assessment from risk management and risk communication is theoretically sound because assessment initially needs to be made without concern for the political, social and financial issues related to management decisions. It must interact with the two other segments of risk analysis, however, and having an evaluation that simply assumes that all implementation and management issues have been handled perfectly is not appropriate. In practice, implementation has repeatedly been shown to be imperfect. True risk assessment requires a transparent audit of the implementation process.

In addition, risk assessment rapidly becomes involved in the problem of risk communication because many of the issues are of intense public concern. Many European governments used to provide simple, understandable messages for consumers, with scientific panels providing a summary of their internal debates. Now, however, civil society not only must be represented in developing the remits and agendas of scientific committees but also should be actively involved before the final opinion is formed. The assessment must be as rigorous and detailed as possible, to reassure the public that the issues have been properly handled. How to express and communicate the degree of complexity of the analysis is a challenge that requires additional expertise to that traditionally involved in risk assessment.

Many of the problems surrounding BSE, for example, arose because management issues and other interests appeared either to modify or to limit the appropriate scientific scrutiny of risk. This is why the need for transparency in independent scientific analysis is now greatly emphasized. Some agencies reinforce this by ensuring that representatives of civil society and other stakeholders formally take part in the assessment process, which had been seen as the domain of scientists alone. It is now recognized that scientists often failed to take account of the public's concerns and may not have addressed the issues in a way that could deal directly with these concerns. The Management Board of the European Food Safety Authority is recognized to require members of civil society, including industrial and other representatives.

The conventional approach to risk analysis specifies a purely scientific basis for assessment. Most pressing food safety problems, however, are characterized by the absence of a complete scientific basis and by the presence of parties with a variety of interests and concerns: commercial, political, economic, legal and religious. This can be seen in the debate over GMOs, in which the EU group contributing to the EU–US Biotechnology Consultative Forum included senior political and consumer interests in addition to the usual range of scientific disciplines. The broader dimensions also need to be included in the debate on many other food safety issues, from the use of hormone growth promoters, pesticides and food irradiation to food additives, labelling and health claims. Scientific knowledge about the hazards and their risks – including their magnitude, extent and rate of change – may be incomplete, and this may reflect earlier priorities in allocating funds to research.

Further, even when the scientific knowledge base appears adequate, the recommendations that emerge from a scientific assessment may be of limited value. The terms of reference for the assessment may be inappropriate or the assessors may be affected by interests such as competition for resources, commercial dependence, theoretical allegiances, personality conflicts or strongly held personal beliefs.

Developing a broader approach to risk analysis

Some types of risk assessment can become very complex when large scientific unknowns and substantial economic interests are involved and major societal issues need to be considered: for example, when assessing the impact of global change. In food safety, this approach has been discussed in documentation submitted to the European Parliament *(94)*. Non-scientific factors should be seen as framing the scientific debate, both before and during risk assessment (Fig. 4.4).

Allowing non-scientific factors to enter the assessment process could do much to ameliorate the concern that present processes neglect consumers' interests. The institutional structures capable of handling this form of risk assessment have yet to be built, but they may prove to be a politically expedient means of encouraging consumer to accept risk assessment techniques.

In the meantime, because of the overwhelming economic importance of having a universally agreed principle on which to base international food regulation, several attempts have been made to improve consumers' acceptance of risk analysis. These include using the precautionary principle and recognizing factors other than science in setting standards for international trade.

The precautionary principle

In both EU and global food policy, the precautionary principle has been introduced or at least affirmed as a guiding principle to be applied when a

Fig. 4.4. Two approaches to risk analysis

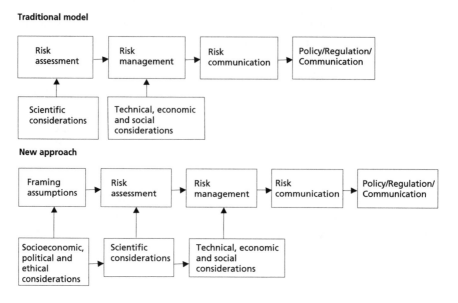

Source: adapted from Millstone *(95)*.

scientific analysis is incomplete. The idea is to let scientific doubt benefit the consumer. A precondition for applying the principle is clear recognition that the science is incomplete, that safety cannot be assured and that precautions should therefore be applied.

From one viewpoint, most food safety policies are precautionary in that risks are assessed in an anticipatory rather than a reactive way. For example, there are positive rather than negative lists for pesticides, veterinary medicines and food additives, and standards are or may be set before overt harm occurs. Thus, having a legislative framework, making routine pre-marketing reviews of new products and processes and operating a regulatory regime amount to the exercise of precaution.

From a second viewpoint, which corresponds to the traditional model shown in Fig. 4.4, precaution is seen as a non-scientific consideration that may be invoked only if there is some clear evidence of a particular risk, a scientific risk assessment has first been conducted and some residual uncertainty is identified. Risk managers (as distinct from risk assessors) may then make judgements on the steps that might be taken to avoid or diminish the risks about that remain uncertain and imprecise. In this model, precautionary judgement is distinct from the risk assessment or scientific studies.

A more valuable but complex approach employs the precautionary principle before, during and after the risk assessment; it is increasingly being adopted. A relatively precautionary risk assessment does not interpret or represent the absence of evidence of risk as if it were evidence of the absence of risk. Precaution, in this model, is also a consideration for risk managers who must make explicit judgements about the extent to which uncertainties may or may not be acceptable and how they may take steps to reduce these uncertainties.

Consumer organizations have emphasized the importance of the precautionary principle when such issues as substantial equivalence arise. The concept of substantial equivalence was seen as a means for justifying little scrutiny of new products or processes if they seemed to be very similar, often as assessed by relatively crude techniques, to a previous product or process. In practice, the assessment of substantial equivalence should be just a preliminary step to framing the analyses that should then be conducted.

Other legitimate factors

Non-scientific factors clearly have a legitimate role in the framing of risk assessment in European risk analysis. For example, in the evaluation of GMOs or pesticides, risk assessment should address not only to the direct effects on human health but also the indirect and secondary effects, such as the risk to animal health and environmental integrity. The EC has accepted that the second approach should prevail: a 2002 regulation on food law (96) stated that "... scientific risk assessment alone cannot, in some cases, provide all the information on which a risk management decision should be based, and ... other factors relevant to the matter under consideration should legitimately be taken into account including societal, economic, traditional, ethical and environmental factors ...".

Non-scientific issues can frame the scientific risk assessment by determining how far the assessment should extend. Should an assessment be confined to the direct effects on human health or include the effects on the non-human participants in food production and on the surrounding ecological systems? For example, the risk assessment of the yield-enhancing hormone bovine somatotrophin for milk production might be limited to the effects of residues in milk and milk products on human health or might be extended to include the effects on the health and welfare of the animals receiving the treatment. Similarly, the risk assessment of a pesticide may be limited to its health effects as a residue in food ingredients or can be extended to include its effect on ecosystems and farmworkers' health. The same questions can be applied to GMOs; should they be assessed for their environmental impact and their potential impact on neighbouring farms? In

Austria, stringent criteria must be satisfied, showing that the use of a proposed GMO will be at least as benign as organic farming and will provide positive environmental benefits compared with currently available alternatives (97).

In all these cases, the risks can be scientifically assessed, but the choice of the scope of the risk assessment may not be a purely scientific judgement. A mechanism for setting the scope of risk assessment needs to be established, and consumer participation in this mechanism should be encouraged (97).

Definition of the scope of such legitimate factors is being studied at the international level, especially in the Codex Alimentarius Commission. In addition to the environmental impact of production methods and animal welfare, examples of such factors include fair trade, consumers' expectations for product quality, appropriate labelling information and claims, and the definition of the essential characteristics of products (98).

This may be the first step in institutionalizing the framing assumptions shown in Fig. 4.4, but a coherent structure and process are lacking. The debate about risk often takes place in the mass media, where risks are made more readily visible and their political consequences are shaped. The mass media may tend to dramatize and oversimplify complex issues. In such a context, risk assessment tends to become intimately linked with risk communication. The mass media also spotlight the role of risk managers, challenging the authorities and their spokespeople to perform roles for which they may not be well prepared.

The risk communication process reinforces the need to consider other legitimate factors at an early stage in setting food safety requirements. Providing correct, relevant and meaningful information about risks to consumers in clear and understandable language is no longer sufficient. The EC noted (99): "Risk communication should not be a passive transmission of information, but should be interactive, involving a dialogue with and feed-back from all stakeholders". Probably very few national food safety authorities in the Region are involved in such interaction.

A continuing problem is that stakeholder groups – including consumers, food workers and local food authorities – may need to develop their skills to ensure they can make constructive and participatory responses to risk communication processes. If stakeholders are to participate constructively, all stages in risk analysis need to accommodate interactions with these groups. Steps are being taken to formalize these relationships in the United States, where a report (100) introduced a new approach to risk management that combines scientific analysis with continuing deliberations with affected parties, such as individuals and interest groups including NGOs.

In the United Kingdom, citizens' juries and other mechanisms have been used to gain insight into consumers' perception of risk and other factors they believe to be legitimate in assessing risk and ensuring food safety and environmental protection *(101)*.

Changes in the responsibility of official food control systems: the use of HACCP

Previously, an official food control system was seen as carrying the major responsibility for securing a supply of safe food for consumers. It relied heavily on certification, testing end products and comparing the results with official standards. This is still the case in many countries, especially the NIS *(24)*.

In contrast, the current trend in international food legislation is to require producers – feed manufacturers, farmers and food operators – to take primary responsibility for food safety. Food control authorities monitor and enforce this responsibility by operating national surveillance and control systems covering the food chain. Further, the focus has shifted from testing end products to risk assessment and food companies' implementation of food safety assurance systems based on HACCP principles.

According to a 1993 directive *(102)*, EU countries should ensure that all food businesses implement their own quality control systems based on HACCP principles. This applies to both small enterprises and large food manufacturers, although it excludes primary producers. In general, large enterprises have established quality control systems and operate them successfully. Large companies have access to highly trained technicians who understand HACCP principles and the language in which regulations are written. This is not the case for many small and medium-sized businesses, and they can have difficulty in fully implementing such quality control systems.

Small and medium-sized businesses are most numerous at both ends of the food chain: farmers and small retail shops and restaurants. Unfortunately, these are where the most serious safety problems in the food chain exist. For instance, foodborne problems with *Salmonella* and *Campylobacter* spp., pesticide residues, dioxin contamination and BSE arise from farming practices. Similarly, hygiene problems are greatest in small retail outlets, restaurants and private homes. It is a problem that the EC's major strategy, HACCP, is not very effective here, where the need for food safety measures is greatest.

In addition, although HACCP deals adequately with well recognized problems in a routine food production process, it deals less well with emerging problems and poorly identified critical control points. BSE is a case in point: there was considerable uncertainty about the nature of the disease, its possible source in the rendering process, its possible presence in sheep populations, the potential contamination of pastureland, the export of meat and bone meal or the infectivity of bovine blood (used for calf feed throughout the 1980s and 1990s). HACCP procedures were not sufficient with this emerging disease;

neither do they prevent the transfer of material from GMOs in experimental crops into the food supply (for example, into honey).

Modernizing food control

Because food control infrastructures in all European countries have developed over decades in response to changing economic and social conditions, experience shows that changing them is difficult. Such systems tend to be large and bureaucratic and have staff accustomed to doing their work in well established routines. One way to start the process of change is to reach agreement on a number of basic principles for strengthening and developing the food control infrastructure, such as the following.

- Food producers and food handlers have the key responsibility for ensuring food safety by establishing effective quality control systems.
- The primary role of public food safety authorities is to ensure compliance with food regulations, which may best be achieved by auditing food handlers' quality control systems.
- The food safety system aims at prevention rather than cure.
- Inspections should be carried out according to need.
- Analytical control functions primarily as a support to food inspections.
- Control activities should attend to both the immediate cause and the original source of a problem.
- The means of enforcement must be necessary, sufficient and proportionate to the risks involved.

The principles must reflect the situation in which the food control infrastructure will have to operate. This means taking account of the important changes in recent decades in consumers' attitudes towards risk and food safety.

Several elements require consideration before a food control infrastructure can be strengthened, including consumer-centred activity, new approaches to enforcement and comprehensive coverage of the food chain.

Consumer-centred activity and the allocation of responsibilities

Food safety measures must not only ensure safe food but also be seen to do so. Consumers need to be assured that controls are in place and are fully and properly implemented.

One move to establish consumer confidence has been removing food safety responsibilities from departments responsible for the trade interests of the food industry and agriculture and giving them to a new independent agency (87,88). Whether independent agencies can really improve food safety remains to be seen.

An alternative approach has been tried in Denmark, where formerly separate departments were combined. In 1997, responsibility for the food control infrastructure was vested in the new Ministry of Food, Agriculture and Fisheries. The old Ministry of Agriculture and Fisheries merged with the National Food Agency, which had previously been within the Ministry of Health, to create a ministry with a clear consumer profile, without losing connections with producers, traders and manufacturers.

This approach does not separate the inherently conflicting interests of consumers and producers, but locates them within one ministry and gives one minister the responsibility for resolving conflicts. In addition, Denmark's Ministry of Food, Agriculture and Fisheries can implement regulations throughout the whole food chain, from farm to fork. The crucial test of this way of organizing the food control system is its ability to maintain the confidence of consumers. This depends on the Ministry's ability to keep the decision-making process open, transparent and honest and to ensure adequate consumer participation.

Some other countries divide food control responsibilities between different ministries or government departments, such as health, agriculture, environment, industry or trade and tourism. Dialogue between these departments may be limited, and activities may easily and unintentionally overlap or be duplicated or omitted. This fragmentation may also lead to confusion over jurisdiction between agencies and their inspectors. As a result, some sectors of the food chain may receive intense scrutiny and others, little or no regulatory supervision or inspection. Both consumers and industry find these arrangements confusing and frustrating, and they do little to improve consumer confidence in the integrity of the food supply.

New, market-oriented means of enforcement
In practice, making food producers and handlers comply with regulations is often difficult for food control authorities. The traditionally available means of enforcement are not particularly strong. Food establishments can typically be ordered to correct things that are not in accordance with regulations. More serious cases may involve the police and courts, but fines and other penalties are usually modest. Food control authorities usually employ more dramatic means only when public health is endangered.

As a consequence, food establishments may be tempted to cut their standards: for example, to to reduce cleaning costs and pay the fines for poor hygiene. The food control system may lack means of enforcement that are strong enough to convince food producers and handlers to improve their practices, and enforcement drains the resources of national food inspection services. These are good reasons to seek innovative, appropriate and more effective means of enforcement.

The classic regulatory approach requires that the regulated activity be reasonably stable; areas undergoing rapid development are not well suited to regulation by rigid rules. Indeed, rules always lag behind problems, and the need for continuously adjusting rules demands many resources. In addition, those who are supposed to follow the rules should know them and perceive them as sensible and relevant. Rules that are not considered relevant will not be carefully followed.

In other sectors of modern society, the use of detailed rules and regulations is in general diminishing and the use of more flexible and less precise framework laws is increasing. The following examples show how food regulations can be adapted to deal with the more flexible activities in modern market economies.

Naming and shaming: publishing inspection results

Food authorities in several countries are already using market forces as a tool by informing consumers of the results of inspection in individual food establishments. Several states in the United States require that restaurants display their latest inspection reports in the customer areas. In certain states the restaurants are classified into categories, such as A–E, according to hygienic performance. The inspection results for all 10 000 restaurants in New York City are published on the Internet (http://www.nyclink.org/html/doh/ html/ rii/index.html, accessed 10 November 2002). In the United Kingdom, the inspection results from all slaughterhouses and meat processors are published according to a special classification system (the Hygiene Assessment Scheme).

In 2001, Denmark's Parliament (*Folketing*) passed an amendment to the food law requiring the Danish Veterinary and Food Administration to publish the results of food inspections. The inspection results include a classification of food establishments into four categories according to performance. An establishment must exhibit the inspection report in the customer area, and all results are published on the Internet. The primary purpose is to enable consumers to select food shops and restaurants according to their hygiene status, to reduce the risk of food poisoning. Compliance with other legislation is also recorded. It is hoped that the practice will influence food establishments to practise good hygiene.

Sticks and carrots: linking costs to behaviour

The idea is to reward the food enterprises that follow the law by giving them a competitive advantage. For example, award schemes, giving accolades for good practice, can be used so that the recipient of an award has a marketing advantage.

Food companies that break the regulations should receive sanctions that can reduce their competitiveness. Fines might be higher and could be more immediately applied, as with road traffic offences. When necessary, business could be suspended with minimal delay.

More proactively, a polluter-pays system may be developed in which food establishments that do not comply with the regulations must pay the cost of the food control system, including their own inspection. For example, they could be charged for inspections, and the cost and frequency of reinspection would be based on the previous inspection results.

Creating a culture of good practice

Norms and knowledge are soft tools that food control authorities can use to enforce national regulations. They require standards for good practice to be set and disseminated to all food establishments. One method may be to give awards to the establishments in a locality with the best practices and to use these to encourage others in the area.

Educating staff is vital to ensure full-hearted compliance. Food establishments should recognize the need to train food handlers, and training should be made available to all employees to ensure a food hygiene culture based on consistent and well understood principles.

Food control authorities need to become centres of knowledge, using norms and knowledge as tools. They should continually gather and disseminate new information. After appropriate interpretation of the information, the authorities could form new norms in dialogue with both consumers and the relevant food industry.

If necessary, a system of licensing might be appropriate, although the numbers of small businesses involved, and their short lifespan, may militate against licensing. Even with a licensing system, surveillance and inspection needs to enforce regulatory compliance.

Product liability

Besides regulation and criminal prosecution, food establishments may be subject to private civil prosecution for damages caused by the products they sell. The EU has introduced generalized product liability to primary producers, including farmers *(103)*.

The opportunities for private prosecution are limited if food is untraceable. This problem is not insurmountable, and improvements in traceability schemes are already being implemented.

Proving liability is difficult if the harmful effects of food occur long after a person was in contact with it. The problems of delayed harm can be dealt with by using insurance schemes that require no-fault compensation.

Insurance schemes that cover food establishments for product liability are available, although ensuring that they cover the use of new technology, such as genetically modified foods, may be difficult.

Food security and sustainable development policy

Existing promotion measures

The latest WHO analysis of policies and practices in nutrition, food safety and food security in 1998–1999 *(24)* indicates that food insecurity is widespread in many countries of the European Region (Table 4.6).

The socioeconomic transition undergone by many eastern countries in the Region has reduced food security. For example, the Baltic countries and other NIS reported that many low-income people depend substantially on subsistence farming and home-grown produce. Declining agricultural production was reported to result from a lack of financial support, expertise and improved agricultural methods. In addition, collaboration between the different sectors involved in producing and distributing food was reported as very poor.

In contrast, western European countries reported abundant food supplies, but several acknowledged the need to reduce farm inputs (fuel, pesticides and antibiotics) and to encourage greater sustainability. There is some evidence that economic concerns may be taking priority over health. For example, Iceland reported the taxation of imported fruits and vegetables to protect local producers, probably resulting in lower intake. An abundant supply of food, however, does not mean equitable distribution and access in many western European countries *(104)* (see Chapter 1, pp. 66–73 and Chapter 3, pp. 158–168).

Inequality in food security has led some countries, such as the Russian Federation and Uzbekistan, to initiate specific programmes or policy measures (Table 4.6). Several western European countries, such as France and Germany, acknowledge that they have few data on the dietary patterns of low-income families. Some countries are approaching inequality through more general measures to improve the income and employment levels among poorer families through social security and training programmes.

Considerations for the future

Food insecurity can be considered as both lack of access to appropriate food and the longer-term impact and sustainability of food production practices. Helping to rectify problems of immediate access is probably easier for ministries than guiding the longer-term environmental impact of food production systems on land use, which involves a substantial number of sectors, such as rural development, trade, agriculture, finance and local government. Assessing food access requires identifying how poor and vulnerable people gain access to high-quality foods and whether foods such as vegetables, fruits and fish are available at reasonable prices throughout the year. Undertaking a series of targeted surveys in particular cities or areas may be more helpful than attempting a comprehensive analysis of a whole country. Health promotion groups can help to solve problems of access by identifying local centres and underemployed

Table 4.6. Examples of policy measures for food security and sustainable development

Country	Measures
Austria	Programmes to support organic production
Czech Republic	Support for sustainable farming in uplands Educational projects in schools and training in higher education on sustainable farming Targeted programme for health promotion among the minority Romanian population, especially children
Estonia	Agriculture act (1997) to encourage sustainable farming practices A council formed in 1999 to develop anti-poverty strategies
Finland	Revision of the social assistance act (1998) Reduced use of pesticides and fertilizers National programmes for managing environmental quality and food production
France	Improved programme for school meals Distribution of reduced-price food to low-income families
Georgia	Centre for Nutrition Studies established to coordinate national programmes and improve legal framework
Germany	Development of guidance on good agricultural practices Federal support for organic farming
Ireland	Rural environment protection scheme to promote rural economies and social cohesion Nutrition education projects for low-income women Scheme for free school lunches Community-run cafés and shops
Kyrgyzstan	Training of health personnel to raise awareness of inequality
Norway	National Council on Nutrition and Physical Activity to advise on agricultural production and pricing policies
Russian Federation	Development of new plant varieties for higher yields in stressful conditions Report of a commission to make policies encouraging healthy nutrition for disadvantaged groups: recommendations being adopted
Ukraine	Assistance to low-income families through housing subsidies and social benefits
United Kingdom	Employment action zones and national minimum wage to boost the incomes of poorer families Health action zones to target health inequality
Uzbekistan	National programme on food security (1997)

Source: Comparative analysis of food and nutrition policies in the WHO European Region 1994–1999. Full report (24).

people who, with suitable support, can develop local facilities to allow poor people to buy food at affordable prices. Several successful schemes have been introduced in European countries *(105)*.

A number of measures can counteract environmental degradation, including policies on replanting and setting aside selected areas to increase the diversity of flora and fauna. In western Europe, schemes have been established to reduce the contamination of rivers and beaches to comply with new standards for water quality. Similar innovation and modern techniques need to be applied to rejuvenating degraded land and limiting soil erosion. For example, CAP reforms need to consider nutritional health as well as environmental protection (see p. 224), as recommended by Sweden's National Institute of Public Health *(2)*.

An integrated approach: food, health and environment

Fortunately, the strategies needed to create desired changes in nutritional and environmental patterns are often complementary and, as a whole, provide cost-effective, sustainable development for agricultural land (see Chapter 3, pp. 197–200, and p. 224). In addition, local strategies that seek to improve the availability of, access to and consumption of locally produced foods, particularly fruits and vegetables, also increase the interdependence and thus the social cohesion between urban and rural dwellers (see Chapter 3, pp. 205–208).

The United Nations projects that about 83% of the population in the European Region (excluding 10 countries: Armenia, Azerbaijan, Georgia, Kazakhstan, Kyrgyzstan, Israel, Tajikistan, Turkey, Turkmenistan and Uzbekistan) will live in cities by 2030 *(106)*. Cities produce enormous amounts of waste, which is usually transported as far away and as inexpensively as possible. Urban and peri-urban horticulture businesses have the potential to recycle organic waste, stormwater and treated grey water (any water used in the home, except water from toilets) for use in food production. Urban organic waste (solid waste and wastewater) is a valuable resource that can help to conserve the limited water supply. Moreover, growing and processing fruits and vegetables locally can reduce the energy used in food packaging and transport *(105)* (see Chapter 3, pp. 178–179).

The current trends in urbanization, combined with the increasing globalization of the food trade, will profoundly affect the sustainability of the food system *(107,108)*. Over the next decade, about 10% of the EU population and 25% of the population in the CCEE will move from rural areas into cities. In 1999, the percentage of the population living in rural areas and working in agriculture was much higher in the CCEE (22.5%) than in the EU (5.5%). Rapid urbanization in the CCEE is therefore likely to be traumatic for both the people left behind and those moving to urban areas in search of jobs. Planners will need to design infrastructure in both urban and rural areas to protect vulnerable people – including unemployed, low-income and elderly people – against food insecurity *(105)*.

A more integrated approach to developing food and environmental plans will help to reduce the stress from rapid urbanization and increased global food trade *(107,108)*. Planners should capitalize on communities' skills, and city authorities should ensure that the appropriate legal, financial, technical and support structures are in place.

Integrated food, health and environmental policies can:

• create opportunities for local employment
• stimulate local economic growth
• strengthen social cohesion
• improve the aesthetics of the city environment
• increase opportunities for more active lifestyles
• improve mental health
• recycle treated water and organic waste for food production
• provide a closer link between consumers and producers
• improve the environment and develop rural areas.

All these advantages lead to more sustainable food, health and environmental systems. In many countries, authorities concerned with community development are beginning to link existing projects or networks, such as Agenda 21 projects; projects of NGOs for poverty alleviation, urban renewal and community and rural development; and networks of the WHO Healthy Cities project.

Identifying the local stakeholders
Successfully developing and implementing local food and nutrition action plans requires the participation of various stakeholders: national authorities, food producers, consumer groups, neighbourhood and environmental groups, schools, community health centres, retailers, markets, banks and authorities responsible for food control and safety. All have a role to play *(109)*. The following questions will help to identify the key stakeholders.

• Who might be affected positively or negatively by the concerns to be addressed?
• What groups may have trouble making their views heard and need special efforts to ensure their inclusion?
• Who are the representatives of those likely to be affected?
• Who is responsible for what is intended?
• Who is likely to mobilize for or against intended action?
• Who can make intended action more effective by participation or less effective by nonparticipation or outright opposition?
• Who can contribute financial and technical resources?
• Whose behaviour must change for the policy to succeed?

Work towards a sustainable future should not be left entirely to policy-makers and technical experts. Broad community involvement is essential in both finding sustainable solutions and facilitating action. Although ensuring such involvement can be daunting, because it consumes both time and re-sources, it is vital to achieving equitable and sustainable solutions. Finding such solutions requires not only public debate but effective interaction be-tween policy-makers, technical and educational institutions, commercial in-terests, community groups and citizens.

Analysing problems and assets

Preparing a new policy requires data to clarify the problems that existing food systems create and to determine which potential changes could improve the situation. Thus, a common starting-point is to analyse the existing situation in relation the production of, access to and consumption of healthy foods. Once this is done, an action plan can be designed to meet the population's needs.

Poor availability of and inequitable access to healthy food among vulner-able groups are common problems that create barriers to increasing consump-tion of a healthy diet, including fruits and vegetables. The best way to increase fruit and vegetable intake is not only to use health education but also to assess and make structural changes to support policy implementation. All action should improve equity, promote local sustainability, empower vulnerable groups and reduce social and health problems and poverty.

Potential opportunity to reduce foodborne risks

Food policies are needed to reduce the spread of foodborne diseases and to reduce the level of perceived health risks. Food production and retailing are increasingly perceived as presenting risks to society in the European Region. Consumers are increasingly concerned about foodborne disease (see Chapter 2) and no longer trust the food supply.

Consumers are increasingly concerned about the microbiological and chemical safety of food, genetically modified foods, novel foods and new processing techniques. Reports of antibiotic resistance, BSE, dioxins and foot-and-mouth disease in animals have damaged their confidence in the safety of what they eat.

Many of the foodborne diseases described in Chapter 2 are associated with intensive agriculture and mass-produced and widely transported and distrib-uted food. Producing more food nearer the consumer could more easily con-trol and perhaps reduce some of the risks. Proper management could elimi-nate or more easily mitigate foodborne diseases. For example, introducing healthy farmers' markets could have several advantages *(105)* (see p. 290). In the CCEE, the sale of local food contributes substantially to food security, particularly the availability of fruits and vegetables, and provides a viable means for local producers to earn extra income.

Barriers to increasing equitable access

Just as the emphasis of food production varies between the CCEE (more subsistence) and western countries in the Region (more commercial or recreational), so do consumers and food consumption patterns. City dwellers in western Europe are predominantly purchasers of value-added processed foods and have little connection with food production. In contrast, about 66% of urban families in the CCEE and NIS produce food. This self-reliance and subsistence farming are likely to change towards the patterns of development in western Europe, with the expansion of the global market *(107,108)* through, for example, supermarkets and standardization of products. This means that people in the CCEE and NIS are likely to become more dependent on the market-driven food distribution systems. This poses a problem for poor people, who cannot buy their way into this system.

Planners facing increases in city populations should therefore consider alternative food distribution systems and not assume that market-driven systems will cover all needs, especially those needs of people who live in rural areas or on low incomes, and other vulnerable groups. Planners should promote scope for subsistence farming and particularly horticulture in both rural and urban areas.

Barriers to increasing the consumption of fruits and vegetables

As discussed in Chapter 1, most people in Europe, and especially poor and disadvantaged people, do not eat enough fruits and vegetables. The exact reasons must be examined in each situation, but the higher intake in populations in the Mediterranean countries than in northern Europe demonstrates that access and availability are key factors to increasing consumption. Many barriers need to be overcome.

- Some communities may have lost confidence in fruits and vegetables because of scares about pesticide use (see Chapter 2, pp. 129–131), soil contamination and air pollution.
- Taste can be a factor; in particular, children may dislike the taste of vegetables (see pp. 248–249).
- Most research has focused on extending the shelf life of non-perishable value-added foods, instead of perishable food.
- Many consumers now prefer food that is processed, pre-packaged and sold in supermarkets.
- City planners perceive food growing and distribution projects as unimportant and not progressive.

- The community may find some foods culturally unacceptable.
- Many people, especially vulnerable groups, eventually lose cooking skills and cannot cook fruits or vegetables.
- Fresh fruits and vegetables may be too expensive.
- Fruits and vegetables may not be available or accessible.
- Spending more time at work and less at home creates the need for time-saving convenience foods.

Partnerships with retailers to improve access

The supermarket revolution has brought both advantages and unexpected challenges (see Chapter 3, pp. 175 and 196), but city authorities can influence supermarkets' policies. For instance, in the United States, local authorities have successfully encouraged supermarkets to enter the poorer areas of large cities, and the concept of neighbourhood supermarkets that sell local produce is being promoted. Good cooperation between supermarkets and the health and voluntary sectors, both in the United States and Europe is leading to increased sales of fruits and vegetables.

Many services provided by supermarkets can greatly improve their customers' access to fruits and vegetables:

- increased variety of fresh fruits and vegetables for sale;
- wheelchairs and walking assistance;
- the availability of small, reasonably priced packs and unpackaged, affordable fruits and vegetables, sold singly for small households;
- free bus service to and from supermarkets;
- loyalty cards or stamps that offer discounts on fruits and vegetables; and
- home delivery service.

Food retailers, especially supermarket chains, are a dominant force in shaping the preferences and demand for goods *(108,109)*. Large retail distribution chains often build very large central terminals for produce from all over the world. From here trucks deliver to the shops belonging to the distribution chain. This does not encourage these shops to stock locally grown produce. Attempts to reverse this trend are being tested in some cities. For example, supermarkets in Mikkeli, Finland, sell locally grown and processed foods that are promoted by special shelf signs advertising "provincial products".

The exponential growth and high-profile promotional campaigns of supermarkets in the CCEE are likely to influence consumption patterns substantially. Such changes are not inevitable (see Chapter 3, Fig. 3.5, p. 166). Several factors shape dietary change: policies on food supply, pricing and technology, activities to promote products and public health messages. A combination of consumer demand and commercial investment in mass production and promotion largely determines the direction of change.

Patterns of change differ with circumstances. For example, 60% of the direct foreign investment in the food sector in the CCEE during the 1990s was in confectionery and soft drink production and less than 6% in fruit and vegetable production. Ministries should attempt to work with food retailers to develop new health promotion strategies to limit the damage from these trends.

Mechanisms to help health ministries set priorities for future action

From science to policy-making

This book depends greatly on scientists' interpretation of available data: material from large-scale surveys, international bodies and peer-reviewed scientific journals. The scientific evidence showing the relationships discussed here forms only part of the argument needed to provide policy-makers with a basis for action.

Scientists have the skills to generate testable theories, develop methods for measuring and evaluating and show statistical relationships. Policy-makers have the skills to negotiate between conflicting interests and to draft, enact and ensure the enforcement of legislation. Between the two lies the problem of how scientific findings are fed into the policy process (Fig. 4.5).

Scientific advisory committees play the key role, interpreting the current scientific evidence and giving opinions for policy purposes, but they have been criticized for biased views, narrowness of focus and a lack of transparency. In response, national and international scientific committees are becoming more open. Members are being asked to declare their commercial as well as their academic interests. Non-scientific members, such as consumer representatives, are being invited to participate. Further, the methods for evaluating scientific evidence are becoming clearer and more tightly structured, and such evaluation is becoming a well developed science. The sensitivity of theories and models can be assessed by checking on the importance of the various assumptions and the robustness of the predictions. Evidence can be ranked in importance according to agreed criteria, such as the methods used in the research, the size of the sample and the replication of the findings.

Decisions, however, are not based on evidence alone. Evidence is often inadequate: for example, there was little evidence of a link between BSE and any human disease during the late 1980s and early 1990s, yet precautions were advised and proved to be greatly needed. Evidence often has significant shortcomings, and more data inevitably accumulate in subsequent years. Thus, a precautionary approach is always recommended.

Fig. 4.5. Steps in developing and implementing policy

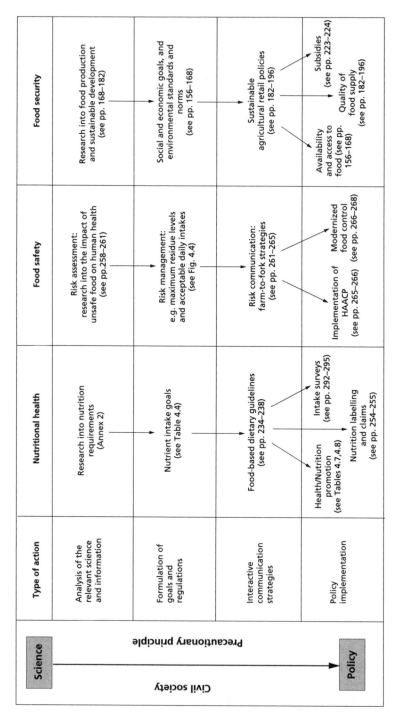

Further, there can only be evidence on what is or what was, not what might be. Scientific evidence can show differences and trends and the results of tests and trials, but not the results of an action before it is taken. Policy decisions cannot therefore be based entirely on evidence but must rely on a combination of the best available evidence with predictions and assumptions. These can be, for example, organized into methods of health impact assessment to evaluate the health effects of proposed policies, programmes and projects (see pp. 289–292).

Some countries have mechanisms for providing information on nutrition, food safety and food security (23,24), but few have explored how best to integrate scientific evidence from the agricultural and environmental sectors with that from health analyses. Agricultural policies since the Second World War have dealt mainly with food production, while health policies have dealt mainly with health care and treatment and health education. Developing integrated policies requires evolving systems for ensuring closer interaction between both scientists and policy-makers in health, agriculture and the environment.

In 1997, the EC developed new mechanisms whereby a scientific committee would evaluate the health aspects of the environment, agriculture and other societal activities, and publish the agendas and minutes of its meetings and its numerous opinions on the Internet and through press conferences. Special scientific bodies are needed to analyse the evidence and to make recommendations for policy ensuring the involvement of civil society. The emergence of a huge range of bodies within civil society means that the mechanisms of developing and implementing policy need to be rethought, as outlined in a publication on the nature of global governance (110).

Fig. 4.5 illustrates some of the steps required between science and policy development and implementation in relation to nutrition, food safety and food security. A similar process is warranted in all three areas: analysis of the relevant science and information, formulation of regulations and control mechanisms and transmission of this information to citizens, using the precautionary principle (see pp. 261–263), in an interactive way involving dialogue and feedback from all stakeholders.

Fig. 4.5 brings together the three main issues that have been discussed individually in previous sections of this chapter. This section illustrates how a ministry can develop an integrated, comprehensive food and nutrition policy that attempts to find sustainable solutions to many of the public health concerns highlighted in Chapters 1–3. Fig. 4.6 outlines a proposed process to help governments set priorities among their activities, recognizing that everything cannot be tackled at once. Nevertheless, a written policy must be developed that comprehensively describes all the problems before policy-makers decide where major new efforts should begin. Identifying national assets and building new policies around them are especially important.

Fig. 4.6. A proposed process for governments to use in setting priorities for action

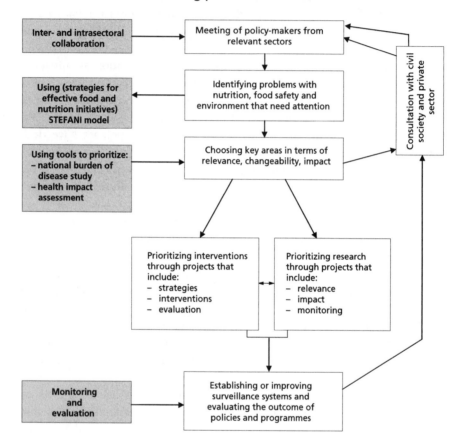

Source: inspired by Swinburn et al. (40).

Fig. 4.6 proposes an approach for health and other relevant ministries to use in developing policies and identifying priority areas within food and nutrition. It involves:

- taking a multisectoral approach;
- identifying problems that call for scientific research or health promotion intervention through the strategies for effective food and nutrition initiatives model (see Table 4.7);

- setting priorities, with the help of such tools as assessment of health impact or the relative burdens of different diseases, and then agreeing on intervention projects or research activities; and
- monitoring and evaluation.

Objective, reliable data are essential for policy-making and should be generated by national health information systems. Mechanisms for process and outcome evaluation must be created to ensure that the policies tackle the problems that place the heaviest burdens on society and individuals.

Intra- and intersectoral collaboration

One of the first steps in developing an integrated and comprehensive food and nutrition policy is to ensure good collaboration between nutrition and food safety experts working in the health sector. The general public perceives food holistically, and sees only academic differences between food safety and nutrition. People want good, wholesome food that they can enjoy without fear.

Interestingly, in the European Region, nutritionists and food safety specialists seem to work more closely together in the CCEE and NIS than in other countries. There may be several reasons for this. For example, nutrition is a relatively new science, and in the CCEE and NIS its evolution is closely linked to hygiene, ecology and the sanitary-epidemiology system. Specialists in nutrition and food hygiene evolve from the same postgraduate medical specialization. Moreover, the responsibility for food safety lies with health ministries in the CCEE and NIS but has been transferred to agriculture or other ministries in many other countries. With the increasing food safety scandals in western Europe, however, health ministries are taking a more proactive role in protecting public health and food safety.

Coordination between public health specialists working in food safety and nutrition is important for many reasons. For example, nutritionists encourage consumers to eat more lean meat, fish, fruits and vegetables, whereas consumers and food safety experts may express concern about increasing levels of *Salmonella* and *Campylobacter* (in chicken), dioxins (fish) and pesticides (fruits and vegetables). Health ministries are responsible for ensuring that all public health specialists deliver the same consistent and reliable information to consumers. Closer cooperation between nutritionists and food safety specialists can prevent the dissemination of conflicting or confusing messages. In addition, the health ministry can build the trust of civil society if it actively seeks citizens' opinions through NGOs and the voluntary sector. The opinions of the private sector must also be included, and one of the difficulties in developing intersectoral policies is stakeholders' level of commitment to public health versus their own economic or other interests. Intersectoral polices will probably not be implemented unless all stakeholders are committed to the process (Fig. 4.7).

Fig. 4.7. Collaboration of sectors in developing and implementing food and nutrition policy

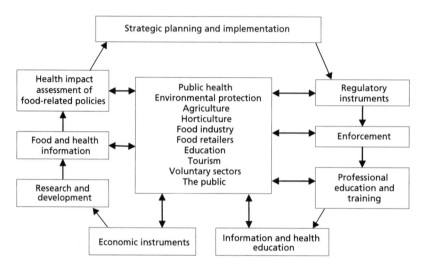

Public health specialists dealing with food safety and nutrition have to learn how best to strengthen their collaboration with other sectors such as agriculture and the food industry, including wholesalers, retailers and caterers. Consumers have an interest in supporting the supply of high-quality, nutritious and safe food, and the food industry has an interest in supplying what consumers want. This gives the health sector a good opportunity to strengthen alliances with NGOs concerned with food and public health. Unfortunately, the WHO comparative analysis of nutrition policies (24) provided little evidence of such alliances, except in Hungary, Norway, Poland and Sweden.

Strategies for effective food and nutrition initiatives (STEFANI)

The STEFANI model is a framework developed for policy-makers to use in setting priorities among intervention projects and research. The model was inspired by the analysis grid for environments linked to obesity (ANGELO) framework (37), which aims to analyse factors that promote overweight and obesity and set priorities among areas for intervention and research. The ANGELO framework is diagnostic, covering elements that influence behaviour. The STEFANI model is a framework for action that includes a wide range of interventions.

The STEFANI model (Table 4.7) examines four main settings – physical, economic, policy and sociocultural – against three main sectors – nutrition, food safety and food security, to determine action that health and other ministries can take.

The physical setting comprises what is available in the infrastructure (such as school canteens or football fields), capacity-building opportunities (such as nutrition and exercise expertise) and information (such as food labels). The economic setting is composed of financial factors: both the related costs (for example, for building bicycle paths or subsidizing fruits and vegetables) and the income available to pay for them (for example, taxing saturated fat (111) and using the additional revenue on public health campaigns). The policy setting covers rules, legislation and recommendations (such as whether the government has endorsed HACCP (see pp. 265–266) or national dietary guidelines have been developed). Finally, the sociocultural setting comprises attitudes, perceptions, values and beliefs that characterize certain societal groups (such as the acceptability of breastfeeding in public or mistakenly feeding infants tea, or the belief that organic food is healthier). All these settings significantly affect the behaviour of individuals and organizations and must be addressed before areas for intervention and research can be identified.

Table 4.8 gives examples of how a health ministry can systematically analyse problems and initiate action by, for example, reassessing funding priorities, making new legislation or developing innovations in public information or citizen participation.

Other ministries may be responsible for many of the required actions, and the health ministry will therefore need strategies for interacting with them. Successful policies in the European Region suggest that health ministries can exert considerable influence if they have the evidence to ensure that the public, professional groups and politicians understand the need for integrated and comprehensive food and nutrition policies.

Table 4.8 includes some aspects of food and nutrition policy that can be carried out by the health sector at the national and local levels. It covers a series of issues relating to the whole lifespan. The policies listed may involve changing physical facilities, reorienting economic priorities or taking educational or sociocultural initiatives. In addition, health professionals need to develop schemes that require multisectoral solutions. Tables 4.7 and 4.8 systematically set out some of the many initiatives that are needed to improve nutritional health, ensure food safety and sustain the environment. This is not a complete portfolio, but it is hoped that this scheme may stimulate discussion on different policy options.

Table 4.7. The STEFANI model: examples of action by ministries in different settings

Settings	Action by health ministry			Action by other ministries		
	Nutritional health	Food safety	Food security and sustainable development	Nutritional health	Food safety	Food security and sustainable development
Physical: what is available?	Appropriately accessible health centres; Promotion of access to appropriate self-monitoring systems, for example, for weight and blood pressure; Providing information on disease prevention	Catering in hospitals; Monitoring facilities; Health information systems; Food control	Systems for clean water; Facilities for monitoring iodized salt; Laboratories for testing air, water and soil quality	Playgrounds in schools, suitable cycling and road systems, urban planning, sports facilities; Designated urban areas for local food production	Appropriate local abattoirs; Proper public toilet and sanitary facilities; Proper catering facilities with stringent hygiene requirements	Urban planning: green spaces, cycle paths, parks, playgrounds, lead-free soil; Facilities for farmers' markets; Facilities to support breastfeeding in shops, etc.
Economic: what are the financial factors?	Primary health care staff paid to give advice on disease prevention	Penalties for providing unsafe food	Investment in health promotion projects	Re-evaluating taxation and subsidy policies; Support for low-income groups	Appropriate penalties for inappropriate hygiene	Reformed agricultural subsidies; Financing of new public transport systems; Promotion of urban agriculture
Policy: what are the rules, legislation, and recommendations?	Baby-friendly hospitals; Dietary guidelines; Fortification policies; Policies on health claims, for example, for functional foods	Assessment of health impact of agricultural policies; Consideration of consumers' concerns in food safety policy	Specific guidelines for toxicants and contaminants in soil, water and primary food products; Assessment of health impact of agrochemical and pesticide use	Assessment of health impact of CAP; Food labelling with appropriate, understandable health-related information	Criteria for ensuring a pathogen- and contaminant-free food chain; HACCPs for the food chain, systematic surveillance and mechanisms for emergency response	Reformed agricultural subsidies; Policies on: soil improvement, clean water, agricultural recycling, planting and use of fertilizer, pesticides and water; Paid maternity leave
Sociocultural: what are the attitudes, perceptions, values and beliefs?	Health education; Community activities; Promoting cycling and walking and building appropriate paths	Promotion of concept of limited clinical antibiotic use; Maximum residue limits and acceptable daily intakes; Publicizing of results of food hygiene inspections	Promoting: • health impact assessment of food policies • urban agriculture • organic food as healthier than non-organic food	Promotion of physical activity in the workplace; Creation of time and space for breastfeeding in the workplace, with the help of NGOs	New criteria excluding antibiotics as growth promoters and specifying veterinary use; Start of educational initiatives for the safety of fast-food outlets, modifying nutrient composition and limiting and ensuring appropriate food waste disposal	Positive attitudes to cycle path use and pedestrian areas; Educational initiatives for caterers, use of school recreational facilities by the community

Table 4.8. Potential action for health ministries

Professional groups	National level			Local level		
	Nutritional health	Food safety	Food security and sustainable development	Nutritional health	Food safety	Food security and sustainable development
Health professionals dealing with the perinatal period, such as obstetricians, gynaecologists, midwives, paediatricians, primary health care physicians and paediatric nurses	Audit of policies on anaemia, weight gain, optimum diet in pregnancy and breastfeeding Initiatives for baby-friendly hospitals Policy on feeding infants and young children	Policies advising pregnant women on such topics as avoiding listeriosis, salmonellosis and toxoplasmosis, and promoting food hygiene Surveillance policies	Policies advising pregnant women on, for example, preventing toxoplasmosis	Optimum techniques for limiting low birth weight, anaemia, pregnancy diabetes and neural tube defects; breast-feeding strategies Breastfeeding within 1 hour of birth Informing parents on complementary feeding	Antenatal education including as food hygiene and preventing listeriosis and salmonellosis	Antenatal education including preventing toxoplasmosis Leaflets and posters to inform the public
Health professionals dealing with children and schools, such as paediatricians, school medical officers, paediatric and school nurses and health visitors	Promoting physical activity in preschools and schools Policies with the education ministry, to monitor children's weight and BMI Training of school nurses and canteen staff on healthy diets	Policies for food and water hygiene for young children Policies to support universal salt iodization	Policies to reduce access to unhealthy food (such as typical food from vending machines) and to increase access to healthy food	Monitoring of iodine levels of the population Promotion of consumption of iodized salt, with education on the need to limit intake Policies to reduce vending machines in schools and to limit availability of soft drinks and sweets	Monitoring of hygiene standards of preschool and school canteens Tackling parasitic diseases (providing anthelmintic treatment)	Comprehensive food and nutrition policies for schools Promoting a network of health promoting schools

Table 4.8 continued

Professional groups	National level			Local level		
	Nutritional health	Food safety	Food security and sustainable development	Nutritional health	Food safety	Food security and sustainable development
Health professionals dealing with adolescents, such as physicians in primary health care, community centres and schools, gynaecologists and school nurses	Policies on weight control, healthy eating and physical activity in schools and community centres, with adolescents as decision-makers. Teachers and health professionals educated on adolescents' dietary and psychosocial needs	Policies for food hygiene in places where adolescents spend time	Policies with the sports industry to promote physical activity among adolescents via the mass media	Projects on diet, physical activity and health. Policies on anaemia in adolescence and in teenage pregnancy	Policies to tackle parasitic diseases (providing anthelmintic treatment)	Policies to create green spaces around schools and community centres. Support for policies to maintain parks and recreational facilities
Health professionals dealing with adults, such as primary health care physicians and adult specialists	Nutrient reference values and food-based dietary guidelines. Health professionals educated on adults' dietary needs	Policies to ensure hygienic canteens at workplaces	–	Consistent information from health professionals on a healthy diet. Monitoring patients' BMI	Support for policies for proper food labelling, especially to inform consumers about GMOs and food additives	Support for policies to improve public transport, particularly to increase accessibility to farmers' markets and shops. Support for urban planning policies that create safe bicycle paths
Health professionals dealing with older people, such as geriatricians and nursing home personnel	Policies to promote physical activity (especially weight bearing) via nursing homes, caregivers and community centres	Geriatricians and nursing home personnel educated on the susceptibility of the immune system in relation to food. Monitoring of food preparation and hygiene in nursing homes and hospitals	Policies to monitor hospital hygiene and nosocomial diseases	Regular monitoring by health professionals of bone density and micronutrient and macronutrient deficiencies	Monitoring of older people for infections and infestations	Clean and safe communal rooms in hospitals for older long-term inpatients

Public health professionals	Start and monitoring of a range of public health initiatives involving both hospital and community policies Policy on nutrition labelling and health claims	Specific responsibilities assigned for dealing with acute food safety problems Food control services Support for farmers' markets	Toxicological monitoring and evaluation of any possible environmental occupational health problem Support for the development of farmers' markets	Promoting demonstration projects, for example, for physical activity and dietary change in the community	Criteria for giving quality marks to companies of various sizes, based on auditing food hygiene practices	Environmental audits for all factories with water effluence, and spot checks on potential lead contamination in local waste disposal centres; and of soil contamination, especially for urban agriculture projects
Public health professionals dealing with refugees, internally displaced persons and migrant populations	Policies for proper training of volunteers and health staff on the particular needs of refugees and internally displaced persons Policies for regularly monitoring nutritional health Health professionals educated on the special dietary needs of migrant populations	Policies to provide refugees with proper tools for food preparation Training of professionals on proper water purification	Support for policies that create a "sustainable" infrastructure in a refugee camp Support for NGOs working to integrate and support refugees in a host country	Policies to provide oral rehydration therapy and nutrient-rich supplements and foods to refugees in camps Monitoring of refugees for anaemia Support for monitoring of BMI and micronutrient deficiencies of migrant populations, especially children	Policies to tackle parasitic diseases: monitoring hookworm and other helminth infestations and providing anthelmintic treatment Provision of chlorine drops or other water purification methods	Support for the creation of community centres and physical activity spaces for children and adults Support for initiatives that provide free language classes and special support services to refugees in a host country
Hospital staff	Consistent policies on food and nutrition during illness Membership of network of health promoting hospitals	Policies to prevent or deal with food poisoning outbreaks	Policies on healthy catering, and places where patients and staff can eat Policies to prevent undernutrition in patients	Consistent information and advice available on diet and physical activity	Implementation of food safety regulations	Monitoring of the eating environment of patients Food purchased from local producers

Policy-makers can identify priorities by asking questions.

- Is the issue a great public health problem?
- Is it amenable to change?
- What is the estimated impact if a solution is found?

They can use the answers to rank each problem and thus identify the top priorities. This may give policy-makers ideas on how to strengthen existing interventions or begin new ones. They may need more data before proceeding to intervention (thereby calling for more research) or decide that further consultation is needed before any priorities can be set.

Suggested methods for setting priorities

The global burden of disease and disability *(112)* can be analysed at the national level to decide the appropriate setting of priorities. In addition, different types of health impact assessment, prospective and retrospective, can be made to help identify which policies need changing *(113)*. These are two structured ways of compiling evidence, evaluating, working in partnership and consulting the public for more explicit decision-making.

Estimating the national burden of disease

Outlining a scheme here for analysing the burden of disease is inappropriate. Interested readers may refer to Murray & Lopez *(114)*, the updated analysis of the global burden of disease (http://www.who.int/oeh/OCHweb/OCHweb/OSHpages/GlobalBurdenProject/WHOProject.htm, accessed 22 October 2002) and established systems for estimating the contribution from important risk factors. WHO has published an overview of the risk assessment methods used to estimate the current and future disease burden *(112)*.

Earlier analyses of the global burden of disease *(114)* excluded issues relating to food safety, except for infant diarrhoeal disease. Infectious diarrhoeal disease is a major global killer, but its total burden in western Europe is about one third of that attributable to diabetes, a sixth of that from stroke and about only one fifteenth of that from CHD. In many countries in the European Region, nutrition-related diseases therefore have a far greater impact than unsafe food on the prevalence and incidence of disease. Nevertheless, health ministries are aware of the political dominance of food safety, which stems principally from two factors:

- the huge economic implications of the public's sudden aversion to eating a particular range of foods as a result of a food scandal; and
- the intense public concern, often perceived as irrational by scientists, that arises as a result of deaths from *E. coli*, botulism, typhoid or vCJD.

The reaction to the *E. coli* and vCJD outbreaks and the intense concern about GMOs (Chapters 2 and 3) are responses from a public that feels it no longer has access to safe food. They are understandable, although scientific analyses indicate that people should be far more concerned about chronic health problems such as CVD and obesity. Health ministries, in addition to dealing with political concerns, are encouraged to ensure that health surveillance systems allow the main causes of premature death and disability in society to be evaluated.

Some European institutions are analysing the national disease burden. A group in the Netherlands *(115)* concluded that the country's burden of disease could be assessed in DALYs (see Chapter 1, pp. 7–8). Ideally, this approach should be carried out in each country in the WHO European Region to enable priorities for health policy to be determined.

Health impact assessment of food-related policies

Interest in addressing the determinants of health that lie outside the health sector is increasing. Health impact assessment is a process that identifies both the positive and negative effects of policies on health and includes recommendations to improve policies to maximize the health benefit to the population *(116)*.

Health impact assessment is a proactive way to improve health, to promote equity in health and to increase the transparency of decision-making. An exciting aspect of a systematic approach to health impact assessment is its potential to prevent future harm and maximize future benefit. The health impact of a proposal can be assessed prospectively, including recommendations on how to adjust policies to enhance health gain *(117)*.

Food production can influence health in many ways besides effects on nutrition and food safety. These other influences may be either beneficial or harmful. For example, food production plays a significant part in local economies, creating employment and social cohesion *(118)*. It may affect transport patterns, either improve or damage the physical environment *(119)* and pose occupational hazards to agricultural and other workers *(120)*. These other influences should be recognized in advocating a healthy food policy. Gaining an understanding of all the ways a policy may influence health requires systematic assessment of the overall health effects *(121)*.

Most policies have different kinds of health effects: some positive and others negative. Health impact assessment should make all these trade-offs explicit and thus make decisions more transparent. An example is the debate on appropriate policies on local food markets. Local markets are important in ensuring a sustainable food supply, safeguarding local employment and minimizing food transport and may strengthen community cohesion *(118,119)*. These are all important health benefits. However, regulating these markets and ensuring that food hygiene procedures are robust are often difficult. This is potentially a serious health hazard *(122)*. This situation can lead to conflict between those responsible for food safety and those trying to promote local farmers' markets. Health impact assessment would identify the potential effects, comparing different policy options and allowing these different effects to be taken into account in policy-making *(123)*.

A consensus paper from a WHO seminar on health impact assessment in Gothenburg, Sweden in 1999 *(116)* aims to create a common understanding of health impact assessment, to clarify some of the main concepts and to suggest an approach to health impact assessment. It defines health impact assessment as a combination of procedures, methods and tools to assess the potential effects of a policy, programme or project on the health of a population and the distribution of these effects within the population. The paper proposes the following core elements of health impact assessment:

- consideration of evidence about the anticipated relationships between a policy, programme or project and the health of a population (both the total population and population groups);
- consideration of the opinions, experience and expectations of those who may be affected by the proposed policy, programme or project;
- provision of more informed understanding by decision-makers and the public regarding the effects of the policy, programme or project on health; and
- proposals for adjustments or options to maximize the positive and minimize the negative health effects.

Fig 4.8 illustrates the main stages in the process of health impact assessment.

An essential first stage is the systematic screening of policies and programme proposals. In practice, the next stage may not be sequential but iterative, with some steps being repeated as questions and potential health effects emerge from the various stages. The appraisal stage includes qualitative and quantitative assessments that cover both risks and hazards to health, and can take the form of rapid appraisal done over a few days or an in-depth appraisal lasting weeks to months. The conclusions are reported to those responsible for the development process. Where appropriate, the effects of a policy or programme on people's health and wellbeing should be monitored *(124)*.

Integrating health impact assessment into the policy cycle

Health impact assessment should be a way to ensure that the health consequences of policies are not overlooked. It should raise awareness of the possible unintended effects of a wide range of policies. For this to happen, assessment should not be ad hoc, but part of everyday policy-making

Fig. 4.8. Overview of the main stages in the process of health impact assessment, their functions and relationship to developing and implementing policy

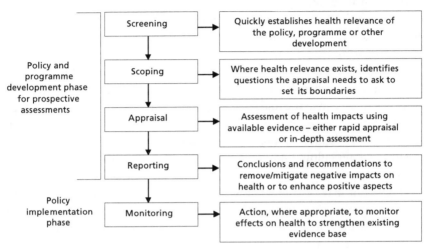

Source: Breeze & Lock *(124).*

(116,121). Mechanisms are needed to identify the policies that should be subjected to health impact assessment and to ensure that it is done when they can still be changed. This implies that awareness of health effects is needed at all stages of the policy-making process. Three main types of health impact assessment *(124)* have been described: prospective, retrospective and concurrent.

Prospective assessment is undertaken during the development of a new or revised policy or development. It aims to consider and, if possible, predict the effects on health and wellbeing that might be expected as a result of implementing the policy and to identify corrective measures that could prevent or mitigate these effects.

Retrospective assessment looks at the consequences of a policy, programme or other development that has already been implemented or the consequences of an unplanned development or event.

Concurrent assessment assesses health effects as the policy or programme is being implemented. It is mainly used when effects are anticipated but their nature and/or magnitude is uncertain. It allows the implementation of a policy or programme to be monitored and the results to be fed back for prompt corrective action.

In food policy, the best known examples are assessments of the health impact of CAP by Sweden's National Institute of Public Health *(2,125).* They show the potential for agricultural policy to affect health and indicates the range of methods and disciplines that are needed in trying to assess the effects. The policy analysts required skills in public health and health policy research, and in consumer affairs, agriculture, food policy and sociology. Further, systematic health impact assessment of food and agriculture policies is urgently needed; Slovenia, in particular, has had a pioneering role *(126)*.

Trends in nutrition and food safety change and vary across the European Region *(127)*. Health impact assessment should take account of the local context, and the evidence should be appropriate to the situation. In addition, new evidence may change the understanding of health. For example, health impact assessment of the agricultural policies after the Second World War would probably have supported most of them: food shortages threatened population health, and agricultural policies were designed to ensure food security *(128)*. As a result, intensive methods of agriculture have lessened the risk of food shortages but may be contributing to food scares and the prevalence of CVD, cancer and obesity. The agricultural policies predominant after the Second World War may not be the best way to improve food security and health in the future (see Chapter 3).

Monitoring and evaluation

Objective, reliable data are essential to compare regions or countries, to provide the basis for testing the impact of change, to monitor progress over time and, ultimately, to be the basis for policy decisions. Health information systems generate data; they should be able to detect the existence of a problem, act as a mechanism for identifying the causes and solutions and provide an effective way to communicate this to the people responsible for taking action (Fig 4.9). For example, steps might include identifying socioeconomic groups with a high prevalence of CVD (assessment), investigating the reasons for elevated rates among these groups (analysis) and recommending appropriate public health programmes targeting them (action) *(129)*.

Monitoring

The limited amount of information included in Chapters 1–3 shows the paucity of data, and the desperate need to improve information on food and health. New national food agencies are emerging all over Europe *(87)*, and they could be asked to collect more health-related food information. National food safety agencies collect intake data to get information on sources of contaminated food. These surveys could also be used to collect information on food and nutrient intake, thus making cost-effective use of limited resources.

A project on the European Food Consumption Survey Method (EFCO-SUM) *(130)*, funded by the EU, was undertaken to contribute to a European

Fig. 4.9. Health information systems

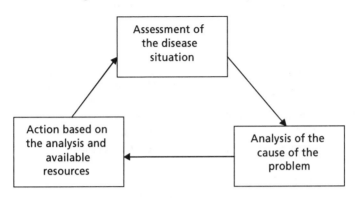

Source: adapted from Jonsson (129).

monitoring system that includes measurement of health status and trends in and determinants of health. A standardized method was defined for monitoring food consumption in nationally representative samples of all age and sex categories in a comparable way. A total of 23 countries in the European Region participated.

The EFCOSUM findings emphasize the need for coordinating surveillance activities in the Region. The project revealed a huge diversity of approaches to assessing dietary intake on an individual level, as do the data collected by WHO (Table 4.9). As a consequence, the data sets on dietary intake available at the country level are not directly comparable.

As a first step in harmonization, the EFCOSUM Group decided that existing data from 15 countries can be made comparable at the food level, but much remains to be done. The data from household budget surveys of 13 European countries (131) can fulfil the needs of the EC's health monitoring system at the food supply level (the software can be found on the Internet (http://www.nut.uoa.gr/english/, accessed 16 September 2003)), but data at an individual level are recommended to study the relationship between diet and health and properly to identify risk groups.

The EFCOSUM project demonstrated a broad European consensus on the basic components of an individually based dietary monitoring system. The consortium of 23 countries not only created a general outline of methods and indicators but also proved the feasibility of carrying out a European survey. It was recommended that any country carrying out a national food consumption survey include the minimum number of 24-hour dietary recalls that allows calibration with other countries (130). The EFCOSUM project provides good recommendations for a standard method for national food consumption surveys in the European Region.

Table 4.9. Methods of collecting dietary information used
in selected European countries

Country	Years of collection	Method
Andorra	1994–1995	Household budget survey linked with individual 7-day records
Austria	1998	24-hour recall
Azerbaijan	1994–1995	24-hour recall
Bulgaria	1998	24-hour recall
Croatia	1990	Household budget survey
Denmark	1995	7-day food record
Estonia	1997	24-hour recall
Finland	1997	24-hour recall
France	1994–1997	24-hour recall
Ireland	1990	Dietary history
Kazakhstan	1996	24-hour recall
Latvia	1997	24-hour recall
Lithuania	1997	24-hour recall
Iceland	1990	Dietary history method
Netherlands	1997–1998	2-day notebook method
Norway	1993–1994	Food frequency questionnaire
Portugal	1980	24-hour recall
Slovenia	1997	24-hour recall and food frequency questionnaire
Sweden	1989	7-day food record
Ukraine	1997	Express 1-day and 7-day questionnaires
United Kingdom	1986–1987, 1992–1993, 1994–1995	4-day weighed intake inventory

Source: Comparative analysis of food and nutrition policies in the WHO European Region 1994–1999. Full report (24).

Surveillance of foodborne diseases is a high priority on the public health agendas of many countries. It is instrumental for estimating the burden of foodborne diseases, assessing their relative impact on health and economics and evaluating programmes to prevent and control them. It allows rapid detection of and response to outbreaks, and is a major source of information for risk assessment, management and communication. Data from foodborne disease surveillance could be integrated with food monitoring data along the entire food chain. This would result in strong surveillance information and could allow appropriate priority setting and public health intervention. Collaboration between sectors and institutions is of paramount importance.

The WHO global strategy on food safety *(132)* and resolution EUR/ RC52/R3 of the WHO Regional Committee for Europe on food safety and quality (http://www.euro.who.int/AboutWHO/Governance/resolutions/2002/ 20021231_10, accessed 16 September 2003) recognize that the surveillance of foodborne diseases should have high priority in the development of food safety infrastructure. Building capacity for public health laboratories to conduct surveillance and for conducting epidemiological surveillance is an important public health objective. A global approach needs to be developed and coordinated to strengthen surveillance at the national, regional and global levels. Foodborne disease reporting should be integrated into the revision of the International Health Regulations.

Evaluation

Surveillance systems can measure whether an intervention produces the desired changes in mortality or morbidity, but results are not achieved until several years after a policy is implemented. In contrast, process evaluation monitors how a policy or intervention is implemented. A process evaluation assesses how a health initiative achieves its effects, and includes evaluating the resources used and describing the activities implemented and outputs achieved (intermediate outcomes and proximal effects) *(133)*.

Several considerations drive the process evaluation of any project or initiative *(133)*:

• the project's overall goal, specific objectives, strategies and target populations;
• the scope and level of the evaluation (national, regional or local); and
• the cost and practicality of gathering various types of data.

Fig. 4.10 shows how process evaluation fits into the broader context of an evaluation framework. Inputs are converted into outputs via implementation strategies, and feedback mechanism among the various processes, inputs and outputs facilitates this process.

A useful tool for policy-makers is a WHO publication *(134)* that summarizes the core features of approaches for the evaluation of health promotion initiatives: participation, multiple methods, capacity building and appropriateness. Table 4.10 presents recommendations to policy-makers.

Fig. 4.10. A framework for process evaluation

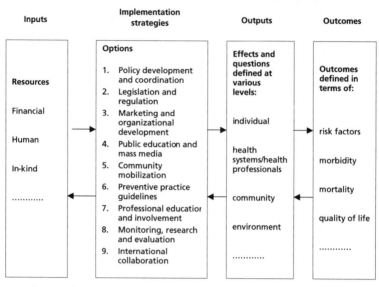

Source: adapted from Handbook for process evaluation in noncommunicable disease prevention (133).

Table 4.10. Health promotion evaluation: conclusions and recommendations to policy-makers

Conclusions	Recommendations
Those who have direct interest in a health promotion initiative need the opportunity to participate in all stages of its planning and evaluation.	Encourage the adoption of participatory approaches to evaluation that provide meaningful opportunities for involvement by everyone with a direct interest in health promotion initiatives.
Adequate resources are needed for the evaluation of health promotion initiatives.	Require that a minimum of 10% of the total financial resources for a health promotion initiative be allocated to evaluation.
Both the processes and outcomes of health promotion initiatives need evaluation.	Ensure that a mixture of process and outcome information is used to evaluate all health promotion initiatives.
The use of randomized controlled trials to evaluate health promotion initiatives is inappropriate, misleading and unnecessarily expensive in most cases.	Support the use of multiple methods to evaluate health promotion initiatives. Support further research into the development of appropriate approaches to evaluating health promotion initiatives.

Table 4.10 continued

Expertise in the evaluation of health promotion initiatives needs to be developed and sustained.	Support the establishment of a training and education infrastructure to develop expertise in the evaluation of health promotion initiatives. Create and support opportunities for sharing information on evaluation methods used in health promotion through conferences, work-shops, networks and other means.

Source: Health promotion evaluation: recommendations to policy makers. Report of the WHO European Working Group on Health Promotion Evaluation (134).

References

1. GRIFFITHS, J. & GRIEVES, K. *Tobacco in the workplace: meeting the challenge. A handbook for employers* (http://www.euro.who.int/document/ e74819.pdf). Copenhagen, WHO Regional Office for Europe, 2002 (accessed 10 November 2003).

2. *Public health aspects of the EU CAP – developments and recommendations for change in four sectors: fruit and vegetables, dairy, wine and tobacco* (http://www.fhi.se/shop/material_pdf/eu_inlaga.pdf). Stockholm, National Institute of Public Health, 2003 (accessed 3 September 2003).

3. *Scrap the CAP! Consumers' Association says abolish the Common Agricultural Policy, as research shows UK food prices are artificially high* (http://www.which.net/media/pr/dec01/general/capscrap.html). London, Consumers' Association, 2001 (accessed 10 November 2003).

4. VALLERON, A.-J. ET AL. Estimation of epidemic size and incubation time based on age characteristics of vCJD in the United Kingdom. *Science*, **294**: 1726–1728 (2001).

5. Commission directive 2001/101/EC of 26 November 2001 amending Directive 2000/13/EC of the European Parliament and of the Council on the approximation of the laws of the Member States relating to the labelling, presentation and advertising of foodstuffs. *Official journal of the European Communities*, L 310(28 November): 19–21.

6. EUROPEAN COMMISSION. *CORINE – soil erosion risks and important land resources in the southern regions of the European Community.* Luxembourg, Office for the Official Publications of the European Communities, 1992 (EU 13233).

7. *Note to the Council of Ministers and to the European Parliament on the olive and olive oil sector (including economic, cultural, regional social and environmental aspects), the current common market organisation, the need for reform and the alternatives envisaged.* Brussels, European Commission, 1997 (COM(97) 57 final).

8. EUROPEAN FORUM ON NATURE CONSERVATION AND PASTORALISM. *The environmental impact of olive oil production in the EU: practical options for improving the environmental impact.* Brussels, European Commission, 2000.

9. BEAUFOY, G. *EU policies for olive farming: unsustainable on all counts.* (http://www.panda.org/resources/programmes/epo/publications/agpub.cfm). Brussels, European Policy Office, World Wildlife Fund/BirdLife International, 2001 (accessed 11 November 2003).

10. *Diet, nutrition and the prevention of chronic diseases. Report of a joint WHO/FAO expert consultation* (http://whqlibdoc.who.int/trs/WHO_TRS_916.pdf). Geneva, World Health Organization, 2003 (WHO Technical Series, No. 916) (accessed 3 September 2003).

11. *Big drop in salt levels in bread* (http://www.foodstandards.gov.uk/news/newsarchive/saltinbread). London, Food Standards Agency, 29 November 2001 (accessed 25 November 2003).

12. WHITEHEAD, R.R., ED. *UK pesticide guide 2000.* Wallingford, British Crop Protection Council, CABI Publishing, 2000.

13. HEALTH AND SAFETY EXECUTIVE. *Annual report of the Working Party on Pesticide Residues 1999.* London, Ministry of Agriculture, Fisheries and Food, 2000.

14. PIETINEN, P. Trends in nutrition and its consequences in Europe: the Finnish experience. *In:* Pietinen, P. et al., ed. *Nutrition and quality of life: health issues for the 21st century.* Geneva: World Health Organization, 1996, pp. 67–71.

15. PUSKA, P. Nutrition and mortality: the Finnish experience. *Acta cardiologica*, 55: 213–220 (2000).

16. *Urban agriculture in St Petersburg, Russian Federation: past, present and future perspectives. Conducted by the Urban Gardening Club* (http://www.euro.who.int/document/e70095.pdf). Copenhagen, WHO Regional Office for Europe, 2000 (document EUR/00/5014688; accessed 10 November 2003).

17. VAIL, D. Sweden's 1990 food policy reform. *In*: McMichael, P., ed. *The global restructuring of agro-food systems.* Ithaca, Cornell University Press, 1994, pp. 53–75.

18. COMMISSION ON ENVIRONMENTAL HEALTH. *Environment for sustainable health development – an action plan for Sweden.* Stockholm, Ministry of Health and Social Affairs, 1996 (Swedish Official Reports Series 1996: 124).

19. MCMICHAEL, A.J. ET AL., ED. *Climate change and human health: an assessment prepared by a Task Group on behalf of the World Health Organization, the World Meteorological Organization, and the United Nations Environment Programme.* Geneva, World Health Organization, 1996 (document WHO/EHG/96.7).

20. CARLSSON-KANYAMA, A. *Consumption patterns and climate change: consequences of eating and travelling in Sweden* [thesis]. Stockholm, Department of Systems Ecology, University of Stockholm, 1999.

21. *Planting the seeds* (http://www.city.toronto.on.ca/food_hunger/index.htm). Toronto, Toronto Food and Hunger Action Committee, 2000 (accessed 10 November 2003).

22. *The growing season* (http://www.city.toronto.on.ca/food_hunger/index.htm). Toronto, Toronto Food and Hunger Action Committee, 2001 (accessed 10 November 2003).

23. *Comparative analysis of food and nutrition policies in the WHO European Region 1994–1999. Summary report.* Copenhagen, WHO Regional Office for Europe (in press).

24. *Comparative analysis of food and nutrition policies in the WHO European Region 1994–1999. Full report.* Copenhagen, WHO Regional Office for Europe (in press).

25. *Food-based dietary guidelines in WHO European Member States.* Copenhagen, WHO Regional Office for Europe, 2002 (unpublished document).

26. *World Health Assembly resolution WHA54.2 on infants and young children.* (http://www.who.int/gb/EB_WHA/PDF/WHA54/ea54r2.pdf). Geneva, World Health Organization, 2001 (accessed 10 November 2003).

27. *Food, nutrition and the prevention of cancer: a global perspective.* Washington, DC, World Cancer Research Fund and American Institute for Cancer Research, 1997.

28. EURODIET WORKING PARTY 1. European diet and public health: the continuing challenge. EURODIET Working Party 1 final report. *Public health nutrition,* 4(2(A)): 275–292 (2001).

29. *Preparation and use of food-based dietary* guidelines: report of a Joint FAO/WHO Consultation. Geneva, World Health Organization, 1998 (WHO Technical Report Series, No. 880).

30. *CINDI dietary guide* (http://www.euro.who.int/document/e70041.pdf). Copenhagen: WHO Regional Office for Europe, 2000 (document EUR/ICP/LVNG 02 07 08; accessed 31 January 2003).

31. *The European health report 2002.* Copenhagen, WHO Regional Office for Europe, 2002 (WHO Regional Publications, European Series, No. 97).

32. *A physically active life through everyday transport with a special focus on children and older people and examples and approaches from Europe* (http://www.euro.who.int/document/e75662.pdf). Copenhagen, WHO Regional Office for Europe, 2002 (accessed 9 July 2003).

33. *Health and development through physical activity and sport* (http://whqlibdoc.who.int/hq/2003/WHO_NMH_NPH_PAH_03.2.pdf). Geneva, World Health Organization, 2003 (accessed 9 July 2003).

34. FOSTER, C. *Guidelines for health-enhancing physical activity promotion pro-grammes.* Tampere, UKK Institute, 2000.

35. UKK INSTITUTE. *Promotion of health-enhancing physical activity* (http://europa.eu.int/comm/health/ph/programmes/health/reports/fp_promotion_2000_frep_09_en.pdf). Brussels, European Commission, 1996 (accessed 10 November 2003).

36. *Status report on the European Commission's work in the field of nutrition in Europe.* Luxembourg, European Commission, 2003.

37. VOGT, T.M. ET AL. Dietary approaches to stop hypertension: rationale, design, and methods. DASH Collaborative Research Group. *Journal of the American Dietetic Association,* **99**(Suppl): S12–S18 (1999).

38. SWINBURN, B. ET AL. Dissecting obesogenic environments: the development and application of a framework for identifying and prioritizing environmental interventions for obesity. *Preventive medicine,* **29**(6): 563–570 (1999).

39. LOBSTEIN, T. ET AL. *Childhood obesity: the new crisis in public health.* London, International Obesity Task Force, 2003.

40. The prevention and treatment of childhood obesity. *Effective healthcare,* 7(6): 1–12 (2002).

41. *Obesity: preventing and managing the global epidemic: report of a WHO Consultation on Obesity, Geneva, 3–5 June 1997.* Geneva, World Health Organization, 2000 (WHO Technical Report Series, No. 894).

42. Eight guidelines for a healthy diet. A guide for nutrition educators. London, Health Education Authority, 1994.

43. US DEPARTMENT OF HEALTH AND HUMAN SERVICES, PUBLIC HEALTH SERVICE, OFFICE OF THE SURGEON GENERAL. *The Surgeon General's call to action to prevent and decrease overweight and obesity 2001.* Washington, DC, US Government Printing Office, 2001.

44. The Diabetes and Nutrition Study Group (DNSG) of the European Association for the Study of Diabetes (EASD), 1999. Recommendations for the nutritional management of patients with diabetes mellitus. *European journal of clinical nutrition,* **54**: 353–355 (2000).

45. BECK, A.M. ET AL. Practices in relation to nutritional care and support – Report from the Council of Europe. *Clinical nutrition,* **21**: 351–354 (2002).

46. *Healthy food and nutrition for women and their families: training course for health professionals. Part 1. Trainers' instructions including overheads and handouts.* (http://www.euro.who.int/document/e73470.pdf). Copenhagen, WHO Regional Office for Europe, 2001 (accessed 31 January 2003).

47. MICHAELSEN, K. ET AL. *Feeding and nutrition of infants and young children. Guidelines for the WHO European Region, with emphasis on the*

former Soviet countries (http://www.euro.who.int/InformationSources/ Publications/Catalogue/20010914_21). Copenhagen, WHO Regional Office for Europe, 2003 (WHO Regional Publications, European Series, No. 87, accessed 25 September 2003).

48. *HIV and infant feeding. Guidelines for decision-makers* (http://www.un-aids.org/publications/documents/mtct/infantpolicy.html). Geneva, Joint United Nations Programme on HIV/AIDS (accessed 10 November 2003).

49. FOWLER, M.G. & NEWELL, M.-L. *Breastfeeding, HIV transmission and options in resource-poor settings* (http://www.who.int/reproductive-health/ rtis/MTCT/mtct_consultation_october_2000/consultation_documents/ breastfeeding_and_HIV_in_resource_poor_settings/breastfeeding_and_ HIV.en.html). Geneva, World Health Organization, 2000 (accessed 31 January 2003).

50. STEINER, J.E. Facial expressions of the neonate infant indicating the he-donics of food-related chemical stimuli. *In*: Weiffenbach, J., ed. *Taste and development: the genesis of sweet preference.* Washington, DC, US Government Printing Office, 1977 (DHEW Publication No. NIH 77-1068).

51. ROSENSTEIN, D. & OSTER, H. Differential facial responses to four basic tastes in newborns. *Child development*, **59**: 1555–1568 (1988).

52. DAVIS, C. Self-selection of diets by newly-weaned infants. *American journal of diseases of children*, **36**: 961–979 (1928).

53. DAVIS, C. Results of the self-selection of diets by young children. *Canadian Medical Association journal*, **41**: 257–261 (1939).

54. ROZIN, P. The role of learning in the acquisition of food preferences by humans. *In*: Sheperd, R., ed. *Handbook of the psychophysiology of human eating.* Chichester, Wiley, 1989, pp. 205–227.

55. BIRCH, L.L. Developmental aspects of eating. *In*: Sheperd, R., ed. *Handbook of the psychophysiology of human eating.* Chichester, Wiley, 1989, pp. 179–204.

56. PLINER, P. The effects of mere exposure on liking for edible substances. *Appetite*, **3**: 283–290 (1982).

57. DUNCKER, K. Experimental modification of children's food preferences through social suggestion. *Journal of abnormal and social psychology*, **33**: 489–507 (1938).

58. BIRCH, L.L. Effects of peer models' food choices and eating behaviors on preschoolers' food preferences. *Child development*, **51**: 489–496 (1980).

59. BIRCH, L.L. & DEYSHER, M. Conditioned and unconditioned caloric compensation: evidence for self-regulation of food intake by young children. *Learning & motivation*, **16**: 341–355 (1985).

60. BIRCH, L.L. ET AL. Clean up your plate: effects of child feeding practices on the conditioning of meal size. *Learning & motivation*, **18**: 310–317 (1987).

61. *Broadcasting bad health* (http://www.foodcomm.org.uk/Broadcasting_ bad_health.pdf). London, Food Commission, 2003 (accessed 3 September 2003).

62. UNITED NATIONS CHILDREN'S FUND, UNITED NATIONS UNIVERSITY AND WORLD HEALTH ORGANIZATION. *Iron deficiency anaemia: assessment, prevention and control. A guide for programme managers* (http:// www.who.int/nut/documents/ida_assessment_prevention_control.pdf). Geneva, World Health Organization, 2001 (document WHO/NHD/ 01.3, accessed 11 November 2003).

63. *Iodine deficiency in Europe: a continuing public health problem.* Geneva, World Health Organization (in press).

64. *Indicators for assessing iodine deficiency disorders and their control programmes: report of a Joint WHO/UNICEF/ICCIDD consultation, 3–5 November 1992* (http://whqlibdoc.who.int/hq/1993/WHO_NUT_93.1.pdf). Geneva, World Health Organization, 1994 (document WHO/NUT/ 94.6; accessed 10 November 2003).

65. DELANGE, F. ET AL., ED. *Elimination of iodine deficiency disorders (IDD) in central and eastern Europe, the Commonwealth of Independent States and the Baltic states. Proceedings of a conference held in Munich, Germany, 3–6 September 1997* (http://whqlibdoc.who.int/hq/1998/WHO_EURO_ NUT_98.1.pdf). Copenhagen, WHO Regional Office for Europe, 1998 (document WHO/EURO/NUT/98.1, accessed 31 January 2003).

66. *Progress towards the elimination of iodine deficiency disorders (IDD)* (http:// whqlibdoc.who.int/hq/1999/WHO_NHD_99.4.pdf). Geneva, World Health Organization, 1999 (document WHO/NHD/99.4, accessed 10 November 2003).

67. DELANGE, F. Administration of iodized oil during pregnancy: a summary of the published evidence. *Bulletin of the World Health Organization*, **74**: 101–108 (1996).

68. GLINOER, D. ET AL. A randomized trial for the treatment of excessive thyroid stimulation in pregnancy: maternal and neonatal effects. *Journal of clinical endocrinology and metabolism*, **80**: 258–269 (1995).

69. DELANGE, F. ET AL. Risks of iodine-induced hyperthyroidism after correction of iodine deficiency by iodized salt. *Thyroid*, **9**: 545–556 (1999).

70. HURREL, R.F. & JACOB, S. The role of the food industry in iron nutrition: iron intake from industrial food products. *In*: Hallberg, L. & Asp, N.G., ed. *Iron nutrition in health and disease*. Lund, Swedish Nutrition Foundation, 1996, pp. 339–345.

71. GILLESPIE, S. & JOHNSON, J.L. *Expert consultation on anaemia determinants and interventions.* Ottawa, Micronutrient Initiative, 1998.

72. BACKSTRAND, J.R. The history and future of food fortification in the United States: a public health perspective. *Nutrition reviews*, **60**: 15–26 (2002).

73. *Report on osteoporosis in the European Community – action on prevention.* Luxembourg, Office of Official Publications of the European Communities, 1998.

74. BERMUDEZ, O.I. & DWYER, J. Identifying elders at risk of malnutrition: a universal challenge. *SCN news*, **19**: 15–17 (1999).

75. *A spoonful of sugar: television food advertising aimed at children – An international survey.* London, Consumers International, 1996.

76. BORZEKOWSKI, D.L. & ROBINSON, T.N. The 30-second effect: an experiment revealing the impact of television commercials on food preferences of preschoolers. *Journal of the American Dietetic Association*, **101**: 42–46 (2001).

77. NESTLE, M. *Food politics – how the food industry influences nutrition and health.* London. University of California Press, 2002, pp. 173–197.

78. LEWIS, M.K. & HILL, A.J. Food advertising on British children's television: a content analysis and experimental study with nine-year-olds. *International journal of obesity and related metabolic disorders*, **22**: 206–214 (1998).

79. SCHMITT, J. ET AL. [Television, advertising, and nutritional behaviour of children.] *Bulletin de l'Academie nationale de medecine*, **173**: 701–707 (1989).

80. GARROW, J.S. ET AL. *Human nutrition and dietetics*, 10th ed. Edinburgh, Churchill Livingstone, 2000.

81. *Proposal for a regulation of the European Parliament and of the Council on Nutrition and health claims made on foods* (http://europa.eu.int/comm/food/fs/fl/fl07_en.pdf). Brussels, Commission of the European Communities, 2003 (accessed 3 September 2003).

82. HILL AND KNOWLTON INTERNATIONAL BELGIUM SA/NV. *Study on nutritional, health and ethical claims in the European Union* (http://europa.eu.int/comm/consumers/policy/developments/envi_clai/envi_clai02_en.html). Brussels, European Commission, 2000 (accessed 7 November 2003).

83. *Report of the 28th session of the Codex Committee on Food Labelling, Ottawa, Canada, 5–9 May 2000.* Rome, Joint FAO/WHO Food Standards Programme, Codex Alimentarius Commission, 2001 (document ALINORM 01/22).

84. PASSCLAIM [process for the assessment of scientific support for claims on foods]. *European journal of clinical nutrition*, **42**(Suppl. 1) (2003).

85. THOMAS, B.W. ET AL. *Food labelling and healthy food choices*. Oxford, British Heart Foundation Health Promotion Research Group, University of Oxford, 1997.

86. *Proposals for new nutrition labelling formats* (http://www.norden.org/pub/velfaerd/konsument/sk/TN02_554.asp). Copenhagen, Nordic Council of Ministers, 2002 (TemaNord 2002: 554) (accessed 3 September 2003).

87. *Systems for improved coordination and harmonization of national food safety control services: report on a joint meeting of the WHO/EURO and Food Safety Authority of Ireland, Dublin, Ireland, 19–20 June 2001*. Copenhagen, WHO Regional Office for Europe, 2001 (document EUR/01/5026000).

88. *Improved coordination and harmonization of national food safety control services* (http://www.euro.who.int/document/E74473.pdf). Copenhagen, WHO Regional Office for Europe, 2001 (accessed 10 November 2003).

89. *HACCP – introducing the hazard analysis and critical control point system* (http://whqlibdoc.who.int/hq/1997/WHO_FSF_FOS_97.2.pdf). Geneva, World Health Organization, 1997 (document WHO/FS/FOS/97.2, accessed 10 November 2003).

90. *Guidelines for strengthening a national food safety programme* (http://whqlibdoc.who.int/hq/1996/WHO_FNU_FOS_96.2.pdf). Geneva, World Health Organization, 1996 (document WHO/FNU/FOS/96.2; accessed 10 November 2003).

91. SLOVIC, P. Perception of risk. *Science*, **236**: 280–285 (1987).

92. SLOVIC, P. The risk game. *Journal of hazardous materials*, **86**: 17–24 (2001).

93. *Application of risk communication to food standards and safety matters: report of a Joint FAO/WHO expert consultation, Rome, 2–6 February 1998*. Rome, Food and Agricultural Organization of the United Nations, 1998 (FAO Food and Nutrition Paper, No. 70).

94. TRICHOPOULOU, A., ED. *European policy on food safety, final study: working document for the STOA Panel*. Luxembourg, European Parliament, 2000 (PE 292.026/Fin.St.).

95. MILLSTONE, E.P. *Risk assessment and risk management – Practical issues for regulators*. (http://www.who.it/docs/fdsaf/fdnataut_pres/EMillstone_files/v3_document.htm). Brighton, Science and Technology Policy Research, University of Sussex, 2001 (accessed 25 November 2003).

96. Regulation (EC) No 178/2002 of the European Parliament and of the Council of 28 January 2002 laying down the general principles and requirements of food law, establishing the European Food Safety Authority and laying down procedures in matters of food safety. *Official journal of the European Communities*, L **31**(1 February): 1–24.

97. TORGESEN, H. & SEIFERT, F. Austria: precautionary blockage of agriculture biotechnology. *Journal of risk research*, **3**: 209–217 (2000).

98. *Report of 16th Session of Codex Committee on General Principles, Paris, France, 23–27 April 2001.* Rome, Joint FAO/WHO Food Standards Programme, Codex Alimentarius Commission, 2001 (document ALINORM 01/33A).

99. *White paper on food safety* (http://europa.eu.int/comm/dgs/health_consumer/library/pub/pub06_en.pdf). Brussels, European Commission, 2000 (COM (1999) 719 final; accessed 9 November 2003).

100. STERN, P.C. & FINEBERG, H.V., ED. *Understanding risk: informing decisions in a democratic society.* Washington, DC, National Academy Press, 1996.

101. GROVE-WHITE, R., ET AL. *Uncertain world: genetically modified organisms, food and public attitudes in Britain.* Lancaster, Centre for the Study of Environmental Change (CSEC), Lancaster University, 1997.

102. EUROPEAN COUNCIL. Council directive 93/43/EEC of 14 June 1993 on the hygiene of foodstuffs. *Official journal of the European Communities,* L 145 (19 June): 1–15 (1993).

103. Directive 1999/34/EC of the European Parliament and of the Council of 10 May 1999 amending Council Directive 85/374/EEC on the approximation of the laws, regulations and administrative provisions of the Member States concerning liability for defective products. *Official journal of the European Communities,* L 141(4 June): 20–21 (1999).

104. HAWKES, C. & WEBSTER, J. *Too much & too little?* London, Sustain, 2000.

105. *Urban and Peri-urban Food and Nutrition Action Plan: elements for community action to promote social cohesion and reduce inequalities through local production for local consumption* (http://www.euro.who.int/document/e72949.pdf). Copenhagen, WHO Regional Office for Europe, 2001 (accessed 10 November 2003).

106. *World urbanization prospects: the 1999 revision* (http://www.un.org/esa/population/publications/wup1999/wup99.htm). New York, Population Division, Department of Economic and Social Affairs, United Nations, 2001 (document ST/ESA/SER.A/194, accessed 11 November 2003).

107. LANG, T. & HEASMAN, M. *Food wars – public health and the battle for mouths, minds and markets.* London, Earthscan, 2003.

108. MILLSTONE, E. & LANG, T. *The atlas of food: who eats what, where and why.* London, Earthscan, 2003.

109. *The World Bank participation sourcebook* (http://www.worldbank.org/wbi/sourcebook/sbintro.pdf). Washington, DC, World Bank, 1996 (accessed 11 November 2003).

110. ANHEIER, H. ET AL., ED. *Global civil society.* Oxford, Oxford University Press, 2001.

111. MARSHALL, T. Exploring a fiscal food policy: the case of diet and ischaemic heart disease. *British medical journal,* **320**: 301–305 (2000).

112. *The world health report 2002: reducing risks, promoting healthy life* (http://whqlibdoc.who.int/publications/2002/9241562072.pdf). Geneva, World Health Organization, 2002 (accessed 3 September 2003).

113. LOCK, K. Health impact assessment. *British medical journal*, **320**: 1395–1398 (2000).

114. MURRAY, C.J.L. & LOPEZ, A.D. *The global burden of disease. A comprehensive assessment of mortality and disability from diseases, injuries, and risk factors in 1990 and projected to 2020.* Cambridge, MA, Harvard School of Public Health, 1996.

115. MELSE, J.M. ET AL. A national burden of disease calculation: Dutch disability-adjusted life-years. Dutch Burden of Disease Group. *American journal of public health*, **90**: 1241–1247 (2000).

116. *Health impact assessment: main concepts and suggested approach* (http://www.euro.who.int/document/PAE/Gothenburgpaper.pdf). Copenhagen, WHO Regional Office for Europe, 1999 (accessed 10 November 2003).

117. SCOTT-SAMUEL, A. Health impact assessment – Theory into practice. *Journal of epidemiology and community health*, **74**: 704–705 (1998).

118. *The employment impact of changing agricultural policy.* Salisbury, Wiltshire, Rural Development Commission, 1996.

119. CLUNIES-ROSS, T. & HILDYARD, N. *The politics of industrial agriculture.* London, Earthscan, 1992.

120. RASMUSSEN, K. ET AL. Incidence of unintentional injuries in farming based on one year of weekly registration in Danish farms. *American journal of industrial medicine*, **38**: 82–89 (2000).

121. DOUGLAS, M.J. ET AL. Developing principles for health impact assessment. *Journal of public health medicine*, **23**: 148–154 (2001).

122. GODLEE, F. Food safety: from plough to plate. *British medical journal*, **315**: 619–620 (1997).

123. *Prospective health impact assessment of proposed South Shields farmers' market. Summary report.* Northumbria, Northumbria University, 2002.

124. BREEZE, C.H. & LOCK, K. ED. *Health impact assessment as part of strategic environmental assessment. A review of health impact assessment concept, methods and practice to support the development of a protocol on strategic environmental assessment to the Espoo Convention, which adequately covers health impacts* (http://www.euro.who.int/document/e74634.pdf). Geneva, World Health Organization, 2001 (accessed 11 November 2003).

125. PETTERSSON, B. Health impact assessment of the European Union Common Agricultural Programme. *In*: Diwan, V. et al., ed. *Health impact assessment: from theory to practice.* Gothenburg, Nordic School of Public Health, 2000.

126. LOCK, K. ET AL. Health impact assessment of agriculture and food policies: lessons learnt from the Republic of Slovenia (www.who.int/bulletin/

volumes/81/6/en/lock.pdf). *Bulletin of the World Health Organization,* **81**(6): 391–398 (2003) (accessed 3 September 2003).

127. ROOS, E. & PRÄTTÄLA, R. *Disparities in food habits – Review of research in 15 European countries.* Helsinki, National Public Health Institute, 1999.

128. NEVILLE-ROLFE, E. *The politics of agriculture in the European Community.* London, Policy Studies Institute and European Centre for Political Studies, 1984.

129. JONSSON, U. Towards an improved strategy for nutrition surveillance. *In:* Wahlqvist, M. et al., ed. *Nutrition in a sustainable environment. Proceeding of the XVth International Congress of Nutrition.* London, Smith-Gordon, 1994.

130. EFCOSUM GROUP. *European Food Consumption Survey Method. Final report.* Zeist, Netherlands, TNO Nutrition and Food Research, 2001.

131. TRICHOPOULOU, A. & LAGIOU, P. *DAFNE II Data Food Networking Network for the pan-European food data bank based on household budget survey (HBS) data. Methodology for the exploitation of HBS food data and results on food availability in six European countries.* Luxembourg, Office for Official Publications of the European Communities, 1998.

132. *Background paper: developing a food safety strategy* (http://www.who.int/fsf/BACKGROUND%20PAPER.pdf). Geneva, World Health Organization, 2001 (accessed 6 October 2003).

133. *Handbook for process evaluation in noncommunicable disease prevention* (http://www.euro.who.int/document/E66338.pdf). Copenhagen, WHO Regional Office for Europe, 1999 (accessed 31 January 2003).

134. *Health promotion evaluation: recommendations to policy makers. Report of the WHO European Working Group on Health Promotion Evaluation* (http://www.euro.who.int/document/e60706.pdf). Copenhagen, WHO Regional Office for Europe, 1998 (accessed 11 November 2003).

Conclusion

One of the challenges for health ministries is that many of the societal developments with the greatest impact on health arise from issues and environmental changes for which these ministries are not responsible. Most health resources are focused on the care and treatment of individuals, but the health of a country partly determines its wellbeing and economic capacity. Individuals may cope with modest degrees of disability, but countries may have to cope with a substantial demand for health care, which has an economic impact in terms of work capacity.

This book addresses the problem of how to change the environment to reduce the level of disease and disability and to optimize health. Chapter 4 presents ways in which a health ministry can assess the priorities for action, including a national analysis of the burden of disease and disability as described by WHO *(1)*, to help ensure that appropriate priorities are set. This raises the problem of how, given the multiple players involved, a ministry can develop a realistic strategy for optimizing the environment so that public health can flourish.

As discussed, factors such as fetal nutrition, birth weight, child growth and subsequent obesity, and disease are shaped by environmental and material circumstances, such as poverty, that may be far beyond the individual's control. The demographic transition – from rural societies with low life expectancy at birth and families with many children to urban societies with higher life expectancy at birth and fewer children – is well known. The epidemiological transition that follows is also fairly well understood: the shift from nutrient deficiency and infectious diseases, mostly in early life, to chronic noncommunicable diseases in later life *(2)* (see Chapter 1, pp. 17–19). In such situations, efforts to improve health by using health education methods alone have limited success.

Nevertheless, the nutritional transition described in this book *(2)* is not inevitable; it is shaped by policies on food supply, pricing and technology, activities to promote products and public health messages (see Chapter 3, Fig. 3.5, p. 166). Government policy built around public health can clearly make measurable changes in the composition and availability of the national food supply by:

- shifting food production subsidies to promote health *(3)*, which includes providing incentives for producing low-fat milk and lean meat, improving the quality of and access to fruits and vegetables, and promoting access to fish;
- improving the content and accuracy of food labelling;
- enlarging and improving public information, as well as nutrition education for health professionals and in schools; and
- expanding nutrition and welfare programmes and policy-related research.

So far, many of the influences on changing dietary patterns have not been anticipated. There has been no satisfactory scheme, at the national level or for the EU and beyond, for considering how to optimize the long-term wellbeing of the population by ensuring integrated assessment of the effects on health of environmental, agricultural and food policies. Mechanisms need to be developed that will allow the countries in the WHO European Region to predict and avoid major problems in food security, food safety and public health nutrition.

In the past, the greatest improvements in people's health have resulted not from health services but from social changes. As the HEALTH21 policy *(4,5)* argues, the origins of most health problems lie deep in society and must be tackled through a broad-based strategy.

Just such a broad strategy is needed for food policy, and it is hoped that this book can indicate a step in that direction. There are many opportunities for preventing food-related diseases, but action must be coherent and consistent to be effective.

Developing consistent and coherent programmes and implementing them in the countries of the European Region are both a challenge and an opportunity for governments and public health officials. As The First Action Plan on Food and Nutrition Policy for the European Region (Annex 1) suggests, this may be done most effectively by giving the task to national bodies that include a range of stakeholders and interests and operate openly and transparently. Through such mechanisms, the people in the Region may begin to improve their health.

References

1. *The world health report 2002: reducing risks, promoting healthy life* (http://whqlibdoc.who.int/publications/2002/9241562072.pdf). Geneva, World Health Organization, 2002 (accessed 3 September 2003).
2. *Globalization, diets and noncommunicable diseases* (http://whqlibdoc.who.int/publications/9241590416.pdf). Geneva, World Health Organization, 2002 (accessed 3 September 2003).

3. *Public health aspects of the EU CAP – developments and recommendations for change in four sectors: fruit and vegetables, dairy, wine and tobacco* (http://www.fhi.se/shop/material_pdf/eu_inlaga.pdf). Stockholm, National Institute of Public Health, 2003 (accessed 3 September 2003).

4. *HEALTH21: an introduction to the health for all policy framework for the WHO European region.* Copenhagen, WHO Regional Office for Europe, 1998 (European Health for All Series, No. 5).

5. *HEALTH21: the health for all policy framework for the WHO European Region.* Copenhagen, WHO Regional Office for Europe, 1999 (European Health for All Series, No. 6).

Annex 1.
The First Action Plan for Food and Nutrition Policy, WHO European Region, 2000–2005[1]

Summary

Access to a safe and healthy variety of food, as a fundamental human right, was stressed by the International Conference on Nutrition in 1992 and by the World Food Summit in 1996. A supply of nutritious and safe food is a prerequisite for health protection and promotion. In spite of commitments expressed and efforts made at national and international levels, there is still a need for policies which reduce the burden of food-related ill health and its cost to society and health services.

It is estimated that each year around 130 million Europeans are affected by episodes of foodborne diseases. Diarrhoea, a major cause of death and growth retardation in young children, is the most common symptom of foodborne illness. New pathogens are emerging, such as the agent of bovine spongiform encephalopathy. The use of antibiotics in animal husbandry and the possible transfer of antibiotic resistance to human pathogens are a major public health concern.

Low breastfeeding rates and poor weaning practices result in malnutrition and disorders such as growth retardation, poor cognitive development, and digestive and respiratory infections in young children. Iodine deficiency disorders affect around 16% of the European population and are a major cause of mental retardation. Iron deficiency anaemia affects millions of people and impairs cognitive development in children and, during pregnancy, increases the risk to women.

The prevalence of obesity is up to 20–30% in adults, with escalating rates in children, increasing the risk of cardiovascular diseases, certain cancers and

---

[1] *The First Action Plan for Food and Nutrition Policy, WHO European Region 2000–2005* (http://www.euro.who.int/Document/E72199.pdf). Copenhagen, WHO Regional Office for Europe, 2000 (document EUR/01/5026013) (accessed 23 October 2002)

diabetes. Obesity is estimated to cost some health services about 7% of their total health care budget. Around one third of cardiovascular disease, the first cause of death in the Region, is related to unbalanced nutrition, and 30–40% of cancers could be prevented through better diet.

In countries of the European Union, a preliminary analysis from the Swedish Institute of Public Health suggests that 4.5% of disability-adjusted life-years (DALYs) are lost due to poor nutrition, with an additional 3.7% and 1.4% due to obesity and physical inactivity. The total percentage of DALYs lost related to poor nutrition and physical inactivity is therefore 9.6%, compared with 9% due to smoking.

This document stresses the need to develop food and nutrition policies which protect and promote health and reduce the burden of food-related disease, while contributing to socioeconomic development and a sustainable environment. It insists on the complementary roles played by different sectors in the formulation and implementation of such policies. It provides a framework within which Member States can begin to address the issue. The framework consists of three interrelated strategies:

- a food safety strategy, highlighting the need to prevent contamination, both chemical and biological, at all stages of the food chain (The potential impact of unsafe food on human health is of great concern, and new food safety systems which take a "arm to fork" perspective are being developed.);
- a nutrition strategy geared to ensure optimal health, especially in low-income groups and during critical periods throughout life, such as infancy, childhood, pregnancy and lactation, and older age;
- a sustainable food supply (food security) strategy to ensure enough food of good quality, while helping to stimulate rural economies and to promote the social and environmental aspects of sustainable development.

An action plan is proposed for the period 2000–2005, with approaches and activities to support Member States who wish to develop, implement and evaluate their food and nutrition policies.

The need for coordination between sectors and organizations will increase as ethics and human rights, in addition to science and economics, play a greater role in decision-making. Countries can consider which mechanisms are needed to facilitate better coordination between sectors and ensure that health and environmental concerns are considered when food and nutrition policies are made.

It is proposed to set up a food and nutrition task force, to facilitate coordination between the European Union, the Council of Europe, United Nations agencies (especially UNICEF and FAO) and environmental and other international, intergovernmental and nongovernmental organizations. The Regional Office is ready to ensure the secretariat of the task force.

Goal and existing political commitments

The goal of food and nutrition policy is to protect and promote health and to reduce the burden of food-related disease, while contributing to socioeconomic development and a sustainable environment. A major objective of the health sector is to promote health through a well balanced diet, the avoidance of nutritional deficiencies and the control of foodborne diseases. A multisectoral approach, including agriculture, the environment, the food industry, transport, advertising and commerce, is therefore essential to help place food and nutrition policy high on the political agenda. Health should be an expected outcome from food and nutrition policies and contribute to the success and profitability of the relevant commercial sectors.

Intersectoral action is needed at the international level. Agenda 21 *(1)*, adopted by governments in 1992 at the United Nations Conference on Environment and Development, included the principle that unsustainable patterns of production and consumption should be reduced. During 2000, the United Nations Commission on Sustainable Development is focusing on agriculture and the environment. As part of its responsibility, WHO addressed the question of "The global nutrition transition: policy implications for health and sustainable agriculture in the twenty-first century", bringing the health, agricultural and environmental aspects of food together.

Other political commitments made over the last ten years (Annex 1) stress the need for comprehensive, intersectoral policies which promote public health. The United Nations Children's Fund (UNICEF) organized the Convention on the Rights of the Child in 1989 and the World Summit for Children in 1990, both of which highlighted the importance of nutrition. After the International Conference on Nutrition (ICN) in 1992 (jointly organized by WHO and the United Nations Food and Agriculture Organization – FAO), a World Health Assembly resolution called for comprehensive plans of action to address both nutrition and food safety. The Regional Office issued a progress report on implementation of the ICN Declaration in Member States in 1995 *(2)*.

Within the European Union (EU), the Treaty of Amsterdam states that "a high level of human health protection shall be ensured in the definition and implementation of all Community policies and activities". Elements of food and nutrition policy are included in the European Commission's white paper on food safety (2000) and the new programme for public health (2001–2006). "Health and nutrition – elements for European action" is a priority for the Commission and the French government during the French presidency

(July–December 2000). The Council of Europe is also active in developing aspects of food and nutrition policy.

The Regional Office also works on food and nutrition policy with the Asian Development Bank and the World Bank. It intends to strengthen these partnerships, particularly through the European Food and Nutrition Task Force proposed in this document.

WHO's commitment is stated in a number of World Health Assembly resolutions on food safety, noncommunicable diseases, infant feeding (notably the International Code of Marketing of Breast-milk Substitutes and subsequent relevant resolutions) and iodine deficiency disorders. HEALTH21 *(3)*, the health policy framework for the European Region adopted by Member States in 1998, highlights the importance of addressing the determinants of health, such as food and nutrition.

In a multisectoral context, the role of WHO in the European Region is to argue for placing health at the centre of all policies and activities which have an impact on people's health; to search for, assess and disseminate scientific evidence on the relation between food and health; to support efforts to assess the health impact and economic consequences of food policies; to provide information and support to Member States in the field of food and nutrition policies; and to promote and facilitate partnerships with all relevant organizations and sectors.

Social inequalities and the burden of food-related ill health

The general public, health professionals and national authorities throughout the European Region all express concern at the increasing incidence of foodborne disease. Food-related ill health, notably malnutrition, obesity and related noncommunicable diseases, place an enormous burden on society, particularly the most vulnerable. The diets of low-income groups are likely to be inadequate. Those with a low income and specific groups such as children, adolescents, pregnant and lactating women, and older people, often face problems gaining access to a healthy variety of safe food. There are examples throughout the Region of how food intake is affected by poverty and social inequalities *(4)*.

Foodborne diseases

In 1995 it was estimated that each year around 130 million Europeans are affected by episodes of foodborne diseases. Sources of contamination of food, both chemical (pesticides, heavy metals and other contaminants) and biological (such as *Salmonella, Campylobacter, Listeria* and *E. coli*), can be found at any stage of the food chain. Diarrhoea, which is the major cause of death and growth retardation in infants and young children, is the most common symptom of foodborne illness. Kidney failure, brain and nervous disorders, arthritis and paralysis are other serious consequences. New types of pathogen, such as prions causing bovine spongiform encephalopathy, are now considered to be the cause of variant Creutzfeldt-Jakob disease in humans.

Food can be contaminated during the various stages of primary agricultural production, storage, transport, processing, packaging and final preparation. Each link in the chain must be as strong as every other if the health of consumers is to be protected (see Fig. 1). In addition, the increase in global food trade creates the potential for very large amounts of food, from one single source, to be distributed over far greater distances than ever before. While this does allow cheaper and more varied foods to be produced, it also creates an increased risk of larger and more widespread outbreaks of foodborne illnesses.

Fig. 1. Principal stages of the food supply chain

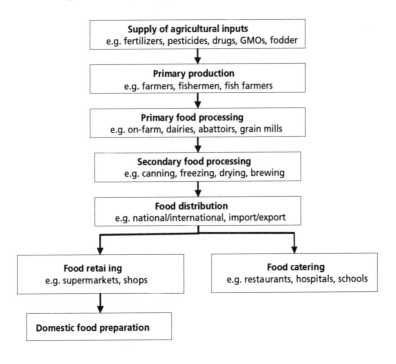

Throughout much of WHO's European Region, the food chain is undergoing substantial changes such as the intensification of agriculture and animal husbandry; increased mass production of food products; increased long-distance food trade; decreased numbers of local shops and street markets; greater difficulty in accessing good quality nutritious food, especially by the poor and disadvantaged groups; and increased consumer concern and lack of consumer confidence, leading to a demand for safe food which is produced in a sustainable way.

In view of the increasing complexity of the food chain and the impact that the food supply has on food safety, there is a need to consider how best to establish effective control mechanisms.

Malnutrition

Low breastfeeding rates and poor weaning practices result in malnutrition and disorders such as growth retardation, poor cognitive development, and digestive and respiratory infections in infants and young children. In 1995, the United Kingdom Department of Health estimated that the savings from reduced incidence of gastroenteritis could amount to £35 million if all infants in the United Kingdom were breastfed (5).

The two major nutrient deficiencies in the European Region are iodine deficiency disorders (IDD) and iron deficiency anaemia (IDA). IDD affect around 16% of the European population and are a major cause of mental retardation. IDA affects millions of people and impairs cognitive development in children and, during pregnancy, increases the risk to women. Other deficiencies, such as those of vitamin A, other antioxidant vitamins and compounds in fruit and vegetables, are linked to increased risks of cancer and cardiovascular disease.

Proven cost-effective public health policies to eliminate IDD are being developed with the support of WHO, UNICEF and the International Council for Control of Iodine Deficiency Disorders (6). Similarly, WHO/UNICEF strategies exist to control IDA (7).

Obesity and noncommunicable diseases

A diet high in saturated fat, energy-dense and low in foods of plant origin, together with a sedentary lifestyle, is the major cause of the pan-European epidemic in obesity and overweight, with increased risks of noncommunicable disease including cardiovascular diseases, certain cancers and diabetes. Other diet-related disorders include dental caries (related to excessive and frequent intake of sugar and poor dental hygiene) and hypertension (related to excessive salt intake in susceptible population groups).

The prevalence of obesity is up to 20–30% in adults, with escalating rates in children. Cardiovascular diseases and cancer, together with diabetes, account for about 30% of the total disability-adjusted life-years (DALYs) lost every year in WHO's European Region (8). Conservative estimates suggest that around one third of all cardiovascular disease is related to unbalanced nutrition, but more analysis is needed. Cancers kill around one million adults each year in the Region, and 30–40% of cancers worldwide could be prevented through a better diet (9).

Obesity is estimated to cost some health services around 7% of their total health care budget. In the early 1990s, the German Ministry of Health estimated that diet-related disorders cost the country approximately DM 113 billion *(10)*. This amounted to 30% of the total cost of treating disease in Germany. The highest cost was generated by treatment of cardiovascular diseases, followed by dental caries and cancer.

Preliminary analysis from the Institute of Public Health in Sweden *(11)* suggests that 4.5% of DALYs are lost in EU countries due to poor nutrition, with an additional 3.7% and 1.4% due to obesity and physical inactivity. The total percentage of DALYs lost related to poor nutrition and physical inactivity is therefore 9.6%, compared with 9% due to smoking. Further analysis, initiated by the Regional Office, is under way to assess the total burden of food-related ill health in the Region.

Food and nutrition strategies

A comprehensive food and nutrition policy comprises three strategies: on nutrition, food safety and a sustainable food supply (food security), based on the principles of HEALTH21 and Agenda 21 (for definitions of selected terms see Annex 2). This framework (see Fig. 2) provides a starting point from which to address the question of how to promote public health through food. The three strategies are interrelated, since the food supply influences both the safety and composition of food. Close collaboration between those responsible for nutrition, food safety and food security is required in order to develop comprehensive, intersectoral policies and concerted action.

**Fig. 2. A comprehensive policy contains nutrition,
food safety and sustainable food supply strategies**

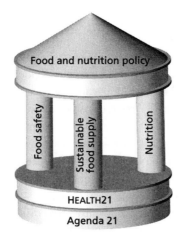

The public wants good, wholesome products it can enjoy without fear, and many consumers do not distinguish between food safety and nutrition. Therefore coordination is essential, to avoid giving consumers conflicting information about which foods are both nutritious and safe. Moreover, increased collaboration can result in better use of resources, if activities for surveillance, risk management and health promotion *(12)* are undertaken jointly by the authorities responsible for food safety and nutrition.

A food safety strategy

A number of government departments or agencies are concerned about the safety of food, including health, agriculture, fisheries, trade, tourism, education, environment, planning and finance. A comprehensive and integrated approach at the national and international levels is required to ensure an effective policy for food control. In 1963, the World Health Assembly approved the establishment of the joint FAO/WHO Codex Alimentarius Commission, which has elaborated many international standards.

In May 2000, the World Health Assembly, recognizing that the health risks from unsafe food are increasing and that these are not being adequately addressed by traditional food hygiene systems, urged Member States (resolution WHA53.15 – Annex 3) to integrate food safety as one of their essential public health functions, and to develop food safety programmes in collaboration with all sectors concerned.

The potential impact of food safety on health is causing increasing public concern and a loss of consumer confidence. A good example is the use of antibiotics in animal husbandry, which is raising fears about the transfer of antibiotic resistance to human pathogens. The application of biotechnology in relation to genetically modified food could dramatically change the food supply. WHO is developing ways to help countries address this dynamic situation and its potential impact on public health.

A nutrition strategy

Nutritional challenges vary as we progress through the life cycle (see Fig. 3). Good nutrition during the first few years pays dividends throughout life *(13)*. This starts with maternal nutrition, because of its importance to the fetus and the evidence that nutritionally related low birth weight raises the risk of cardiovascular disease in later life. The failure of pregnant women to obtain a safe and healthy variety of food has long-term social and economic consequences. The Regional Office, with UNICEF, has developed training materials to help health professionals improve the health of women and their children with safe food and good nutrition.

Analyses demonstrate that exclusive breastfeeding and the introduction of safe and adequate complementary foods from the age of about six months,

Fig. 3. Life cycle: the proposed causal links

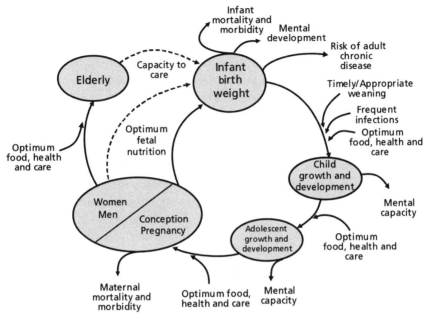

Source: Adapted from *Commission on the Nutrition Challenges of the 21st Century (2000). Final Report to the ACC/SCN.*

but not before four, while breastfeeding continues, can reduce the short- and long-term burden of ill health. The Innocenti Declaration on the protection, promotion and support of breastfeeding was adopted as a basis for policy by the World Health Assembly in 1991 (Annex 1), and the Regional Office monitors its implementation in Member States *(14)*. More recently the Office, together with UNICEF and with support from the governments of the Netherlands and the United Kingdom, has published new feeding guidelines for infants and young children *(15)*.

In adolescence, the health impact of nutrition is pronounced. During their periods of rapid growth, adolescents have increased energy needs. Many of them, especially those in low-income groups, choose relatively cheap sources of energy, such as large amounts of fat and sugar, potentially leading to micronutrient deficiency, obesity and dental caries. Increasingly, there is evidence that poor nutrition due to income inequalities results in health disparities *(16)*. The European Network of Health Promoting Schools, in collaboration with the Regional Office and the EU Commission, has produced a training manual for teachers *(17)*. In addition, an extensive survey, carried out regularly in almost 30 countries, includes results on adolescents' eating habits and their attitudes towards their body image *(18)*.

In adulthood, the main challenge is to avoid premature death from cardio-vascular diseases and cancers. To prevent these, the dietary guide issued by WHO's countrywide integrated noncommunicable disease intervention (CINDI) programme, recommends "Twelve steps to healthy eating" including eating at least 400 g of vegetables and fruit daily (19). WHO has also developed guidelines to encourage increased physical activity as part of regular daily living (20). The aim is to make daily physical activity an easy choice and thus to prevent obesity, as well as reduce the risk of diabetes, heart disease and stroke and promote good health and wellbeing.

The issue of healthy aging is also of major concern. With decreasing activity levels energy needs are reduced, so the food eaten by older people should be rich in micronutrients in order to compensate for the reduction in food intake. Again, 400 g of vegetables and fruits is the daily intake for older people recommended by WHO. Degeneration of eyesight, lower resistance to infection and other micronutrient-related deficiencies can coexist with obesity, making the health management of older people difficult for professionals.

A sustainable food supply strategy (food security)

Food is both an agricultural and an industrial commodity. The contribution of food to global trade has become so great that in 1994 it was included in the World Trade Agreement. Although methods of food production or distribution are not within the expertise or mandate of WHO, the impact of food on public health is a legitimate concern of the health sector. In the United Nations Commission on Sustainable Development, WHO has called for closer links between the agriculture and health sectors. The health sector can stimulate debate on how a sustainable food supply can prevent disease and promote health.

A sustainable food supply should ensure enough food of good quality, while helping to stimulate rural economies and promote social cohesion within rural societies. In Hungary, for example, development of the labour-intensive fruit sector (farming and processing) could provide jobs for 5–10% of the population in areas of high unemployment. Similar developments were carried through in Finland over the past twenty years. With increasing urbanization, there is a need for food and nutrition policies which set out how best to feed large urban populations in a sustainable way. The Regional Office is developing an urban food and nutrition action plan to help local authorities address this (21).

Food policies that promote high levels of meat and dairy products, combined with policies that destroy large quantities of fruit and vegetables, are both environmentally unfriendly and contrary to nutrition goals (22). Nutrition goals, in contrast, emphasize a high consumption of vegetables and fruit, along with a low intake of saturated fats from meat and dairy products. Public health and environmental impact assessments have been carried out by environmentalists within the World Bank, in Sweden (23) and by the EU Commission (24). These assessments provide the evidence that growing the right kind of food for a sustainable environment can also help to promote health. As has already been done in Sweden (25), countries can identify the models of sustainable food supply that are most appropriate for them. WHO will support Member States by enabling them to exchange information on how best to carry out health impact assessments of different types of food supply.

The Regional Office has developed surveillance methods to assess the level of food and nutrition security during disasters and emergencies (26). Based on the data collected, policies have been developed specifically for the European Region (10). This emergency work started in the former Yugoslavia in 1992 and is now being integrated into food and nutrition policies in south-east Europe (28) thus linking humanitarian and development work.

Proposed Action Plan

Approaches
Developing a comprehensive approach
It is recognized that agriculture and other non-health sectors have prime responsibility for the food chain. Contradictory opinions may be held by the various parties involved: food producers and consumers; ministers of the economy and those responsible for social matters; representatives of domestic consumption and export markets; and those advocating traditional food values or modern trends. To be effective, a food and nutrition policy will need to harmonize these opinions as far as possible. Evidence which illustrates the impact of food and nutrition on public health is one way of stimulating harmonization and consensus.

Finding a consensus among potentially conflicting interests is a challenge. Strengthening partnerships between sectors is one way forward (see Fig. 4). To help Member States, and ministries of health in particular, the Regional Office, jointly with WHO headquarters, is developing guidelines on intersectoral policy development for decision-makers, in collaboration with Thames Valley University, London. Intersectoral workshops on policy-making are being carried out for a considerable number of countries in central and south-east Europe and the Baltic region during 2000, with support from the French government. UNICEF and FAO are collaborating with WHO in this initiative.

Monitoring health information
Only a limited number of countries have a comprehensive system for monitoring food and nutrient intake, nutritional status and the incidence of foodborne diseases. The Regional Office will encourage the development of these

Fig. 4. An integrated approach to food and public health

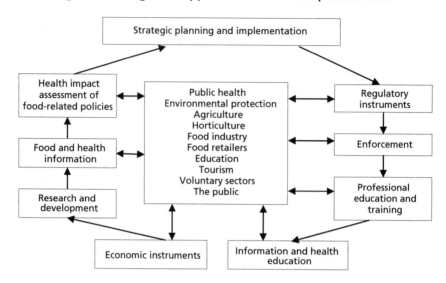

systems and propose cost-effective indicators to help countries assess their policies. A good example exists in the Baltic countries, initiated by the Regional Office with assistance from the London School of Hygiene and support from the government of Luxembourg. Also lacking are data on the cost of food-related ill health and the burden this places on society. The Regional Office has initiated research into this new area.

Improving knowledge

One of the most important roles of the health sector and WHO will be to provide scientific evidence of the positive or negative impact of food and food habits on health. There is a need to gather, assess and disseminate existing knowledge, and to identify areas where the links require clarification and further research.

Mobilizing partners

Partnerships at local, national and European levels are the key to reducing food-related ill health. The Regional Office already collaborates with United Nations bodies, notably UNICEF and FAO (as well as the United Nations Development Programme – UNDP – in Kazakhstan), investment banks, the European Commission and other organizations working on food and nutrition policy. The Office will seek to strengthen and expand these partnerships and to share its information, networking capabilities and experience with these and new partners.

Many health professionals do not receive enough training in food hygiene, nutrition and the benefits of physical activity. WHO will support their undergraduate and postgraduate education by providing information and training materials. In addition, policies are needed to clearly define the role and required training of different health specialists in relation to food safety and nutrition, in order to promote health throughout the life cycle. Health professionals, collectively through their organizations, represent a considerable force for change and provide good examples to help promote this. The Regional Office will use its relations with these organizations to increase the involvement of the health sector in all aspects of food and health.

Consumers need consistent and non-conflicting information in order to make the correct choices about what constitutes a safe and healthy diet. Ensuring that children make healthy choices may require counteracting some of the conflicting messages that are presented when high-fat or energy-dense snack food and soft drinks are marketed. Some countries have adopted laws to prevent television advertisements targeting children under 12 years of age. In others, health promotion campaigns, in collaboration with the media, are organized by health authorities to provide consistent information on healthy food choices. The education sector has an important role to play in ensuring that children have the appropriate skills to promote their health through food.

Nongovernmental organizations have experience in advocating better food and nutrition policies. More specifically, public awareness can be heightened by those organizations concerned with the health of infants and young children, the prevention of cardiovascular disease, cancer and diabetes, the management of food intolerances, and the protection of the environment through a sustainable food supply, as well as (more generally) by public health alliances and consumer organizations.

Food and agriculture industries have formed national and international bodies. Through them, national authorities and international organizations can maintain a dialogue with the sectors producing and selling food. The private sector is probably the major determinant of the food supply – it is thus in the interest of that sector to participate in developing and implementing policies that promote health.

Formulating national food and nutrition action plans

A comparative analysis in WHO's European Member States shows that many countries have developed very effective national action plans (29). Action plans which are firmly based on the national situation, which have a clear timetable for implementation and that are adequately funded are the most successful. The Regional Office is helping a considerable number of Member States, working together in networks, to build on the process launched at the

International Conference on Nutrition and to strengthen their plans of action. This started following a consultation in 1999, organized jointly with WHO headquarters and hosted by the Maltese Ministry of Health, that was attended by representatives of 46 European Member States, with UNICEF, FAO, the European Commission, the World Bank and the World Trade Organization also invited to participate *(30)*.

Promoting the establishment of advisory and coordination mechanisms

Based on a new analysis carried out by the Regional Office, it appears that countries where national coordination mechanisms exist are the most effective in developing and implementing food and nutrition policies. The key role of this mechanism, such as a food and nutrition council, is to advise the government on developing, implementing, monitoring and evaluating comprehensive, intersectoral policies, guidelines and action plans. In addition, such a national body can be responsible for ensuring consistency of the information given to the general public by different agencies; facilitating the creation of a "think-tank" to respond to public concern about food; and advising the government on how to meet its international commitments. Experience from countries, notably the Nordic countries, demonstrates that these mechanisms are effective, particularly where a technical secretariat draws on and coordinates the expertise from the different sectors.

Coordinating activities within the WHO Secretariat

Several WHO programmes, including those on food safety, child health and development, CINDI, national environmental health action plans (NEHAPs), country health, and nutrition policy, infant feeding and food security are working together, and in close collaboration with WHO headquarters, on the development and implementation of food and nutrition policy. This gives added value to countries, by permitting more efficient use of resources to achieve maximum impact through synergistic activities. These in turn stimulate the different specialists, within the health sector, to collaborate more effectively on ensuring the consistency of information at the national level.

Planned activities

In order to promote and support the development and implementation of comprehensive food and nutrition policies, the WHO Regional Office for Europe will act along the lines described above. Some activities are of a general nature and will be carried out throughout the period 2000–2005. More specific activities are also listed mostly for 2000–2001. For the two subsequent biennia, the list is tentative and will be completed on the basis of progress made, emerging needs, requests of Member States and opportunities for collaboration with partners.

Throughout the period 2000–2005, the Regional Office will:

- collate existing knowledge and scientific evidence to support food and nutrition policy development and implementation;
- stimulate research in those areas where the evidence is lacking;
- develop innovative ways to communicate scientific knowledge and information;
- collaborate with countries, at their request, in translating knowledge into action, working with national counterparts and providing information, experience and expertise as required;
- develop cost-effective indicators for surveillance and for reporting on food and nutrition policy;
- regularly produce an updated list of new information, documents and training materials;
- facilitate surveillance and information-sharing, using modern communication tools, and maintain a mechanism for rapid updating.

More specifically the Regional Office will:

1. in 2000–2001:
   - develop and promote the case for a food and nutrition policy and action plan for the European Region;
   - strengthen, with WHO headquarters, national capacity for intersectoral food and nutrition policy-making using the guidelines on intersectoral policy development for decision-makers, in countries of south-east Europe and the Baltic region;
   - present, in 2000, a comparative analysis of the regional situation with regard to food and nutrition policies, so that Member States have a baseline against which to measure their progress over the next five years;
   - collaborate with the EU Commission and the French government during its presidency of the EU Council (July–December 2000) on the development of "Health and nutrition – elements for European action";
   - provide dietary guidelines on the feeding and nutrition of infants, young children and adults;
   - provide training manuals and tools for primary health care workers and other health professionals (*Healthy food and nutrition for women, Food safety for nutritionists, Skills for dietary change*, etc.);
   - publish a book setting out the scientific basis for a food and nutrition policy, provisionally entitled *Food and health in Europe: a basis for action*;

- initiate an analysis on the burden of food-related ill health in the European Region of WHO and present preliminary results;
- establish a food and nutrition task force for the European Region of WHO (see below);

2. in 2002–2003:
   - stimulate the development of new methods to assess the impact of food policies on public health;
   - publish case studies on the development and implementation of food and nutrition policies in WHO's European Region;
   - finalize guidelines for local authorities on regional and urban food and nutrition action plans;
   - organize a meeting of government counterparts to carry out a mid-term evaluation of progress in implementing the Action Plan for the European Region of WHO;

3. in 2004–2005:
   - evaluate the achievements and impact of the Action Plan for the European Region;
   - organize a ministerial conference on food and nutrition policy, to review the evaluation and orient future action.

A Food and Nutrition Task Force for the WHO European Region

The public health sector has not been involved enough in making food policy. Mechanisms are needed to ensure that public health is not overlooked within an increasingly global economy. To do this, a new task force could facilitate better coordination between bodies or organizations such as the European Union, the Council of Europe, United Nations agencies (especially UNICEF and FAO) and environmental and other international, intergovernmental and nongovernmental agencies. The need for coordination will increase as ethics and human rights, in addition to science and economics, are taken more fully into account in decision-making.

The aims of the Food and Nutrition Task Force for the European Region of WHO would be to:

- facilitate collaboration between international agencies and European organizations working on food and nutrition policy;
- create a forum where countries can voice public health concerns regarding international food policies and identify steps to promote health and prevent crises, such as food scares;

- ensure that development agencies support countries synergistically. During their economic transition, the newly independent states and countries of central and eastern Europe (including those in the process of acceding to membership of the EU) need support to keep food and nutrition policy a priority;
- strengthen political commitment to food and nutrition policy at the European level and recommend how to reduce the burden of food-related ill health in the European Region of WHO.

The Task Force will comprise representatives of the different organizations working in the European Region on food and nutrition policy. Skilled scientists will be called on by the Task Force, depending on the public health concerns raised. The Task Force will be set up by the WHO Regional Office for Europe, which will draw up its terms of reference jointly with all partners.

References

1. *Earth Summit Agenda 21: the United Nations Programme of Action from Rio.* New York, United Nations Department of Public Information, 1992.
2. *Nutrition policy in WHO European Member States: progress report following the 1992 International Conference on Nutrition.* Copenhagen, WHO Regional Office for Europe, 1995 (document EUR/ICP/LVNG 94 01/ PB04).
3. *HEALTH21: the health for all policy framework for the WHO European Region. Copenhagen.* WHO Regional Office for Europe, 1999 (European Health for All Series, No. 6).
4. SHAW, M. ET AL. Poverty, social exclusion and minorities. *In*: Marmot, M. & Wilkinson, R.G., ed. *Social determinants of health.* Oxford, Oxford University Press, 1999.
5. DEPARTMENT OF HEALTH. *Review of the Welfare Foods Scheme.* London, The Stationery Office (in press).
6. *Comparative analysis of progress on the elimination of iodine deficiency disorders.* Copenhagen, WHO Regional Office for Europe, 2000 (document EUR/ICP/LVNG/01 01 01).
7. *Prevention and control of iron deficiency anaemia in women and children: report of the UNICEF/WHO regional consultation.* New York, United Nations Children's Fund, 1999.
8. *Obesity – preventing and managing the global epidemic: report on a WHO Consultation.* Geneva, World Health Organization, 1998 (document WHO/NUT/NCD/98.1).
9. *Food, nutrition and the prevention of cancer – a global perspective.* Washington, American Institute for Cancer Research, 1997.

10. KOHLMEIER, L. ET AL. *Ernährungsabhängige Krankheiten und ihre Kosten* [Nutrition-dependent diseases and their costs]. Baden Baden, Nomos, 1993.

11. *Determinants of the burden of disease in the European Union.* Stockholm, National Institute of Public Health, 1997.

12. NARHINEN, M. ET AL. Healthier choices in a supermarket – municipal food control can promote health. *British food journal,* 101(2): 99–107 (1999).

13. HEAVER, R.A. & HUNT, J.M. *Improving early childhood development: an integrated program for the Philippines.* Washington, DC, International Bank for Reconstruction and Development, 1995.

14. *Comparative analysis of implementation of the Innocenti Declaration in WHO European Member States.* Copenhagen, WHO Regional Office for Europe, 1999 (document EUR/ICP/LVNG 01 01 02).

15. MICHAELSEN, K. ET AL. *Feeding and nutrition of infants and young children. Guidelines for the WHO European Region, with emphasis on the former Soviet countries* (http://www.euro.who.int/InformationSources/Publications/Catalogue/20010914_21). Copenhagen, WHO Regional Office for Europe, 2000 (WHO Regional Publications, European Series, No. 87, accessed 28 January 2003).

16. ROOS, G. & PRATTALA, R. *Disparities in food habits – review of research in 15 European countries.* Helsinki, Hakapaino Oy, 1999.

17. DIXEY, R. ET AL. *Healthy eating for young people in Europe: a school-based nutrition education guide.* Copenhagen, WHO Regional Office for Europe, 1999.

18. *Health and health behaviour among young people.* Copenhagen, WHO Regional Office for Europe, 2000 (document EUR/ICP/IVST 06 03 05(A)).

19. *CINDI dietary guide.* Copenhagen, WHO Regional Office for Europe, 2000 (document EUR/00/5018028).

20. *Active living: physical activity for health.* Geneva, World Health Organization, 1997 (document HPR/97.8).

21. *Draft urban food and nutrition action plan.* Copenhagen, WHO Regional Office for Europe, 1999 (document EUR/ICP/LVNG 03 01 02).

22. LOBSTEIN, T. & LONGFIELD, J. *Improving diet and health through European Union food policies.* London, Health Education Authority, 1999.

23. DAHLGREN, G. ET AL., ED. *Health impact assessment of the European Union Common Agricultural Policy.* Stockholm, Swedish National Institute of Public Health, 1996.

24. *Agriculture, environment, rural development: facts and figures – a challenge for agriculture.* Luxembourg, Office for Official Publications of the European Communities, 1999.

25. *A sustainable food supply chain – a Swedish case study.* Stockholm, Swedish Environmental Protection Agency, 1999.

26. ROBERTSON, A. & JAMES, P. War in former Yugoslavia. *In*: Mann, J. & Stewart Truswell, A., ed. *Essentials of human nutrition.* Oxford, Oxford University Press, 1998.

27. *Infant feeding in emergencies.* Copenhagen, WHO Regional Office for Europe, 1997 (document EUR/ICP/LVNG 01 02 08).

28. HAJRULAHOVIC, H. ET AL. *Land of opportunities: fostering health, local economy and peace through food and nutrition policy in Bosnia and Herze-govina and other south European countries.* Copenhagen, WHO Regional Office for Europe, 2001 (document EUR/01/5030563).

29. *Comparative analysis of policies in WHO European Member States – second analysis of policies.* Copenhagen, WHO Regional Office for Europe, 2000.

30. *Development of the First Food and Nutrition Action Plan for the WHO European Region: report on a WHO consultation, Malta, 8–10 November 1999.* Copenhagen, WHO European Regional Office for Europe, 2000 (document EUR/ICP/LVNG 01 02 10).

Annex 1. Policy agreements over the past ten years

Resolution WHA53.15 – Food safety (2000) – see Annex 3

The adoption of this resolution by the World Health Assembly is a move towards developing sustainable, integrated food safety systems for the reduction of health risk along the entire food chain, from the primary producer to the consumer.

European Commission white paper on food safety (2000)

The European Commission has proposed a series of measures to organize food safety in a more coordinated and integrated manner, with a view to achieving the highest possible level of health protection. A number of policy initiatives are described, including the establishment of a European food authority and the development of EU dietary guidelines and an EU nutrition policy. The document also proposes making an EU-wide survey of food consumption patterns.

Resolutions WHA51.18 and WHA53.17 on noncommunicable disease prevention and control (1998 and 2000)

HEALTH21 (1998)

In 1998, the WHO Regional Committee for Europe approved HEALTH21, the health for all policy framework for the WHO European Region. At least

12 of the 21 targets call on Member States to increase intersectoral activities. The development and implementation of food and nutrition action plans provide a concrete example of how HEALTH21 should be translated into practice.

Aarhus Convention (1998)

The signatories to the Aarhus Convention, adopted at the fourth Ministerial Conference "Environment in Europe", organized by the United Nations Economic Commission for Europe, agree to improve public access to information, public participation in decision-making and access to justice on environmental matters. At WHO's Third Ministerial Conference on Environment and Health, London, 1999, ministers of health and the environment jointly reaffirmed their commitment to improving public access to information, securing the role of the public in decision-making, and providing access to social justice for health and environment issues. This includes food policies.

Amsterdam Treaty (1997)

The Amsterdam Treaty of the European Union states that health considerations will be considered in all EU policies and that public health should be ensured. The Treaty provides Member States with an opportunity to call for health impact assessments to be made of EU policies relating to food production, distribution and control.

World Food Summit (1996)

At the World Food Summit, the international community reaffirmed the commitment it had made at the International Conference on Nutrition to stepping up efforts to eliminate hunger and malnutrition, and to achieve food and nutrition security for all.

Convention on the Rights of the Child (1989), World Summit for Children (1990) and Fourth World Conference on Women (1995)

These international conferences dealt among other things with the importance of food and nutrition security, information and education and promoting, protecting and supporting breastfeeding.

International Conference on Nutrition (1992)

In 1992, the International Conference on Nutrition adopted the World Declaration and Plan of Action for Nutrition. Since then, action has been supported by over 30 resolutions of the World Health Assembly. A follow-up consultation was held in the European Region in 1996 to review progress, and the Regional Office has issued reports evaluating the progress being made by Member States on policy implementation.

Agenda 21 and the United Nations Conference on Environment and Development (1992)

Sustainable development was defined in 1992 as development that meets the needs of the present without compromising the ability of future generations to meet their own needs. Many food and health policies can be incorporated into Agenda 21 activities in Member States. WHO, as task manager for Chapter 6 of Agenda 21, has been playing a key role in addressing the health objectives of Agenda 21.

Innocenti Declaration on Protection, Promotion and Support of Breastfeeding (1990)

The Innocenti Declaration sets a number of goals for achieving optimal health for infants and mothers in Member States, including:

- appoint a national breastfeeding coordinator of appropriate authority, and establish a multisectoral national breastfeeding committee composed of representatives from relevant government departments, NGOs and health professional associations;
- ensure that every facility providing maternity services becomes "baby-friendly" and fully practises all ten steps to successful breastfeeding, as set out in the joint WHO/UNICEF statement on "Protecting, promoting and supporting breastfeeding: the special role of maternity services";
- enact imaginative legislation protecting the breastfeeding rights of working women and establish means for its enforcement;
- take action to give effect to the principles and aim of all articles of the International Code of Marketing of Breast-milk Substitutes and subsequent relevant World Health Assembly resolutions in their entirety (see below).

The International Code of Marketing of Breast-milk Substitutes and subsequent World Health Assembly resolutions

The Code and subsequent Health Assembly resolutions are designed to limit the promotion of commercial baby milks and associated products that could undermine breastfeeding. Provisions include:

- no advertising of any breast-milk substitutes (any product marketed or represented to replace breast-milk) or feeding bottles or teats;
- no free samples or free or low-cost supplies to mothers;
- no promotion of products in or through health care facilities;

- no contact between marketing personnel and mothers (mothercraft nurses or nutritionists paid by companies to advise or teach);
- no gifts or personal samples to health workers or their families;
- product labels should be in an appropriate language, with no words or pictures idealizing artificial feeding;
- only scientific and factual information to be given to health workers;
- governments should ensure that objective and consistent information is provided on infant and young child feeding;
- all information on artificial infant feeding, including labels, should clearly explain the benefits of breastfeeding and warn of the costs and hazards associated with artificial feeding;
- unsuitable products, such as sweetened condensed milk, should not be promoted for babies;
- all products should be of a high quality and take account of the climatic and storage conditions of the country where they are used;
- manufacturers and distributors should comply with the Code [and all the resolutions], independent of any government action to implement it.

Annex 2. Definitions of selected terms

Food policy: a policy which does not necessarily explicitly incorporate public health concerns.

Food and nutrition policy: an umbrella term used to incorporate public health concerns into food policy, in order to lead to more concerted intersectoral action.

Food and nutrition action plan: a plan which shows how to develop and implement food and nutrition policy.

Food and nutrition council (or equivalent mechanism): a national mechanism which oversees the development, implementation and evaluation of national action plans through an intersectoral approach.

Food control: a mandatory regulatory activity of enforcement by national or local authorities to provide consumer protection and ensure that all foods during production, handling, storage, processing and distribution are safe, wholesome and fit for human consumption; conform to quality and safety requirements; and are honestly and accurately labelled as prescribed by law.

Food safety: assurance that food will not cause harm to the consumer when it is prepared and/or eaten according to its intended use.

Food security
- All people at all times have both physical and economic access to enough food for an active, healthy life.
- The ways and means by which food is produced and distributed are respectful of the natural processes of the earth and are thus sustainable.

- Both the consumption and production of food are grounded in and governed by social values that are just and equitable, as well as moral and ethical.
- The ability to acquire food is assured.
- The food itself is nutritionally adequate and personally and culturally acceptable.
- The food is obtained in a manner that upholds human dignity.

Annex 3. World Health Assembly resolution WHA53.15 on food safety

The Fifty-third World Health Assembly,

Deeply concerned that foodborne illnesses associated with microbial pathogens, biotoxins and chemical contaminants in food represent a serious threat to the health of millions of people in the world;

Recognizing that foodborne diseases significantly affect people's health and well-being and have economic consequences for individuals, families, communities, businesses, and countries;

Acknowledging the importance of all services – including public health services – responsible for food safety, in ensuring the safety of food and in harmonizing the efforts of all stakeholders throughout the food chain;

Aware of the increased concern of consumers about the safety of food, particularly after recent foodborne-disease outbreaks of international and global scope and the emergence of new food products derived from biotechnology;

Recognizing the importance of the standards, guidelines and other recommendations of the Codex Alimentarius Commission for protecting the health of consumers and assuring fair trading practices;

Noting the need for surveillance systems for assessment of the burden of foodborne disease and the development of evidence-based national and international control strategies;

Mindful that food safety systems must take account of the trend towards integration of agriculture and the food industry and of ensuing changes in farming, production, and marketing practices and consumer habits in both developed and developing countries;

Mindful of the growing importance of microbiological agents in foodborne-disease outbreaks at international level and of the increasing resistance of some foodborne bacteria to common therapies, particularly because of the widespread use of antimicrobials in agriculture and in clinical practice;

Aware of the improvements in public health protection and in the development of sustainable food and agricultural sectors that could result from the enhancement of WHO's food safety activities;

Recognizing that developing countries rely for their food supply primarily on traditional agriculture and small- and medium-sized food industry, and that in most developing countries, the food safety systems remain weak,

1. URGES Member States:

(1) to integrate food safety as one of their essential public health and public nutrition functions and to provide adequate resources to establish and strengthen their food safety programmes in close collaboration with their applied nutrition and epidemiological surveillance programmes;

(2) to develop and implement systematic and sustainable preventive measures aimed at reducing significantly the occurrence of foodborne illnesses;

(3) to develop and maintain national, and where appropriate, regional means for surveillance of foodborne diseases and for monitoring and controlling relevant microorganisms and chemicals in food; to reinforce the principal responsibility of producers, manufacturers, and traders for food safety; and to increase the capacity of laboratories, especially in developing countries;

(4) to integrate measures in their food safety policies aimed at preventing the development of microbial agents that are resistant to antibiotics;

(5) to support the development of science in the assessment of risks related to food, including the analysis of risk factors relevant to foodborne disease;

(6) to integrate food safety matters into health and nutrition education and information programmes for consumers, particularly within primary and secondary school curricula, and to initiate culture-specific health and nutrition education programmes for food handlers, consumers, farmers, producers and agro-food industry personnel;

(7) to develop outreach programmes for the private sector that can improve food safety at the consumer level, with emphasis on hazard prevention and orientation for good manufacturing practices, especially in urban food markets, taking into account the specific needs and characteristics of micro- and small-food industries, and to explore opportunities for cooperation with the food industry and consumer associations in order to raise awareness regarding the use of good and ecologically safe farming and good hygienic and manufacturing practices;

(8) to coordinate the food safety activities of all relevant national sectors concerned with food safety matters, particularly those related to the risk assessment of foodborne hazards, including the influence of packaging, storage and handling;

(9) to participate actively in the work of the Codex Alimentarius Commission and its committees, including activities in the emerging area of food-safety risk analysis;

(10) to ensure appropriate, full and accurate disclosure in labelling of food products, including warnings and best-before dates where relevant;

(11) to legislate for control of the reuse of containers for food products and for the prohibition of false claims;

2. REQUESTS the Director-General:

(1) to give greater emphasis to food safety, in view of WHO's global leadership in public health, and in collaboration and coordination with other international organizations, notably the Food and Agriculture Organization of the United Nations (FAO), and within the Codex Alimentarius Commission, and to work towards integrating food safety as one of WHO's essential public health functions, with the goal of developing sustainable, integrated food safety systems for the reduction of health risk along the entire food chain, from the primary producer to the consumer;

(2) to support Member States in the identification of food-related diseases and the assessment of foodborne hazards, and storage, packaging and handling issues;

(2 bis) to provide developing countries with support for the training of their staff, taking into account the technological context of production in these countries;

(3) to focus on emerging problems related to the development of antimicrobial-resistant microorganisms stemming from the use of antimicrobials in food production and clinical practice;

(4) to put in place a global strategy for the surveillance of foodborne diseases and for the efficient gathering and exchange of information in and between countries and regions, taking into account the current revision of the International Health Regulations;

(5) to convene, as soon as practicable, an initial strategic planning meeting of food safety experts from Member States, international organizations, and nongovernmental organizations with an interest in food safety issues;

(6) to provide, in close collaboration with other international organizations active in this area, particularly FAO and the International Office of Epizootics (OIE), technical support to developing countries in assessing the burden on health and prioritizing disease-control strategies through the development of laboratory-based surveillance systems for major foodborne pathogens, including antimicrobial-resistant bacteria, and in monitoring contaminants in food;

(7) in collaboration with FAO and other bodies as appropriate, to strengthen the application of science in the assessment of acute and long-term health risks related to food, and specifically to support the establishment of an expert advisory body on microbiological risk assessment and to strengthen the expert advisory bodies that provide scientific guidance on food safety issues related to chemicals, and to maintain an updated databank of this scientific evidence to support Member States in making health-related decisions in these matters;

(8) to ensure that the procedures for designating experts and preparing scientific opinions are such as to guarantee the transparency, excellence and independence of the opinions delivered;

(9) to encourage research to support evidence-based strategies for the control of foodborne diseases, particularly research on risk factors related to emergence and increase of foodborne diseases and on simple methods for the management and control of health risks related to food;

(10) to examine the current working relationship between WHO and FAO, with a view to increasing the involvement and support of WHO in the work of the Codex Alimentarius Commission and its committees;

(11) to support Member States in providing the scientific basis for health-related decisions regarding genetically modified foods;

(12) to support the inclusion of health considerations in international trade in food and food donations;

(13) to make the largest possible use of information from developing countries in risk assessment for international standard-setting, and to strengthen technical training in developing countries by providing them with a comprehensive document in WHO working languages, to the extent possible;

(14) to proactively pursue action, on behalf of developing countries, so that the level of technological development in developing countries is taken into account in the adoption and application of international standards on food safety;

(15) to respond immediately to international and national food safety emergencies and to assist countries in crisis management;

(16) to call upon all stakeholders – especially the private sector – to take their responsibility for the quality and safety of food production, including environmental protection awareness throughout the food chain;

(17) to support capacity building in Member States, especially those from the developing world, and facilitate their full participation in the work of the Codex Alimentarius Commission and its different committees, including activities in food safety risk analysis processes.

Annex 4. WHO Regional Committee for Europe resolution EUR/RC50/R8 on the impact of food and nutrition on public health and the case for a Food and Nutrition Policy and an Action Plan for the European Region of WHO, 2000–2005

The Regional Committee,

Concerned by the threat to public health from the lack of safe and healthy food;

Recognizing the roles of other international organizations and sectors with an interest in food;

Recalling Health Assembly resolution WHA46.7, which called for implementation of comprehensive plans of action on nutrition and which endorsed the goals of the fourth United Nations Development Decade and the World Summit for Children;

Further recalling previous Health Assembly resolutions and particularly WHA49.15 on infant and young child nutrition and WHA52.24 on the prevention and control of iodine deficiency, which demonstrate the need for comprehensive food and nutrition policies;

Having considered document EUR/RC50/8, entitled *The impact of food and nutrition on public health – The case for a food and nutrition policy and action plan for the European Region of WHO 2000–2005*;

1. ENDORSES the Action Plan for the European Region of WHO for 2000–2005;

2. RECOMMENDS that Member States take steps to carry out the Action Plan, taking account of differences in their cultural, social, legal and economic environments;

3. REQUESTS European integrational, intergovernmental and nongovernmental organizations to undertake joint action with Member States and the Regional Office to maximize Region-wide efforts to promote public health through food and nutrition policy;

4. REQUESTS the Regional Director:

(a) to ensure appropriate support for the Action Plan from the WHO Regional Office for Europe;

(b) to cooperate with and support Member States and other organizations in comprehensive efforts to promote public health through appropriate food and nutrition policies;

(c) to examine the possibility of setting up, in collaboration with international agencies, the European Commission and the Council of Europe, a Task Force for Food and Nutrition Policies in the European Region of WHO;

(d) to organize a ministerial conference in 2005 to evaluate the implementation of comprehensive food and nutrition policies at regional and country levels;

5. URGES Member States to report on steps taken to promote the health of their population through a food and nutrition policy at the ministerial conference to be held in 2005;

6. REQUESTS the Regional Director to report to the Regional Committee in 2002 on the progress made in implementing the Action Plan.

Annex 2.
International and selected national recommendations on nutrient intake values

Sources

The following are the sources for tables on recommended intakes of: protein, vitamin A, vitamin D, vitamin E, vitamin K, thiamine, riboflavin, niacin, vitamin B_6, folate, vitamin B_{12}, biotin, pantothenic acid, calcium, phosphorus, magnesium, iron, zinc, selenium and iodine:

- FOOD AND NUTRITION CENTER. *Dietary reference intakes (DRI) and recommended dietary allowances (RDA)* (http://www.nal.usda.gov/fnic/etext/000105.html). Beltsville, MD, National Agricultural Library, 2003 (accessed 17 September 2003);
- GARROW, J.S. ET AL. *Human nutrition and dietetics*, 10th ed. Edinburgh, Churchill Livingstone, 2000; and
- *Human vitamin and mineral requirements: report of a joint FAO/WHO expert consultation, Bangkok, Thailand* (http://www.fao.org/DOCREP/004/Y2809E/Y2809E00.HTM). Rome, Food and Agriculture Organization of the United Nations and World Health Organization, 2002 (accessed 17 September 2003).

The sources for the table on recommended intake of energy are:
- GARROW, J.S. ET AL. *Human nutrition and dietetics*, 10th ed. Edinburgh, Churchill Livingstone, 2000; and
- *Human vitamin and mineral requirements: report of a joint FAO/WHO expert consultation, Bangkok, Thailand* (http://www.fao.org/DOCREP/004/Y2809E/Y2809E00.HTM). Rome, Food and Agriculture Organization of the United Nations and World Health Organization, 2002 (accessed 17 September 2003).

Recommended intake of energy (MJ per day)

Groups	WHO/FAO Males	WHO/FAO Females	EU Males	EU Females	Nordic countries	Russian Federation (kcal/day)	United Kingdom Males	United Kingdom Females	United States (AI[a]) Males	United States (AI[a]) Females
Overall Males, RDA[b] Females, RDA	–	–	–	–	–	3300 2600	–	–	–	–
Infants										
0–3 months	2.28	2.16	2.2[c,d]	2.1[c,d]			2.28	2.16	2.7	2.7
4–6 months	2.89	2.69	3.0[c,d]	2.8[c,d]			2.89	2.69	2.7	2.7
7–9 months	3.44	3.20	3.5[c,d]	3.3[c,d]			3.44	3.20	3.5	3.5
10–12 months	3.85	3.61	3.9[c,d]	3.7[c,d]			3.85	3.61	3.5	3.5
Children										
1–3 years	5.15	4.86	5.1[c,d]	4.8[c,d]			5.15	4.86	5.4	5.4
4–6 years	7.16	6.46	7.1[c,d]	6.7[c,d]			7.16	6.46	7.5	7.5
7–9 years	8.24	7.28	8.3[c,d]	7.4[c,d]			8.24	7.28	8.3	8.3
Adolescents										
10–13 years	9.27	7.92	9.8[c]	8.4[c,d]			9.27	7.92	10.4	9.2
14–18 years	11.51	8.83	11.8[c]	8.9[c,d]			11.51	8.83	12.5	9.2
Adults										
19–30 years	10.60	8.10	11.3–12.0[e]	8.4–9.0[e]			10.60	8.10	12.1	9.2
31–50 years	10.60	8.10	11.3–12.0[e]	8.4–9.0[e]			10.60	8.10	12.1	9.2
51–59 years	10.60	8.00	11.3–12.0[e]	8.4–9.0[e]			10.60	8.00	9.6	9.2
60–64 years	9.93	7.99	8.5–9.2[e]	7.2–7.8[e]			9.93	7.99	9.6	9.2
65–74 years	9.71	7.96	8.5–9.2[e]	7.2–7.8[e]			9.71	7.96	9.6	9.2
Elderly people ≥75 years	8.77	7.61	7.5–8.5[e]	6.7–7.6[e]			8.77	7.61	9.6	9.2
Pregnant women										
First trimester	–	–	–	+0.75			–	–	–	–
Second trimester		–	–	–				–		–
Third trimester		+0.80	–	–				+0.80		+1.2
Lactating women	–	+1.9–2.0	–	+1.5–1.9			–	+1.9–2.0	–	+2.1

a AI = average energy allowance.
b RDA = recommended daily allowance of nutrient.
c Values are estimated average nutritional requirement.
d No physical activity and desirable weight for children and adolescents.
e Range represents energy intakes with no physical activity and desirable physical activity, and desirable body weight for adults.

Recommended intake of protein (g per day)

Groups	WHO/FAO	EU	Nordic countries	Russian Federation	United Kingdom EAR[a]	United Kingdom RNI[b]	United States (RDA[c])
Overall							
Males, RDA	52.5	–	–	94	–	55	63
Males, EAR	–						–
Males, minimum[d]	–						–
Females, RDA	45			76		45.5	50
Females, EAR	–			–			–
Females, minimum	–			–			–
Infants							
0–3 months		–	–	–	–	12.5	13.0
4–6 months		14.0			10.6	12.7	13.0
7–9 months		14.5			11.0	13.7	14.0
10–12 months		14.5			11.2	14.9	14.0
Children							
1–3 years	–	14.7	–	–	11.7	14.5	16.0
4–6 years		19.0			14.8	19.7	24.0
7–9 years		27.3			22.8	28.3	28.0
Adolescents	–		–	–			
Males, 10–13 years		42.0			33.8	42.1	45.0
Males, 14–18 years		48.5			46.1	55.2	59.0
Females, 10–13 years		38.7			33.1	41.2	46.0
Females, 14–18 years		51.4			37.1	45.0	44.0
Adults	–		–	–			
Males, 19–30 years		56.0			44.4	55.5	60.0
Males, 31–50 years		56.0			44.4	55.5	60.0
Males, 51–64 years		55.0			42.6	55.3	63.0
Males, 65–70 years		55.0			42.6	55.3	63.0
Females, 19–30 years		47.0			36.0	45.0	46.0
Females, 31–50 years		47.0			36.0	45.0	46.0
Females, 51–64 years		47.0			37.2	46.5	50.0
Females, 65–70 years		47.0			37.2	46.5	50.0

Elderly people	—					
Males, > 70 years	55.0	—	—	42.6	55.3	63.0
Females, > 70 years	47.0	—	—	37.2	46.5	50.0
Pregnant women	+10	—	—	—	+6	60.0
Lactating women	+16	—	—	—	+11	65.0

[a] EAR = estimated average requirement of nutrient.
[b] RNI = required nutritional intake.
[c] RDA = recommended daily allowance of nutrient.
[d] Minimum = minimum required nutritional intake to prevent deficiency.

Recommended intake of vitamin A (µg retinol equivalents[a] per day)

Groups	WHO/FAO	EU	Nordic countries	Russian Federation	United Kingdom			United States	
					LRNI[b]	EAR[c]	RNI[d]	EAR	RDA[e]
Overall									
Males, RDA	600	–	900	1000	–	–	700	–	1000
Males, EAR	–		750	–			–		–
Males, minimum[f]	–		600	–			–		–
Females, RDA	500		800	1000			600		800
Females, EAR	–		700	–			–		–
Females, minimum	–		600	–			–		–
Infants		–	–	–	–	–		–	
0–6 months	375				150	250	350	400[g]	
7–12 months	400				150	250	350	500[g]	
Children			–	–					
1–3 years	400	400			200	300	400	210	300
4–6 years	450	400			200	300	400	275	400
7–9 years	500	450			250	350	500	275	400
Adolescents			–	–					
Males, 10–13 years	600	600			250	400	600	445	600
Males, 14–18 years	600	700			300	500	700	640	900
Females, 10–13 years	600	600			250	400	600	420	600
Females, 14–18 years	600	600			250	400	600	485	700
Adults			–	–					
Males, 19–30 years	600	700			300	500	700	625	900
Males, 31–50 years	600	700			300	500	700	625	900
Males, 51–64 years	600	700			300	500	700	625	900
Males, 65–70 years	600	700			300	500	700	625	900
Females, 19–30 years	500	600			250	400	600	500	700
Females, 31–50 years	500	600			250	400	600	500	700
Females, 51–64 years	500	600			250	400	600	500	700
Females, 65–70 years	500	600			250	400	600	500	700
Elderly people			–	–					
Males, > 70 years	600	700			300	500	700	625	900
Females, > 70 years	600	600			250	400	600	500	700

Pregnant women							
14–18 years	800	+100	–	–	+100	530	750
19–30 years			–	–		550	770
31–50 years			–	–		550	770
Lactating women							
14–18 years	850	+350	–	–	+350	880	1200
19–30 years			–	–		900	1300
31–50 years			–	–		900	1300

a 1 retinol equivalent = 1 µg retinol; 1 µg beta-carotene = 0.167 µg retinol equivalent; 1 µg of other provitamin A carotenoids = 0.084 µg retinol equivalent.

b LRNI = lowest recommended nutritional intake to prevent deficiency.

c EAR = estimated average requirement of nutrient.

d RNI = recommended nutritional intake.

e RDA = recommended daily allowance of nutrient.

f Minimum = minimum required nutritional intake to prevent deficiency.

g Adequate nutritional intake.

Recommended intake of vitamin D (µg per day)

Groups	WHO/FAO	EU	Nordic countries	Russian Federation	United Kingdom (RNI)[a]	United States (AI)[b]
Overall						
Males, RDA[c]	–	–	5	2.5	–	5.0
Males, EAR[d]			–	–		–
Males, minimum[e]			–			
Females, RDA			5	2.5		5.0
Females, EAR			–	–		–
Females, minimum			–	–		–
Infants						
0–6 months	5	10–25			8.5	5.0
7–12 months	5	10			7.0	5.0
Children						
1–3 years	5	0–10	–		0[f]	5.0
4–6 years	5	0–10			0[f]	5.0
7–9 years	5	0–10			0[f]	5.0
Adolescents						
Males, 10–13 years	5	0–15	–	–	0[f]	5.0
Males, 14–18 years	5	0–15			0[f]	5.0
Females, 10–13 years	5	0–15			0[f]	5.0
Females, 14–18 years	5	0–15			0[f]	5.0
Adults						
Males, 19–30 years	5	0–15	–	–	0[f]	5.0
Males, 31–50 years	5	0–10			0[f]	5.0
Males, 51–64 years	10	0–10			0[f]	10.0
Males, 65–70 years	15	10			0[f]	10.0
Females, 19–30 years	5	0–10			0[f]	5.0
Females, 31–50 years	5	0–10			0[f]	5.0
Females, 51–64 years	10	0–10			0[f]	10.0
Females, 65–70 years	15	10			0[f]	10.0

Elderly people					
Males, > 70 years	15	10	—	10	15.0
Females, > 70 years	15	10	—	10	15.0
Pregnant women					
14–18 years	5	10	—	10	5.0
19–30 years					5.0
31–50 years					5.0
Lactating women					
14–18 years	5	10	—	10	5.0
19–30 years					5.0
31–50 years					5.0

[a] RNI = recommended nutritional intake.
[b] AI = adequate nutritional intake.
[c] RDA = recommended daily allowance of nutrient.
[d] EAR = estimated average requirement of nutrient.
[e] Minimum = minimum required nutritional intake to prevent deficiency.
[f] If exposed to the sun.

Recommended intake of vitamin E (mg alpha-tocopherol equivalent per day)

Groups	WHO/FAO	EU	Nordic countries	Russian Federation	United Kingdom (safe intake)	United States EAR[a]	United States RDA[b]
Overall							
Males, RDA	–	–	10	10	–	–	10
Males, EAR			–	–			–
Males, minimum[c]			4	–			–
Females, RDA			8	8			8
Females, EAR			–	–			–
Females, minimum			3	–			–
Infants							
0–6 months	2.7	0.4[b]			0.4[b]	4[d]	–
7–12 months	2.7	0.4[b]			0.4[b]	5[d]	–
Children							
1–3 years	5	0.4[b]	–	–	0.4[b]	5	6
4–6 years	5	–			–	6	7
7–9 years	7	–			–	6	7
Adolescents							
Males, 10–13 years	10	> 4	–	–	> 4	9	11
Males, 14–18 years	10	> 4			> 4	12	15
Females, 10–13 years	7.5	> 3			> 3	9	11
Females, 14–18 years	7.5	> 3	–		> 3	12	15
Adults							
Males, 19–30 years	10	> 4		–	> 4	12	15
Males, 31–50 years	10	> 4			> 4	12	15
Males, 51–64 years	10	> 4			> 4	12	15
Males, 65–70 years	10	> 4			> 4	12	15
Females, 19–30 years	7.5	> 3			> 3	12	15
Females, 31–50 years	7.5	> 3			> 3	12	15
Females, 51–64 years	7.5	> 3			> 3	12	15
Females, 65–70 years	7.5	> 3			> 3	12	15

Elderly people						
Males, > 70 years	10	> 4	—	—	12	15
Females, > 70 years	7.5	> 3	—	—	12	15
Pregnant women						
14–18 years	—	—	—	—	12	15
19–30 years					12	15
31–50 years					12	15
Lactating women						
14–18 years	—	—	—	—	16	19
19–30 years					16	19
31–50 years					16	19

[a] EAR = estimated average requirement of nutrient.
[b] RDA = recommended daily allowance of nutrient.
[c] Minimum = minimum required nutritional intake to prevent deficiency.
[d] mg/g polyunsaturated fatty acid.

Recommended intake of vitamin K (µg per day)

Groups	WHO/FAO[a]	EU[b]	Nordic countries	Russian Federation	United Kingdom (safe intake)[b]	United States (AI)[c]
Overall						
Males, RDA[d]	—	—	—	—	—	80
Males, EAR[e]						—
Males, minimum[f]						—
Females, RDA						65
Females, EAR						—
Females, minimum						—
Infants						
0–6 months	5[g]	—	—	—	10	2.0
7–12 months	10				10	2.5
Children						
1–3 years	15	—	—	—	—	30
4–6 years	20					55
7–9 years	25					55
Adolescents						
Males, 10–13 years	35–65	1	—	—	1	60
Males, 14–18 years	35–65	1			1	75
Females, 10–13 years	35–55	1			1	60
Females, 14–18 years	35–55	1	—	—	1	75
Adults						
Males, 19–30 years	65	1			1	120
Males, 31–50 years	65	1			1	120
Males, 51–64 years	65	1			1	120
Males, 65–70 years	65	1			1	120
Females, 19–30 years	55	1			1	90
Females, 31–50 years	55	1			1	90
Females, 51–64 years	55	1			1	90
Females, 65–70 years	55	1			1	90

Elderly people				
Males, > 70 years	65	1	—	120
Females, > 70 years	55	1		90
Pregnant women				
14–18 years		1	—	75
19–30 years				90
31–50 years				90
Lactating women				
14–18 years	55	1	—	75
19–30 years				90
31–50 years				90

a Based on 1 mg/kg body weight/day of phylloquinone intake.
b Calculation based on mg/kg body weight.
c AI = adequate nutritional intake.
d RDA = recommended daily allowance of nutrient.
e EAR = estimated average requirement of nutrient.
f Minimum = minimum required nutritional intake to prevent deficiency.
g Exclusively breastfed infants should be administered vitamin K supplementation at birth since this intake level cannot be met.

Recommended intake of vitamin C (mg per day)

Groups	WHO/FAO	EU	Nordic countries	Russian Federation	United Kingdom LRNi[a]	United Kingdom EAR[b]	United Kingdom RNi[c]	United States EAR	United States RDA[d]
Overall									
Males, RDA	30	–	60	80	–	–	–	–	60
Males, EAR	–		30	–					–
Males, minimum[e]	–		10	–					–
Females, RDA	30		60	80					60
Females, EAR	–		30	–					–
Females, minimum	–		10	–					–
Infants									
0–6 months	25	–	–	–	6	15	25	40[f]	
7–12 months	30	20			6	15	25	50[f]	
Children									
1–3 years	30	25	–	–	8	20	30	13	15
4–6 years	30	25			8	20	30	22	25
7–9 years	35	30			8	20	30	22	25
Adolescents									
Males, 10–13 years	40	35	–	–	9	22	35	39	45
Males, 14–18 years	40	45			10	25	40	63	75
Females, 10–13 years	40	35			9	22	35	39	45
Females, 14–18 years	40	40			10	25	40	56	65
Adults									
Males, 19–30 years	45	45	–	–	10	25	40	75	90
Males, 31–50 years	45	45			10	25	40	75	90
Males, 51–64 years	45	45			10	25	40	75	90
Males, 65–70 years	45	45			10	25	40	75	90
Females, 19–30 years	45	40			10	25	40	60	75
Females, 31–50 years	45	40			10	25	40	60	75
Females, 51–64 years	45	40			10	25	40	60	75
Females, 65–70 years	45	40			10	25	40	60	75
Elderly people									
Males, > 70 years	45	45	–	–	10	25	40	75	90
Females, > 70 years	45	40			10	25	40	60	75

Pregnant women							
14–18 years	55	–	–	–	+10	66	80
19–30 years	55	–	–	–	+10	70	85
31–50 years	55	–	–	–	+10	70	85
Lactating women							
14–18 years	70	–	–	–	+30	96	115
19–30 years	70	–	–	–	+30	100	120
31–50 years	70	–	–	–	+30	100	120

a LRNI = lowest recommended nutritional intake to prevent deficiency.
b EAR = estimated average requirement of nutrient.
c RNI = recommended nutritional intake.
d RDA = recommended daily allowance of nutrient.
e Minimum = minimum required nutritional intake to prevent deficiency.
f Adequate nutritional intake.

Recommended intake of thiamine (mg per day)

Groups	WHO/FAO	EU	Nordic countries	Russian Federation	United Kingdom LRNI[a]	United Kingdom EAR[b]	United Kingdom RNI[c]	United States EAR	United States RDA[d]
Overall									
Males, RDA	–		1.4	1.6	–	–	1.0	–	1.5
Males, EAR			1.1						–
Males, minimum[e]			0.6						–
Females, RDA			1.1	1.3			1.0		1.1
Females, EAR			0.9						–
Females, minimum			0.5						–
Infants									
0–6 months	0.2	–	–	–	0.2	0.23	0.2	0.2[f]	
7–12 months	0.3	0.3			0.2	0.23	0.3	0.3[f]	
Children									
1–3 years	0.5	0.5	–	–	0.23	0.3	0.5	0.4	0.5
4–6 years	0.6	0.7			0.23	0.3	0.7	0.5	0.6
7–9 years	0.9	0.8			0.23	0.3	0.7	0.5	0.6
Adolescents									
Males, 10–13 years	1.2	1.0	–	–	0.23	0.3	0.9	0.7	0.9
Males, 14–18 years	1.2	1.1			0.23	0.3	0.9	1.0	1.2
Females, 10–13 years	1.1	0.9			0.23	0.3	0.7	0.7	0.9
Females, 14–18 years	1.1	0.9			0.23	0.3	0.8	0.9	1.0
Adults									
Males, 19–30 years	1.2	1.1	–	–	0.23	0.3	0.9	1.0	1.2
Males, 31–50 years	1.2	1.1			0.23	0.3	0.9	1.0	1.2
Males, 51–64 years	1.2	1.1			0.23	0.3	0.9	1.0	1.2
Males, 65–70 years	1.2	1.1			0.23	0.3	0.9	1.0	1.2
Females, 19–30 years	1.1	0.9			0.23	0.3	0.8	0.9	1.1
Females, 31–50 years	1.1	0.9			0.23	0.3	0.8	0.9	1.1
Females, 51–64 years	1.1	0.9			0.23	0.3	0.8	0.9	1.1
Females, 65–70 years	1.1	0.9			0.23	0.3	0.8	0.9	1.1
Elderly people									
Males, > 70 years	1.2	1.1	–	–	0.23	0.3	0.9	1.0	1.2
Females, > 70 years	1.1	0.9			0.23	0.3	0.8	0.9	1.1

Pregnant women	1.4	1.0	–	0.23	0.3	+0.1		
14–18 years							1.2	1.4
19–30 years							1.2	1.4
31–50 years							1.2	1.4
Lactating women	1.5	1.1	–	0.23	0.3	+0.2		
14–18 years							1.2	1.4
19–30 years							1.2	1.4
31–50 years							1.2	1.4

[a] LRNI = lowest recommended nutritional intake to prevent deficiency.
[b] EAR = estimated average requirement of nutrient.
[c] RNI = recommended nutritional intake.
[d] RDA = recommended daily allowance of nutrient.
[e] Minimum = minimum required nutritional intake to prevent deficiency.
[f] Adequate nutritional intake.

Recommended intake of riboflavin (mg per day)

Groups	WHO/FAO	EU	Nordic countries	Russian Federation	United Kingdom			United States	
					LRNI[a]	EAR[b]	RNI[c]	EAR	RDA[d]
Overall									
Males, RDA	–	–	1.6	2.0	–	–	1.3	–	1.7
Males, EAR			1.4						–
Males, minimum[e]			0.8	–					–
Females, RDA			1.3	1.5			1.1		1.3
Females, EAR			1.1						–
Females, minimum			0.8	–					–
Infants									
0–6 months	0.3	–	–	–	0.2	0.3	0.4	0.3[f]	–
7–12 months	0.4	0.4			0.2	0.3	0.4	0.4[f]	–
Children									
1–3 years	0.5	0.8	–	–	0.3	0.5	0.6	0.4	0.5
4–6 years	0.6	1.0			0.4	0.6	0.8	0.5	0.6
7–9 years	0.9	1.2			0.5	0.8	1.0	0.5	0.6
Adolescents									
Males, 10–13 years	1.3	1.4	–	–	0.8	1.0	1.2	0.8	0.9
Males, 14–18 years	1.3	1.6			0.8	1.0	1.3	1.1	1.3
Females, 10–13 years	1.0	1.2			0.8	0.9	1.1	0.8	0.9
Females, 14–18 years	1.0	1.3			0.8	0.9	1.1	0.9	1.0
Adults									
Males, 19–30 years	1.3	1.6	–	–	0.8	1.0	1.3	1.1	1.3
Males, 31–50 years	1.3	1.6			0.8	1.0	1.3	1.1	1.3
Males, 51–64 years	1.3	1.6			0.8	1.0	1.3	1.1	1.3
Males, 65–70 years	1.3	1.6			0.8	1.0	1.3	1.1	1.3
Females, 19–30 years	1.1	1.3			0.8	0.9	1.1	0.9	1.1
Females, 31–50 years	1.1	1.3			0.8	0.9	1.1	0.9	1.1
Females, 51–64 years	1.1	1.3			0.8	0.9	1.1	0.9	1.1
Females, 65–70 years	1.1	1.3			0.8	0.9	1.1	0.9	1.1
Elderly people									
Males, > 70 years	1.3	1.6	–	–	0.8	1.0	1.3	1.1	1.3
Females, > 70 years	1.1	1.3			0.8	0.9	1.1	0.9	1.1

Pregnant women	1.4	1.6	–	–	–	+0.3		
14–18 years							1.2	1.4
19–30 years							1.2	1.4
31–50 years							1.2	1.4
Lactating women	1.5	1.7	–	–	–	+0.5		
14–18 years							1.3	1.6
19–30 years							1.3	1.6
31–50 years							1.3	1.6

[a] LRNI = lowest recommended nutritional intake to prevent deficiency.
[b] EAR = estimated average requirement of nutrient.
[c] RNI = recommended nutritional intake.
[d] RDA = recommended daily allowance of nutrient.
[e] Minimum = minimum required nutritional intake to prevent deficiency.
[f] Adequate nutritional intake.

Recommended intake of niacin (mg niacin equivalent per day)

Groups	WHO/FAO	EU[a]	Nordic countries	Russian Federation	United Kingdom			United States	
					LRNI[b]	EAR[c]	RNI[d]	EAR	RDA[e]
Overall									
Males, RDA	–	–	18	26	–	–	17	–	19
Males, EAR			15	–			–		–
Males, minimum[f]			11	–					
Females, RDA			15	17			13		15
Females, EAR			12	–			–		–
Females, minimum			9	–			–		–
Infants									
0–6 months	2[g]	–	–	–	4.4	5.5	3	2[h]	–
7–12 months	4	5			4.4	5.5	5	4[h]	
Children									
1–3 years	6	9	–	–	4.4	5.5	8	5	6
4–6 years	8	11			4.4	5.5	11	6	8
7–9 years	12	13			4.4	5.5	12	6	8
Adolescents									
Males, 10–13 years	16	15	–	–	4.4	5.5	15	9	12
Males, 14–18 years	16	18			4.4	5.5	18	12	16
Females, 10–13 years	16	14			4.4	5.5	12	9	12
Females, 14–18 years	16	14			4.4	5.5	14	11	14
Adults									
Males, 19–30 years	16	18	–	–	4.4	5.5	17	12	16
Males, 31–50 years	16	18			4.4	5.5	17	12	16
Males, 51–64 years	16	18			4.4	5.5	16	12	16
Males, 65–70 years	16	18			4.4	5.5	16	12	16
Females, 19–30 years	14	14			4.4	5.5	13	11	14
Females, 31–50 years	14	14			4.4	5.5	13	11	14
Females, 51–64 years	14	14			4.4	5.5	12	11	14
Females, 65–70 years	14	14			4.4	5.5	12	11	14

Elderly people								
Males, > 70 years	16	18	–	4.4	5.5	16	12	16
Females, > 70 years	14	14	–	4.4	5.5	12	11	14
Pregnant women	18	–	–	–	–	–		
14–18 years							14	18
19–30 years							14	18
31–50 years							14	18
Lactating women	17	+2	–	–	–	+2		
14–18 years							13	17
19–30 years							13	17
31–50 years							13	17

a Calculation based on 1.6 mg/MJ.
b LRNI = lowest recommended nutritional intake to prevent deficiency.
c EAR = estimated average requirement of nutrient.
d RNI = recommended nutritional intake.
e RDA = recommended daily allowance of nutrient.
f Minimum = minimum required nutritional intake to prevent deficiency.
g Preformed niacin.
h Adequate nutritional intake.

Recommended intake of vitamin B_6 (mg per day)

Groups	WHO/FAO	EU[a]	Nordic countries	Russian Federation	United Kingdom[b] LRNI[c]	United Kingdom[b] EAR[d]	United Kingdom[b] RNI[e]	United States EAR	United States RDA[f]
Overall									
Males, RDA	–	–	1.5	2.0	–	–	1.4	–	2.0
Males, EAR			1.3	–			–		–
Males, minimum[g]			1.0	–			–		–
Females, RDA			1.2	1.8			1.2		1.8
Females, EAR			1.0	–			–		–
Females, minimum			0.9	–			–		–
Infants									
0–6 months	0.1		–	–	3.5	6	0.2	0.1[h]	–
7–9 months	0.3	0.4			6	8	0.3	0.3[h]	
10–12 months	0.3	0.4			8	10	0.4	0.3[h]	
Children									
1–3 years	0.5	0.7	–	–	8	10	0.7	0.4	0.5
4–6 years	0.6	0.9			8	10	0.9	0.5	0.6
7–9 years	1.0	1.1	–	–	8	10	1.0	0.5	0.6
Adolescents									
Males, 10–13 years	1.3	1.3			11	13	1.2	0.8	1.0
Males, 14–18 years	1.3	1.5			11	13	1.5	1.1	1.3
Females, 10–13 years	1.2	1.1			11	13	1.0	0.8	1.0
Females, 14–18 years	1.2	1.1	–	–	11	13	1.2	1.0	1.2
Adults									
Males, 19–30 years	1.3	1.5			11	13	1.4	1.1	1.3
Males, 31–50 years	1.3	1.5			11	13	1.4	1.1	1.3
Males, 51–64 years	1.7	1.5			11	13	1.4	1.4	1.7
Males, 65–70 years	1.7	1.5			11	13	1.4	1.4	1.7
Females, 19–30 years	1.3	1.1			11	13	1.2	1.1	1.3
Females, 31–50 years	1.3	1.1			11	13	1.2	1.1	1.3
Females, 51–64 years	1.5	1.1			11	13	1.2	1.3	1.5
Females, 65–70 years	1.5	1.1			11	13	1.2	1.3	1.5

Elderly people								
Males, > 70 years	1.7	1.5	–	11	13	1.4	1.4	1.7
Females, > 70 years	1.5	1.1	–	11	13	1.2	1.3	1.5
Pregnant women								
14–18 years	1.9	1.3	–	–	–	–	1.6	1.9
19–30 years							1.6	1.9
31–50 years							1.6	1.9
Lactating women								
14–18 years	2.0	1.4	–	–	–	–	1.7	2.0
19–30 years							1.7	2.0
31–50 years							1.7	2.0

a 15 mg/g protein.
b Calculations based on mg/g protein.
c LRNI = lowest recommended nutritional intake to prevent deficiency.
d EAR = estimated average requirement of nutrient.
e RNI = recommended nutritional intake.
f RDA = recommended daily allowance of nutrient.
g Minimum = minimum required nutritional intake to prevent deficiency.
h Adequate nutritional intake.

Recommended intake of folate (µg dietary folate equivalent per day)

Groups	WHO/FAO	EU	Nordic countries	Russian Federation	United Kingdom LRNI[a]	United Kingdom EAR[b]	United Kingdom RNI[c]	United States EAR	United States RDA[d]
Overall									
Males, RDA	200	–	300	200	–	–	200	–	200
Males, EAR	–		140	–			–		–
Males, minimum[e]	–		100	–					
Females, RDA	170		300	200			200		180
Females, EAR	–		120	–			–		–
Females, minimum	–		100	–			–		–
Infants									
0–6 months	80	50	–	–	30	40	50	65[f]	–
7–12 months	80	50			30	40	50	80[f]	–
Children									
1–3 years	160	100	–	–	35	50	70	120	150
4–6 years	200	130			50	75	100	160	200
7–9 years	330	150			75	110	150	160	200
Adolescents									
Males, 10–13 years	400	180	–	–	100	150	200	250	300
Males, 14–18 years	400	200			100	150	200	330	400
Females, 10–13 years	400	180			100	150	200	250	300
Females, 14–18 years	400	200			100	150	200	330	400
Adults									
Males, 19–30 years	400	200	–	–	100	150	200	320	400
Males, 31–50 years	400	200			100	150	200	320	400
Males, 51–64 years	400	200			100	150	200	320	400
Males, 65–70 years	400	200			100	150	200	320	400
Females, 19–30 years	400	200			100	150	200	320	400
Females, 31–50 years	400	200			100	150	200	320	400
Females, 51–64 years	400	200			100	150	200	320	400
Females, 65–70 years	400	200			100	150	200	320	400
Elderly people									
Males, > 70 years	400	200	–	–	100	150	200	320	400
Females, > 70 years	400	200			100	150	200	320	400

Pregnant women	600	400	–	–	–	+100		
14–18 years							520	600
19–30 years							520	600
31–50 years							520	600
Lactating women	500	350	–	–	–	+60		
14–18 years							450	500
19–30 years							450	500
31–50 years							450	500

[a] LRNI = lowest recommended nutritional intake to prevent deficiency.
[b] EAR = estimated average requirement of nutrient.
[c] RNI = recommended nutritional intake.
[d] RDA = recommended daily allowance of nutrient.
[e] Minimum = minimum required nutritional intake to prevent deficiency.
[f] Adequate nutritional intake.

Recommended intake of vitamin B_{12} (μg per day)

Groups	WHO/FAO	EU	Nordic countries	Russian Federation	United Kingdom			United States	
					LRNI[a]	EAR[b]	RNI[c]	EAR	RDA[d]
Overall									
Males, RDA	–	–	2.0	3	–	–	1.5	–	2
Males, EAR			1.4	–			–		–
Males, minimum[e]			1.0	–			–		–
Females, RDA			2.0	3			1.5		2
Females, EAR			1.4	–			–		–
Females, minimum			1.0	–			–		–
Infants									
0–6 months	0.4	–	–	–	0.1	0.25	0.3	0.4[f]	–
7–12 months	0.5	0.5			0.25	0.35	0.4	0.5[f]	
Children									
1–3 years	0.9	0.7	–	–	0.3	0.4	0.5	0.7	0.9
4–6 years	1.2	0.9			0.5	0.7	0.8	1.0	1.2
7–9 years	1.8	1.0			0.6	0.8	1.0	1.0	1.2
Adolescents									
Males, 10–13 years	2.4	1.3	–	–	0.8	1.0	1.7	1.5	1.8
Males, 14–18 years	2.4	1.4			1.0	1.25	2.0	2.0	2.4
Females, 10–13 years	2.4	1.2			0.8	1.0	1.2	1.5	1.8
Females, 14–18 years	2.4	1.4			1.0	1.25	1.5	2.0	2.4
Adults									
Males, 19–30 years	2.4	1.4	–	–	1.0	1.25	2.0	2.0	2.4
Males, 31–50 years	2.4	1.4			1.0	1.25	2.0	2.0	2.4
Males, 51–64 years	2.4	1.4			1.0	1.25	2.0	2.0	2.4
Males, 65–70 years	2.4	1.4			1.0	1.25	2.0	2.0	2.4
Females, 19–30 years	2.4	1.4			1.0	1.25	1.5	2.0	2.4
Females, 31–50 years	2.4	1.4			1.0	1.25	1.5	2.0	2.4
Females, 51–64 years	2.4	1.4			1.0	1.25	1.5	2.0	2.4
Females, 65–70 years	2.4	1.4			1.0	1.25	1.5	2.0	2.4
Elderly people									
Males, > 70 years	2.4	1.4	–	–	1.0	1.25	2.0	2.0	2.4
Females, > 70 years	2.4	1.4			1.0	1.25	1.5	2.0	2.4

Pregnant women	2.6	1.6	–	–	–	–	
14–18 years						2.2	2.6
19–30 years						2.2	2.6
31–50 years						2.2	2.6
Lactating women	2.8	1.9	–	–	+0.5	–	
14–18 years						2.4	2.8
19–30 years						2.4	2.8
31–50 years						2.4	2.8

[a] LRNI = lowest recommended nutritional intake to prevent nutritional deficiency.
[b] EAR = estimated average requirement of nutrient.
[c] RNI = recommended nutritional intake.
[d] RDA = recommended daily allowance of nutrient.
[e] Minimum = minimum required nutritional intake to prevent deficiency.
[f] Adequate nutritional intake.

Recommended intake of biotin (µg per day)

Groups	WHO/FAO	EU[a]	Nordic countries	Russian Federation	United Kingdom[b]	United States[c]
Overall						
Males, RDA[d]	—	15–24	—	—	10–20	—
Males, EAR[e]		—		—	—	
Males, minimum[f]		—			—	
Females, RDA		15–24			10–20	
Females, EAR		—			—	
Females, minimum		—	—	—	—	
Infants						
0–6 months	5	—	—	—	—	5
7–12 months	6					6
Children						
1–3 years	8	—	—	—	—	8
4–6 years	12					12
7–9 years	20					12
Adolescents						
Males, 10–13 years	25	15–100	—	—	10–20	20
Males, 14–18 years	25	15–100			10–20	25
Females, 10–13 years	25	15–100			10–20	20
Females, 14–18 years	25	15–100			10–20	25
Adults						
Males, 19–30 years	30	15–100	—	—	10–20	30
Males, 31–50 years	30	15–100			10–20	30
Males, 51–64 years	30	—			—	30
Males, 65–70 years	30	—			—	30
Females, 19–30 years	30	15–100			10–20	30
Females, 31–50 years	30	15–100			10–20	30
Females, 51–64 years	30	—			—	30
Females, 65–70 years	30	—			—	30

Elderly people						
Males, > 70 years	30	–	–	–	–	30
Females, > 70 years	30	–	–	–	–	30
Pregnant women						
14–18 years	30	–	–	–	–	30
19–30 years					–	30
31–50 years					–	30
Lactating women						
14–18 years	35	–	–	–	–	35
19–30 years					–	35
31–50 years					–	35

[a] Acceptable range of nutrient intake.
[b] Safe range of nutrient intake.
[c] Adequate nutritional intake.
[d] RDA = recommended daily allowance of nutrient.
[e] EAR = estimated average requirement of nutrient.
[f] Minimum = minimum required nutritional intake to prevent deficiency.

Recommended intake of pantothenic acid (mg per day)

Groups	WHO/FAO	EU[a]	Nordic countries	Russian Federation	United Kingdom[b]	United States[c]
Overall						
Males, RDA[d]	–	3–12	–	–	–	–
Males, EAR[e]		–				
Males, minimum[f]		–				
Females, RDA		3–12				
Females, EAR		–				
Females, minimum		–				
Infants						
0–6 months	1.7	–	–	–	1.7	1.7
7–12 months	1.8				1.7	1.8
Children						
1–3 years	2	–	–	–	1.7	2
4–6 years	3				1.7	3
7–9 years	4				3–7	3
Adolescents						
Males, 10–13 years	5	3–12	–	–	3–7	4
Males, 14–18 years	5	3–12			3–7	5
Females, 10–13 years	5	3–12			3–7	4
Females, 14–18 years	5	3–12			3–7	5
Adults						
Males, 19–30 years	5	3–12	–	–	3–7	5
Males, 31–50 years	5	3–12			3–7	5
Males, 51–64 years	5	–			–	5
Males, 65–70 years	5	–			–	5
Females, 19–30 years	5	3–12			3–7	5
Females, 31–50 years	5	3–12			3–7	5
Females, 51–64 years	5	–			–	5
Females, 65–70 years	5	–			–	5

Elderly people					
Males, > 70 years	5	–	–	–	5
Females, > 70 years	5	–	–	–	5
Pregnant women					
14–18 years	6	–	–	–	6
19–30 years					6
31–50 years					6
Lactating women					
14–18 years	7	–	–	–	7
19–30 years					7
31–50 years					7

a Acceptable range of nutrient intake.
b Safe range of nutrient intake.
c Adequate nutritional intake.
d RDA = recommended daily allowance of nutrient.
e EAR = estimated average requirement of nutrient.
f Minimum = minimum required nutritional intake to prevent deficiency.

Recommended intake of calcium (mg per day)

Groups	WHO/FAO	EU	Nordic countries	Russian Federation	United Kingdom EAR[a]	United Kingdom RNI[b]	United States (AI[c])
Overall							
Males, RDA[d]	–	–	800	800	–	–	800
Males, EAR			600	–			–
Males, minimum[e]			400	–			–
Females, RDA			800	800			800
Females, EAR			600	–			–
Females, minimum			400	–			–
Infants							
Premature	–	–	–		–	–	–
0–6 months	–	–		–	–	–	–
0–6 months, breastfed	300	400			400	525	210
0–6 months, formula-fed	400	–			–	–	–
7–12 months	400	400	–	–	400	525	270
Children							
1–3 years	500	400	–	–	275	350	500
4–6 years	600	450			350	450	800
7–9 years	700	550			425	550	800
Adolescents							
Males, 10–14 years	1300	1000	–	–	750	1000	1300
Males, 15–18 years	1300	1000			750	1000	1300
Females, 10–14 years	1300	800			625	800	1300
Females, 15–18 years	1300	800	–	–	625	800	1300
Adults							
Males, 19–65 years	1000	700			525	700	–
Males, 19–24 years	1000	700			525	700	1000
Males, 25–50 years	1000	700			525	700	1000
Males, 51–65 years	1000	700			525	700	1200
Females, 19–65 years	–	700			525	700	–
Females, 19–24 years	1000	700			525	700	1000
Females, 25–50 years	1000	700			525	700	1000
Females, 51–65 years	1300	700			525	700	1200

Elderly people							
Males, > 65 years	1300	700	–	–	525	700	1200
Females, > 65 years	1300	700	–	–	525	700	1200
Pregnant women							
First trimester	–				–		–
Second trimester	–						
Third trimester	1200				–		–
14–18 years							1300
19–30 years							1000
31–50 years							1000
Lactating women	+500				–	+550	
0–3 months	1000						
3–6 months	1000						
7–12 months	1000						
14–18 years							1300
19–30 years							1000
31–50 years							1000

[a] EAR = estimated average requirement of nutrient.
[b] RNI = recommended nutritional intake.
[c] AI = adequate nutritional intake.
[d] RDA = recommended daily allowance of nutrient.
[e] Minimum = minimum required nutritional intake to prevent deficiency.

Recommended intake of phosphorus (mg per day)

Groups	WHO/FAO	EU	Nordic countries	Russian Federation	United Kingdom (RNI[a])	United States EAR[b]	United States RDA[c]
Overall	–					–	–
Males, RDA			600	1200	550		
Males, EAR			450	–	–		
Males, minimum[d]			300				
Females, RDA			600	1200	550		
Females, EAR			450	–	–		
Females, minimum			300	–	–		
Infants	–		–	–	–	–	–
Premature		–			–		
0–3 months		300			400	100[e]	
4–6 months		300			400	100[e]	
7–9 months		300			400	275[e]	
10–12 months		300			400	275[e]	
Children	–		–	–			
1–3 years		350–450			270	380	460
4–6 years		350–450			350	405	500
7–9 years		350–450			350	405	500
Adolescents	–		–	–			
Males, 10–13 years		775			775	1055	1250
Males, 14–18 years		775			775	1055	1250
Females, 10–13 years		625			625	1055	1250
Females, 14–18 years		625			625	1055	1250
Adults	–		–	–			
Males, 19–65 years		550			550	–	–
Males, 19–24 years		550			550	580	700
Males, 25–50 years		550			550	580	700
Males, 51–65 years		550			550	580	700
Females, 19–65 years		550			550	–	–
Females, 19–24 years		550			550	580	700
Females, 25–50 years		550			550	580	700
Females, 51–65 years		550			550	580	700

Elderly people					
Males, > 65 years	–	550	550	580	700
Females, > 65 years	–	550	550	580	700
Pregnant women					
First trimester	–	550	–	–	–
Second trimester	–	–	–	–	–
Third trimester	–	–	–	–	–
14–18 years				1055	1250
19–30 years				580	700
31–50 years				580	700
Lactating women	–	+400	+440	–	–
0–3 months				–	–
3–6 months				–	–
7–12 months				–	–
14–18 years				1055	1250
19–30 years				580	700
31–50 years				580	700

[a] RNI = recommended nutrient intake set equal to calcium in molar terms.
[b] EAR = estimated average requirement of nutrient.
[c] RDA = recommended daily allowance of nutrient.
[d] Minimum = minimum required nutritional intake to prevent deficiency.
[e] Adequate nutrient intake.

Recommended intake of magnesium (mg per day)

Groups	WHO/FAO	EU[a]	Nordic countries	Russian Federation	United Kingdom EAR[b]	United Kingdom RNI[c]	United States EAR	United States RDA[d]
Overall								
Males, RDA	–		350	400	–	300	–	350
Males, EAR			–	–		–		–
Males, minimum[e]			–	–				–
Females, RDA		–	280	400		270		280
Females, EAR			–	–		–		–
Females, minimum			–	–		–		–
Infants								
Premature	–		–		–	–	–	
0–6 months	26				–	–	30[f]	
0–6 months, breastfed							–	
0–6 months, formula-fed	36							
0–3 months					40	55	30[f]	
4–6 months					50	60	30[f]	
7–9 months	53				60	75	75[f]	
10–12 months	53			–	60	80	75[f]	
Children								
1–3 years	60	–			65	85	65	80
4–6 years	73				90	120	110	130
7–9 years	100		–		150	200	110	130
Adolescents								
Males, 10–14 years	250	–		–	230	280	200	240
Males, 15–18 years	250				250	280	340	410
Females, 10–14 years	230				230	280	200	240
Females, 15–18 years	230				250	300	300	360

Adults							
Males, 19–65 years	260	150–500	—	250	300	330	400
Males, 19–24 years	260	150–500		250	300	350	420
Males, 25–50 years	260	150–500		250	300	350	420
Males, 51–65 years	260	150–500		250	300	350	420
Females, 19–65 years	220	150–500		—	—	—	—
Females, 19–24 years	220	150–500		300	300	255	310
Females, 25–50 years	220	150–500		300	300	265	320
Females, 51–65 years	220	150–500		270	270	265	320
Elderly people							
Males, > 65 years	230	150–500	—	300	300	350	420
Females, > 65 years	190	150–500		270	270	265	320
Pregnant women							
First trimester		—	—	—	—	+35	—
Second trimester			—			—	—
Third trimester		—				—	—
14–18 years	220					335	400
19–30 years	220					290	350
31–50 years	220					300	360
Lactating women							
0–3 months		—	—	—	+550	—	—
3–6 months						—	—
7–12 months						—	—
14–18 years	270					300	360
19–30 years	270					255	310
31–50 years	270					265	320

a Acceptable range of nutrient intake.
b EAR = estimated average requirement of nutrient.
c RNI = recommended nutritional intake.
d RDA = recommended daily allowance of nutrient.
e Minimum = minimum required nutritional intake to prevent deficiency.
f Adequate nutritional intake.

Recommended intake of iron (mg per day)

Groups	WHO/FAO[a]				EU[a]	Nordic countries	Russian Federation	United Kingdom			United States	
	15%	12%	10%	5%	(15%)			LRNI[b]	EAR[c]	RNI[d]	EAR	RDA[e]
Overall	–	–	–	–	–			–	–	–	–	–
Males, RDA						10	10			8.7		
Males, EAR						8.5	–			–		
Males, minimum[f]						7	–			–		
Females, RDA						12	18			14.8		
Females, EAR						18 (10[g])	–			–		
Females, minimum						10 (6[g])	–			–		
Infants	–[h]	–[h]	–[h]	–[h]								
0–3 months					–			0.9	1.3	1.7	0.27[i]	–
4–6 months					–			2.3	3.3	4.3	0.27[i]	–
7–12 months	[6[j]]	[8[j]]	[9[j]]	[19[j]]	6			4.2	6.0	7.8	6.9	11.0
Children												
1–3 years	4	5	6	13	4			3.7	5.3	6.9	3.0	7.0
4–6 years	4	5	6	13	4			3.3	4.7	6.1	4.1	10.0
7–9 years	6	7	9	18	6			4.7	6.7	8.7	4.1	10.0
Adolescents												
Males, 10–13 years	10	12	15	29	10			6.1	8.7	11.4	5.9	8.0
Males, 14–18 years	12	16	19	38	13			6.1	8.7	11.4	7.7	11.0
Females, 10–13 years	9[g]/22	12[g]/28	14[g]/33	28[g]/65	18–22[k]			8.0	11.4	14.8[l]	5.7	8.0
Females, 14–18 years	21	26	31	62	17–21[k]			8.0	11.4	14.8[l]	7.9	15.0
Adults												
Males, 19–30 years	9	11	14	27	9			4.7	6.7	8.7	6.0	8.0
Males, 31–50 years	9	11	14	27	9			4.7	6.7	8.7	6.0	8.0
Males, 51–64 years	9	11	14	27	9			4.7	6.7	8.7	6.0	8.0
Males, 65–70 years	9	11	14	27	9			4.7	6.7	8.7	6.0	8.0
Females, 19–30 years	20	24	29	59	17–21[k]			4.7	6.7	8.7	8.1	18.0
Females, 31–50 years	20	24	29	59	17–21[k]			4.7	6.7	8.7	8.1	18.0
Females, 51–64 years	8	9	11	23	8			4.7	6.7	8.7	5.0	8.0
Females, 65–70 years	8	9	11	23	8			4.7	6.7	8.7	5.0	8.0

Elderly people												
Males, > 70 years	9	11	14	27	9	—	—	4.7	6.7	8.7	6.0	8.0
Females, > 70 years	8	9	11	23	8	—	—	4.7	6.7	8.7	5.0	8.0
Pregnant women												
14–18 years	_m	_m	_m	_m	—	—	—	—	—	—	23.0	27.0
19–30 years											22.0	27.0
31–50 years											22.0	27.0
Lactating women												
14–18 years	40	40	48	95	10	—	—	—	—	—	7.0	10.0
19–30 years											6.5	9.0
31–50 years											6.5	9.0

a Bioavailability of dietary iron.
b LRNI = lowest recommended nutritional intake to prevent nutritional deficiency.
c EAR = estimated average requirement of nutrient.
d RNI = recommended nutritional intake.
e RDA = recommended daily allowance of nutrient.
f Minimum = minimum required nutritional intake to prevent deficiency.
g Non-menstruating adolescents.
h Premature and low-birth-weight infants require additional iron.
i Adequate nutritional intake.
j The bioavailability of dietary iron greatly varies during this period.
k Lower value for 90% of the population, upper value for 95% of the population.
l Insufficient for women with high menstrual losses who may need iron supplements.
m Iron supplements in tablet form are recommended for all pregnant women because correctly evaluating iron status in pregnancy is difficult. In non-anaemic pregnant women, daily supplements of 100 mg iron given during the second half of pregnancy are adequate.

Recommended intake of zinc (mg per day)

Groups	WHO/FAO[a]			EU	Nordic countries	Russian Federation	United Kingdom			United States	
	High	Moderate	Low				LRNI[b]	EAR[c]	RNI[d]	EAR	RDA[e]
Overall											
Males, RDA	–	–	–	–	9	15	–	–	9.5	–	15
Males, EAR					6	–			–		–
Males, minimum[f]					5	–			–		–
Females, RDA					7	15			7.0		12
Females, EAR					5	–			–		–
Females, minimum					4	–			–		–
Infants											
0–3 months	1.1	2.8	6.6	–	–	–	2.6	3.3	4.0	2.0[g]	–
4–6 months	1.1	2.8	6.6	–			2.6	3.3	4.0	2.0[g]	–
7–12 months	0.8/2.5[h]	4.1	8.3	4.0			3.0	3.8	5.0	2.2	3.0
Children											
1–3 years	2.4	4.1	8.3	4.0	–	–	3.0	3.8	5.0	2.2	3.0
4–6 years	3.1	5.1	10.3	6.0			4.0	5.0	6.5	4.0	5.0
7–9 years	3.3	5.6	11.0	7.0			4.0	5.4	7.0	4.0	5.0
Adolescents											
Males, 10–13 years	5.7	9.7	19.2	9.0	–	–	5.3	7.0	9.0	7.0	8.0
Males, 14–18 years	5.7	9.7	19.2	9.0			5.5	7.3	9.5	8.5	11.0
Females, 10–13 years	4.6	7.8	15.5	9.0			5.3	7.0	9.0	7.0	8.0
Females, 14–18 years	4.6	7.8	15.5	7.0			4.0	5.5	7.0	7.5	9.0
Adults											
Males, 19–30 years	4.2	7.0	14.0	9.5	–	–	5.5	7.3	9.5	9.4	11.0
Males, 31–50 years	4.2	7.0	14.0	9.5			5.5	7.3	9.5	9.4	11.0
Males, 51–64 years	4.2	7.0	14.0	9.5			5.5	7.3	9.5	9.4	11.0
Males, 65–70 years	4.2	7.0	14.0	9.5			5.5	7.3	9.5	9.4	11.0
Females, 19–30 years	3.0	9.8	9.8	7.0			4.0	5.5	7.0	6.8	8.0
Females, 31–50 years	3.0	4.9	9.8	7.0			4.0	5.5	7.0	6.8	8.0
Females, 51–64 years	3.0	4.9	9.8	7.0			4.0	5.5	7.0	6.8	8.0
Females, 65–70 years	3.0	4.9	9.8	7.0			4.0	5.5	7.0	6.8	8.0

Elderly people												
Males, > 70 years	4.2	7.0	14.0	9.5	—		5.5	7.3	9.5		9.4	11.0
Females, > 70 years	3.0	4.9	9.8	7.0			4.0	5.5	7.0		6.8	8.0
Pregnant women												
First trimester	3.4	5.5	11.0	—	—	—	—	—	—		—	—
Second trimester	4.2	7.0	14.0									
Third trimester	6.0	10.0	20.0									
14–18 years	—	—	—								10.5	13.0
19–50 years	—	—	—								9.5	11.0
Lactating women												
0–3 months	5.8	9.5	19.0	+5.0	—		—		+6.0		—	—
4–6 months	5.3	8.8	17.5	+5.0					+2.5		—	—
7–12 months	4.3	7.2	14.4	+5.0					+2.5		—	—
14–18 years	—	—	—	—					—		11.6	14.0
19–50 years	—	—	—	—					—		10.4	12.0

a Based on bioavailability of nutrient.
b LRNI = lowest recommended nutritional intake to prevent deficiency.
c EAR = estimated average requirement of nutrient.
d RNI = recommended nutritional intake.
e RDA = recommended daily allowance of nutrient.
f Minimum = minimum required nutritional intake to prevent deficiency.
g Adequate nutritional intake.
h Higher value for formula-fed infants.

Recommended intake of selenium (µg per day)

Groups	WHO/FAO	EU[a]	Nordic countries	Russian Federation	United Kingdom LRNI[b]	United Kingdom RNI[c]	United States EAR[d]	United States RDA[e]
Overall								
Males, RDA	–	–	50	–	–	75	–	70
Males, EAR			35			–		–
Males, minimum[f]			20			–		–
Females, RDA			40			75		55
Females, EAR			30			–		–
Females, minimum			20			–		–
Infants								
Premature			–	–	–	–	–	–
0–6 months	6	–			–	–	2.1[g]	
0–6 months, breastfed	–	–			–	–		
0–6 months, formula-fed	–	–			–	–		
0–3 months	–	–			4	10	2.1[g]	
4–6 months	–	–			5	13	2.1[g]	
7–9 months	10	8			5	10	2.2[g]	
10–12 months	10	8			6	10	2.2[g]	
Children								
1–3 years	17	10	–	–	7	15	17	20
4–6 years	21	15			10	20	23	30
7–9 years	21	25			16	30	23	30
Adolescents								
Males, 10–14 years	34	35			25	45	35	40
Males, 15–18 years	34	45			40	70	45	55
Females, 10–14 years	26	35			25	45	35	40
Females, 15–18 years	26	45			40	60	45	55

Adults							
Males, 19–65 years	34	55	–	40	75	45	55
Males, 19–24 years	34	55		40	75	45	55
Males, 25–50 years	34	55		40	75	45	55
Males, 51–65 years	34	55		40	75	45	55
Females, 19–65 years	26	55		40	60	45	55
Females, 19–24 years	26	55		40	60	45	55
Females, 25–50 years	26	55		40	60	45	55
Females, 51–65 years	26	55	–	40	60	45	55
Elderly people							
Males, > 65 years	34	55		40	75	45	55
Females, > 65 years	26	55	–	40	60	45	55
Pregnant women							
First trimester	–	–	–	–	–	–	–
Second trimester	28						
Third trimester	30						
14–18 years						49	60
19–30 years						49	60
31–50 years						49	60
Lactating women							
0–3 months	35	+15	–	+15	+15		55
3–6 months	35						
7–12 months	42						
14–18 years						59	70
19–30 years						59	70
31–50 years						59	70

a Acceptable range of nutrient intake.
b LRNI = lowest recommended nutritional intake.
c RNI = recommended nutritional intake.
d EAR = estimated average requirement of nutrient.
e RDA = recommended daily allowance of nutrient.
f Minimum = minimum required nutritional intake to prevent deficiency.
g Adequate intake based on mg/kg body weight.

Recommended intake of iodine (µg per day)

Groups	WHO/FAO	EU[a]	Nordic countries	Russian Federation	United Kingdom LRNI[b]	United Kingdom RNI[c]	United States EAR[d]	United States RDA[e]
Overall								
Males, RDA	–	–	150	150	–	140	–	150
Males, EAR			100	–		–		–
Males, minimum[f]			70	–				
Females, RDA			150	150	–	140		150
Females, EAR			100	–		–		–
Females, minimum			70	–		–		–
Infants								
Premature	30[g]		–					
0–3 months	15[g]	–			40	50	110[h]	
4–6 months	15[g]	–			40	60	110[h]	
7–9 months	135	50			40	60	130[h]	
10–12 months	135	50			40	60	130[h]	
Children								
1–3 years	75	70	–	–	40	70	65	90
4–6 years	110	90			50	90	65	90
7–9 years	100	100			55	120	65	90
Adolescents								
Males, 10–11 years	135	120	–	–	65	130	73	120
Males, 12–14 years	110	120			65	130	73	120
Males, 15–18 years	110	130			70	140	95	150
Females, 10–11 years	135	120			65	130	73	120
Females, 12–14 years	110	120			65	130	73	120
Females, 15–18 years	110	130			70	140	95	150

	1	2	3	4	5	6	7	8
Adults			—					
Males, 19–65 years	130	130			70	140	95	150
Males, 19–24 years	130	130			70	140	95	150
Males, 25–50 years	130	130			70	140	95	150
Males, 51–65 years	130	130			70	140	95	150
Females, 19–65 years	110	130			70	140	95	150
Females, 19–24 years	110	130			70	140	95	150
Females, 25–50 years	110	130			70	140	95	150
Females, 51–65 years	110	130			70	140	95	150
Elderly people			—					
Males, > 65 years	130	130			70	140	95	150
Females, > 65 years	110	130			70	140	95	150
Pregnant women			—			140		
First trimester	200						—	—
Second trimester	200						—	—
Third trimester	200						—	—
14–18 years	—						160	220
19–30 years	—						160	220
31–50 years	—						160	220
Lactating women		160	—			—		
0–3 months	200						—	—
3–6 months	200						—	—
7–12 months	200						—	—
14–18 years	—						209	290
19–30 years	—						209	290
31–50 years	—						209	290

a Acceptable range of nutrient intake.
b LRNI = lowest recommended nutritional intake.
c RNI = recommended nutritional intake.
d EAR = estimated average requirement of nutrient.
e RDA = recommended daily allowance of nutrient.
f Minimum = minimum required nutritional intake to prevent deficiency.
g Adequate intake based on mg/kg body weight.
h Adequate nutrient intake.